The Slimming Foodie

ULTIMATE COMFORT FOOD

hamlyn

First published in Great Britain in 2025 by Hamlyn, an imprint of
Octopus Publishing Group Ltd
Carmelite House
50 Victoria Embankment
London EC4Y 0DZ
www.octopusbooks.co.uk

An Hachette UK Company
www.hachette.co.uk

The authorized representative in the EEA is Hachette Ireland,
8 Castlecourt Centre, Dublin 15, D15 XTP3, Ireland (email: info@hbgi.ie)

Distributed in the US by Hachette Book Group,
1290 Avenue of the Americas, 4th and 5th Floors, New York, NY 10104

Distributed in Canada by Canadian Manda Group,
664 Annette St., Toronto, Ontario, Canada M6S 2C8

ISBN: 978 1 78325 567 2
eISBN: 978 1 78325 566 5

A CIP catalogue record for this book is available from the British Library.

Printed and bound in Italy.

10 9 8 7 6 5 4 3 2

Editorial Director: Natalie Bradley
Senior Managing Editor: Sybella Stephens
Art Director: Yasia Williams
Photographer: Chris Terry
Food Stylist: Lizzie Harris
Props Stylist: Tamsin Weston
Production: Lucy Carter & Nic Jones

Publisher's note
The information contained in this book is not intended to replace any dietary advice
from your own qualified nutritionist or dietician. Any application of the ideas and
information contained in this book is at the reader's sole discretion and risk.

Both imperial and metric measurements have been given in all recipes. Use one set
of measurements only and not a mixture of both.

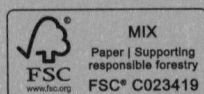

MIX
Paper | Supporting
responsible forestry
FSC® C023419

The Slimming Foodie

ULTIMATE COMFORT FOOD

Simple, healthy, filling meals under 600 calories

PIP PAYNE

hamlyn

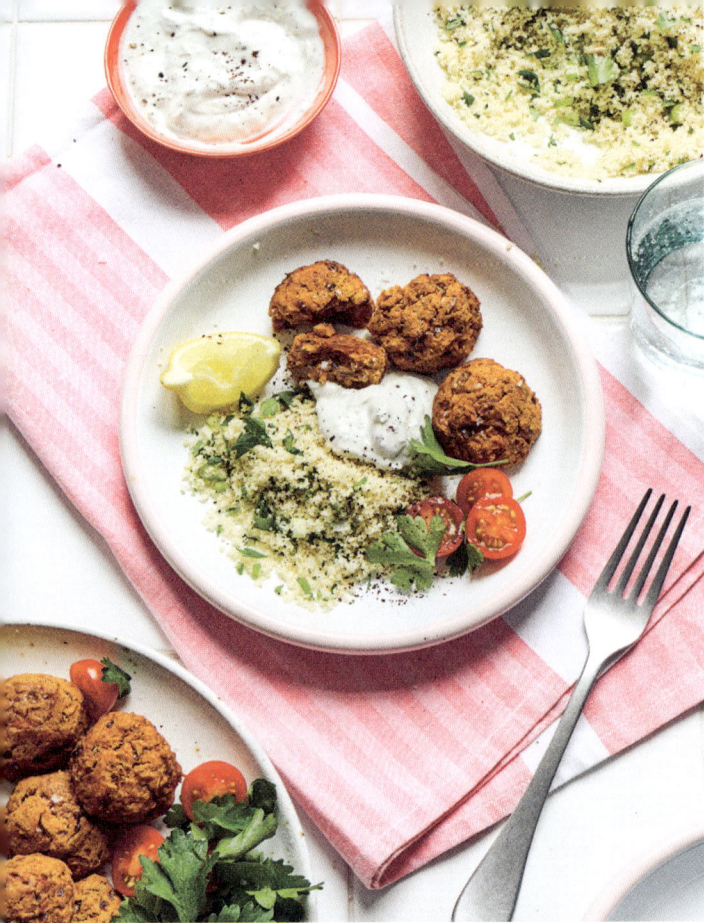

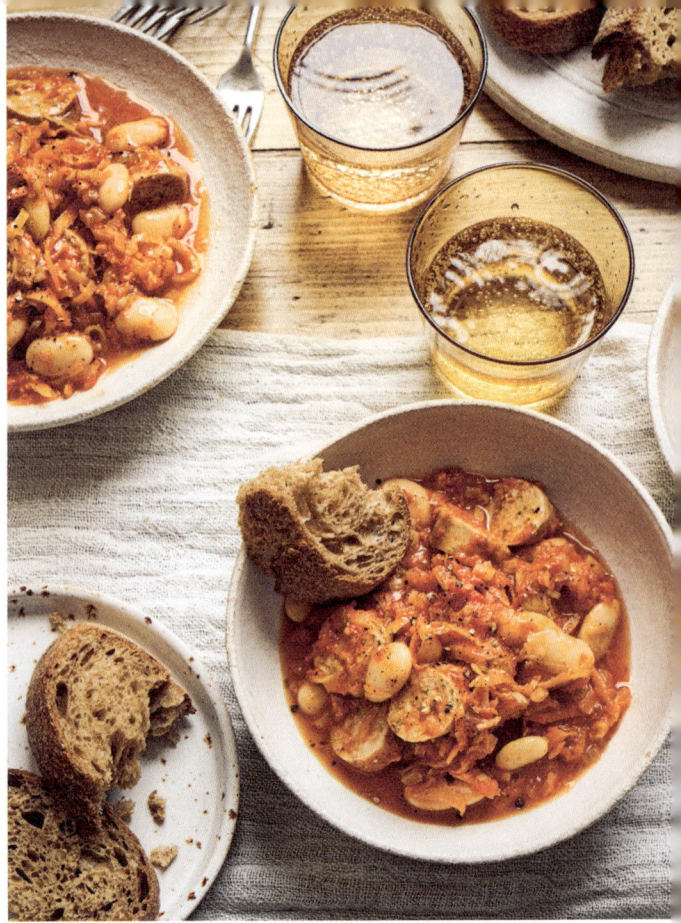

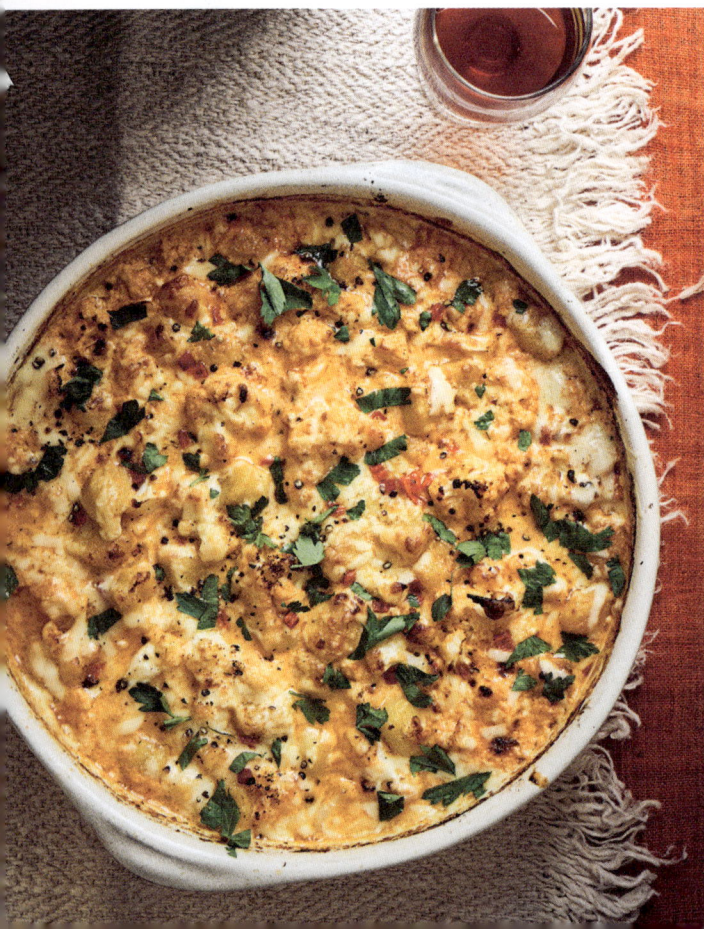

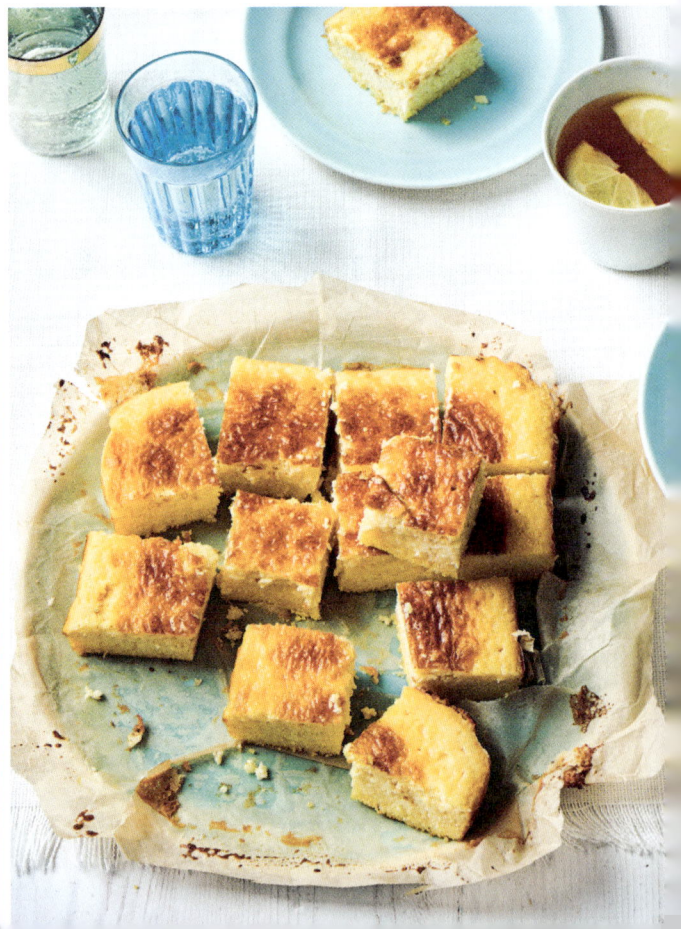

Contents

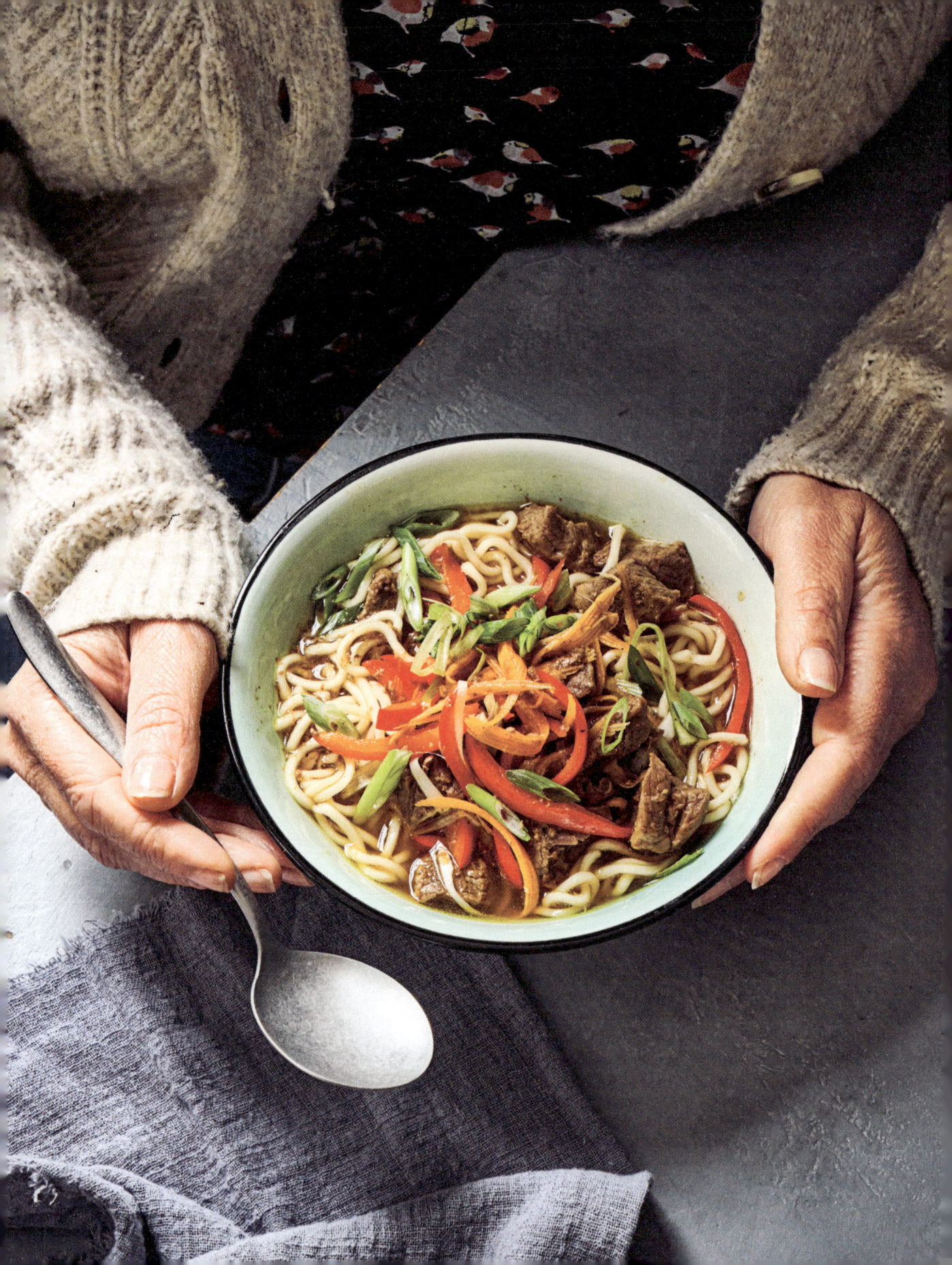

INTRODUCTION

Hi! If you haven't come across The Slimming Foodie before, I'm Pip, a passionate home cook who has been sharing recipes online for 10 years and writing cookbooks for more than half of those. For me, cooking has always been a way to bring joy into my daily life and I love helping others to do the same, creating simple, delicious and comforting recipes that fit into busy schedules, while keeping the food balanced and healthy, too.

For me, comfort food isn't about indulgence for its own sake. Rather, it is about the meals that make us feel good, whether that's a steaming bowl of soup on a cold day, a nostalgic childhood classic, a takeaway-style favourite or a cosy dinner shared with loved ones. This book is all about celebrating the joy of comforting food that is accessible, fuss-free and satisfying.

A daily back-and-forth with my blog readers and social media followers keeps me tuned in to what home cooks really want, from budget-friendly ideas to meals that bring families together. That means I get real-time feedback on my recipes from thousands of home cooks, so I'm always listening, adapting and refining. This connection with my community is what drives me to create dishes for you that truly work in your real-life kitchen.

With this, my sixth book, I wanted to reflect on a year of comfort in my own kitchen, those go-to meals that bring warmth, ease and satisfaction to every season. From family-friendly classics to easy batch-cook favourites, through cosy slow-cooker meals and even dishes perfect for feeding a table full of friends, my goal is to inspire you with comforting recipes for every occasion.

STORE CUPBOARD & KITCHEN KIT

A well-equipped store cupboard is an essential for an effective home cook, and, as you become more seasoned (literally!) in the kitchen, yours will build up naturally. When you read the recipes in this book, you'll see that there are many herbs, spices and ingredients I use repeatedly in different dishes. If I suggest an ingredient that is more specialist, I try to ensure that it is used in at least one more recipe in the book (or you may find it's used in previous

Slimming Foodie books), so you can make the most out of it and it isn't wasted. You will find an index at the back of the book where you can look up ingredients and find recipes that use them. I'm not going to list everything I think you need, because it will very much depend on which recipes you fancy trying first. I suggest the best approach is to mark which recipes you are going to try and build up your store cupboard from there.

In terms of kitchen kit for the recipes in this book, other than the basics (good knives and pans, a mini chopper, stick blender, slow-cooker and so on), I specify only a few more specialist items: a 25cm (10 inch) quiche dish for the Herby Mushroom Quiche (see page 14); a 6cm (2½ inch) round pastry cutter for the Crunchy Chocolate Clusters and Gingerbread Thins (see pages 225 and 234); a 24cm (9½ inch) square cake tin for the Raspberry & White Chocolate Yogurt Cake (see page 229), and a 20cm (8 inch) square cake tin for the Lemon Polenta Cake (see page 230). I also recommend you invest in a meat thermometer (see below).

GENERAL NOTES

Prep & cook times
My prep times do not include the time spent rummaging through cupboards trying to find ingredients! They are for the time it takes to chop, grate or mix. I'm not a pro chopper, so these timings are for an intermediate home cook. If cooking is new to you, it may take a little longer, but you'll soon speed up with practice.

Salt
I often specify 'coarse salt', which just means I'm not using table salt, as that will give a saltier taste. I buy Cornish sea salt flakes, as I like the way you can crumble them between your fingers.

Ovens, hobs & thermometers
Ovens and hobs vary hugely, though I have used a budget induction hob and fan oven to test every single recipe in this book. I keep a thermometer in my oven to make sure that the temperatures I'm cooking at are accurately reflected. If you want to get the same results as me, you could buy an in-oven thermometer, but

remember that variations in the oven dishes you use – even the outside temperature – can affect cooking times, as can how often you open your oven during the cooking process. I have done my best to provide guidance on checking when your food is cooked, indicating what you should look for in both taste and appearance. However, the failsafe to check when meat is cooked properly is to use a meat thermometer.

Oil

I mainly use spray oil in my cooking. Some shop-bought sprays include additives, such as emulsifiers and propellants, which means they're classed as ultra-processed. If you'd prefer to keep things simpler, I recommend picking up a food-grade refillable spray bottle. I use one every day – just filled with olive oil – and it works a treat for frying or sautéing. In some recipes, I'll suggest a spoon of oil, because sometimes that little extra just makes everything work better. Once the meal is split between four, the calorie difference is usually tiny and the boost in taste or texture is worth it.

Eggs

All eggs used are large and free-range.

Food prep

The best way to cook a successful meal is to prep your ingredients in advance, and to quickly read through the full recipe before you start cooking, to make sure there aren't any surprises!

Calories

The calorie counts included in the recipes are for a single portion, and please bear in mind that there is often some variation between the same food item, such as between different brands of light (reduced-fat) coconut milk. I do not include serving suggestions or side dishes in the calorie count unless they are listed with the other ingredients.

Pans & dishes

If I think it matters, I will suggest a certain type of pan or dish. If you use something different, your cooking times may vary.

Portion sizes

This is a very hard thing to generalize about: all families are different, and a family with two small children is going to have very different requirements from those of a family with two hungry teenagers! I base my portion sizes on recommended amounts and my experience of making the dish or what I consider to be a satisfying portion. Of course, this is very subjective and you may need to adjust things to work for you and your family (I think it's always worth cooking some extra vegetables on the side). I also realize that not everyone who buys this book is living with family or cooking for four people, so you will find that many of the recipes are easy to scale up or down.

Freezing

I make suggestions for freezer-friendly food based on what I know will defrost well. There are other recipes in this book that you may be able to freeze, but they may lose consistency when reheated, which is why I have not marked them as freezer friendly. For example, with most of the pasta dishes, I might happily freeze the sauce element, but I wouldn't freeze the actual pasta, so I have not marked those as freezer friendly. When freezing meals, always allow the food to fully cool before placing it in the freezer. Transfer leftovers into airtight plastic containers or freezer bags, then label them with the contents and date. Make sure that food is thoroughly defrosted before reheating.

Light & reduced-fat ingredients

These recipes are designed to be lower in fat and calories, but I know that many of the people who enjoy cooking from my books are not watching either of those. Please feel free to use the whole version of any low-fat or lower-calorie ingredient I suggest, such as sausages, coconut milk and cream cheese; I love the fact that my recipes are enjoyed by all! Note: with cheeses, such as Cheddar or mozzarella, I always use the full-fat versions, as I think they both taste and melt better.

Key to symbols

❄ **FREEZER-FRIENDLY**

🌿 **VEGETARIAN**

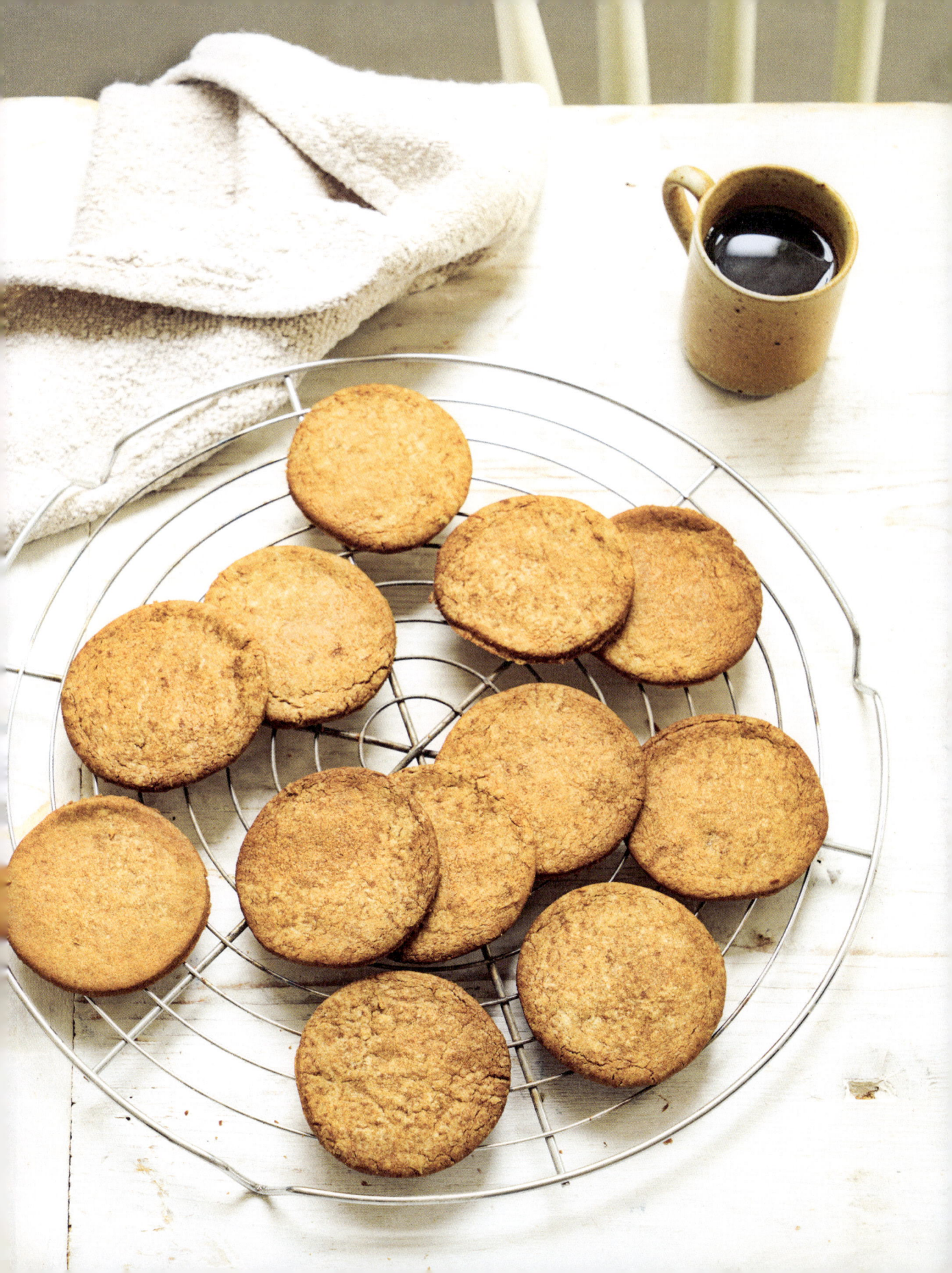

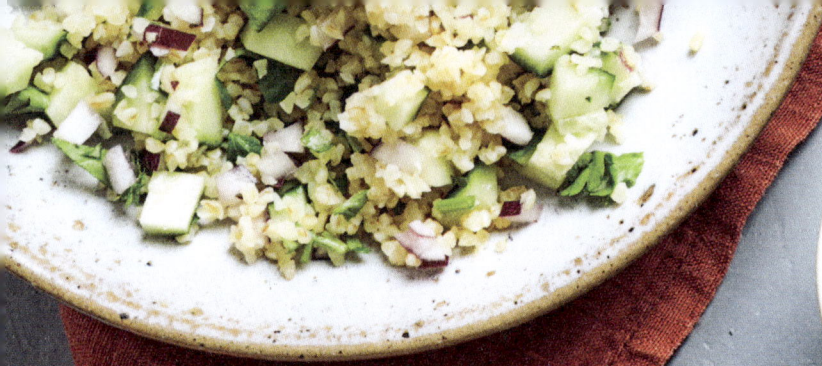

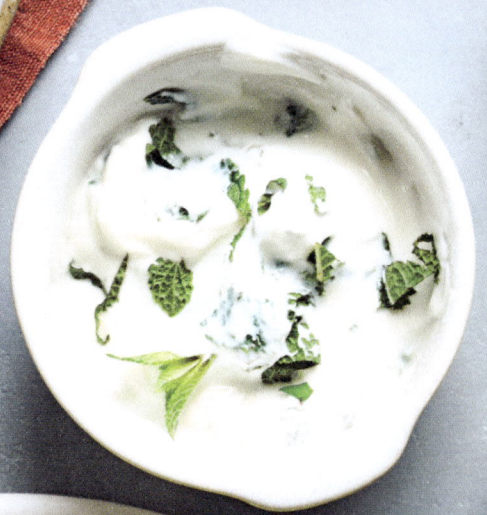

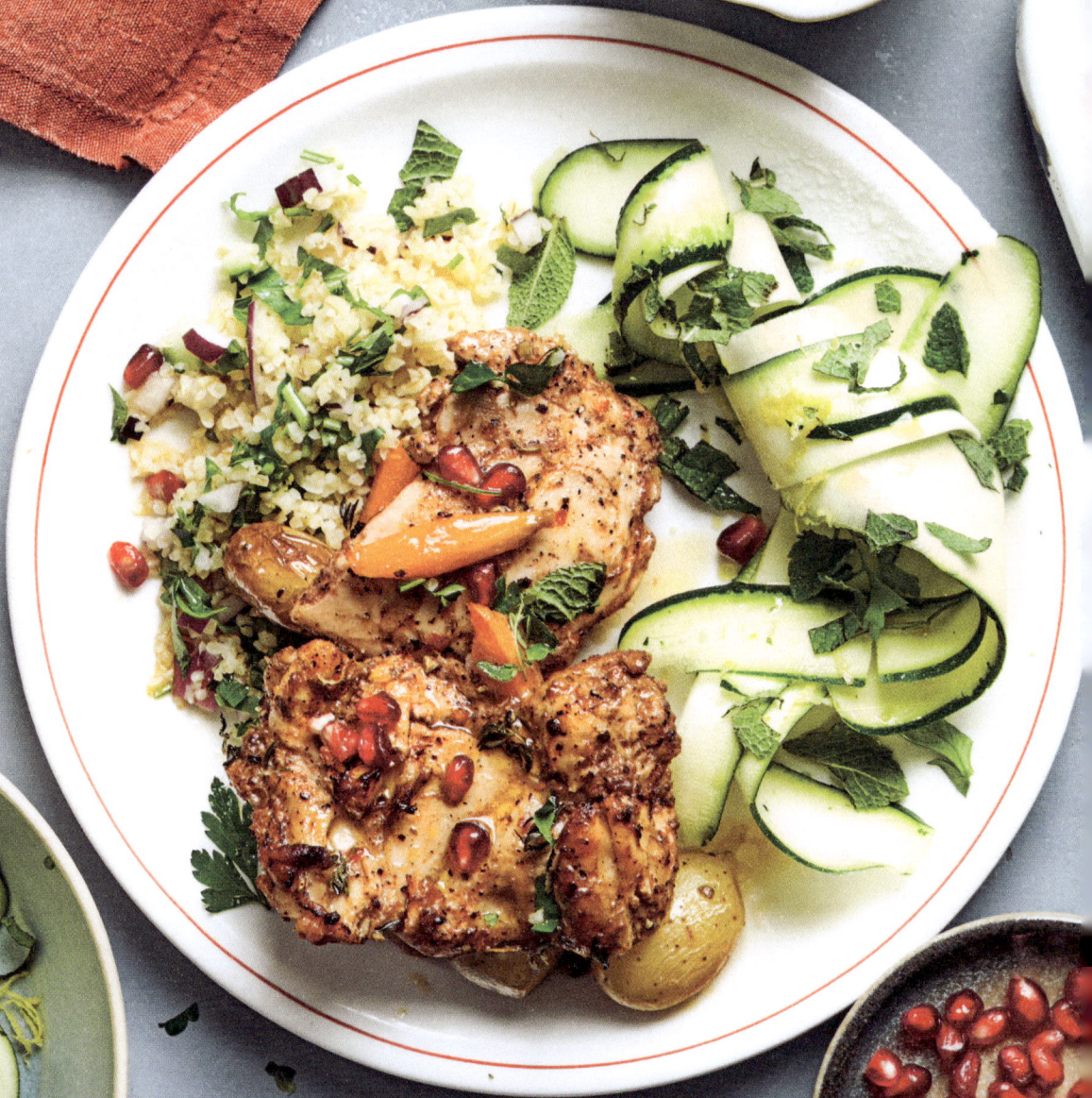

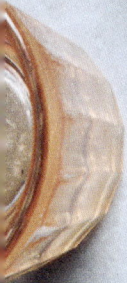

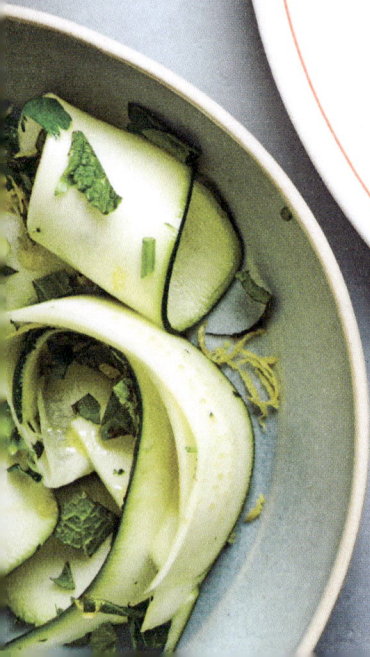

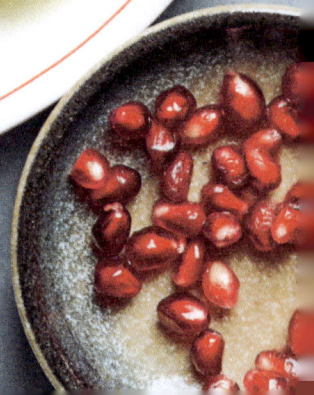

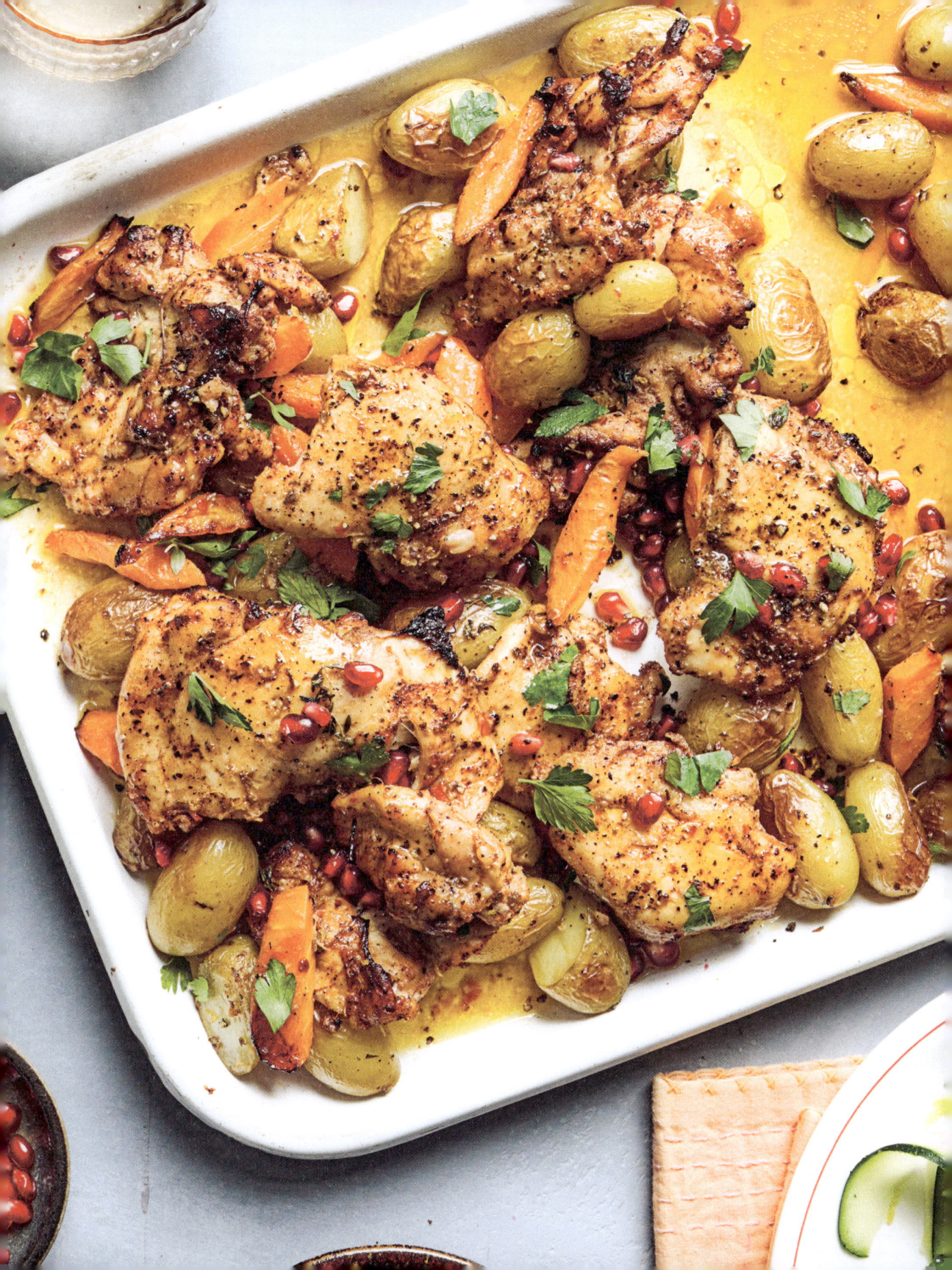

EASY
LUNCHES

1

HERBY MUSHROOM QUICHE WITH SWEET POTATO & OAT CRUST

SERVES 6
PREP TIME 10 minutes
COOK TIME 40 minutes

1 medium (250g/9oz) sweet
   potato, peeled and roughly
   chopped
120g (4¼oz) oats
7 eggs
spray oil
90g (3¼oz) Cheddar cheese,
   grated
2 tablespoons dried mixed herbs
250g (9oz) chestnut mushrooms,
   sliced
30g (1oz) Parmesan-style
   vegetarian cheese, finely grated
salt and pepper

This crust is great when you don't want to have regular pastry.
The recipe still gives you a filling crust with a crisp to the edge
of it, which I find much more satisfying than a crustless quiche.
I like to serve this with salad.

1   Preheat the oven to 200°C/180°C fan (400°F), Gas Mark 6.

2   Put the sweet potato and oats into a food processor and whizz them up
    until they are very finely chopped. Crack in 1 egg, season with salt and
    pepper and blend again to combine.

3   Spray a 25cm (10 inch) quiche dish with spray oil, then spoon in the
    mixture. First use a spatula to spread the crust out evenly over the
    base and sides of the dish, then your fingers to help press it in around
    and up the edges, right to the top of the rim, and ensure you have
    even coverage.

4   Bake in the oven for 15 minutes.

5   Meanwhile, lightly beat the remaining 6 eggs in a bowl, then add the
    Cheddar, 1 tablespoon of the mixed herbs and salt and pepper.
    Pour the egg mixture into the sweet potato crust, then evenly spread
    the mushrooms over the top. Sprinkle all over with the Parmesan-style
    cheese, then with the remaining tablespoon of mixed herbs. Spray with
    spray oil, then bake on the middle shelf of the oven for 25 minutes.

6   Allow to cool for 10 minutes before slicing. You can enjoy this hot or
    cold.

NOTE

Finely chopped bacon or chorizo works well in this quiche, just add it to
the egg mixture at step 5.

PER SERVING

CALORIES	FAT	SAT FAT	CARBS	SUGARS	FIBRE	PROTEIN	SALT
305	14.7G	6.3G	23.3G	3.2G	3.1G	18G	0.8G

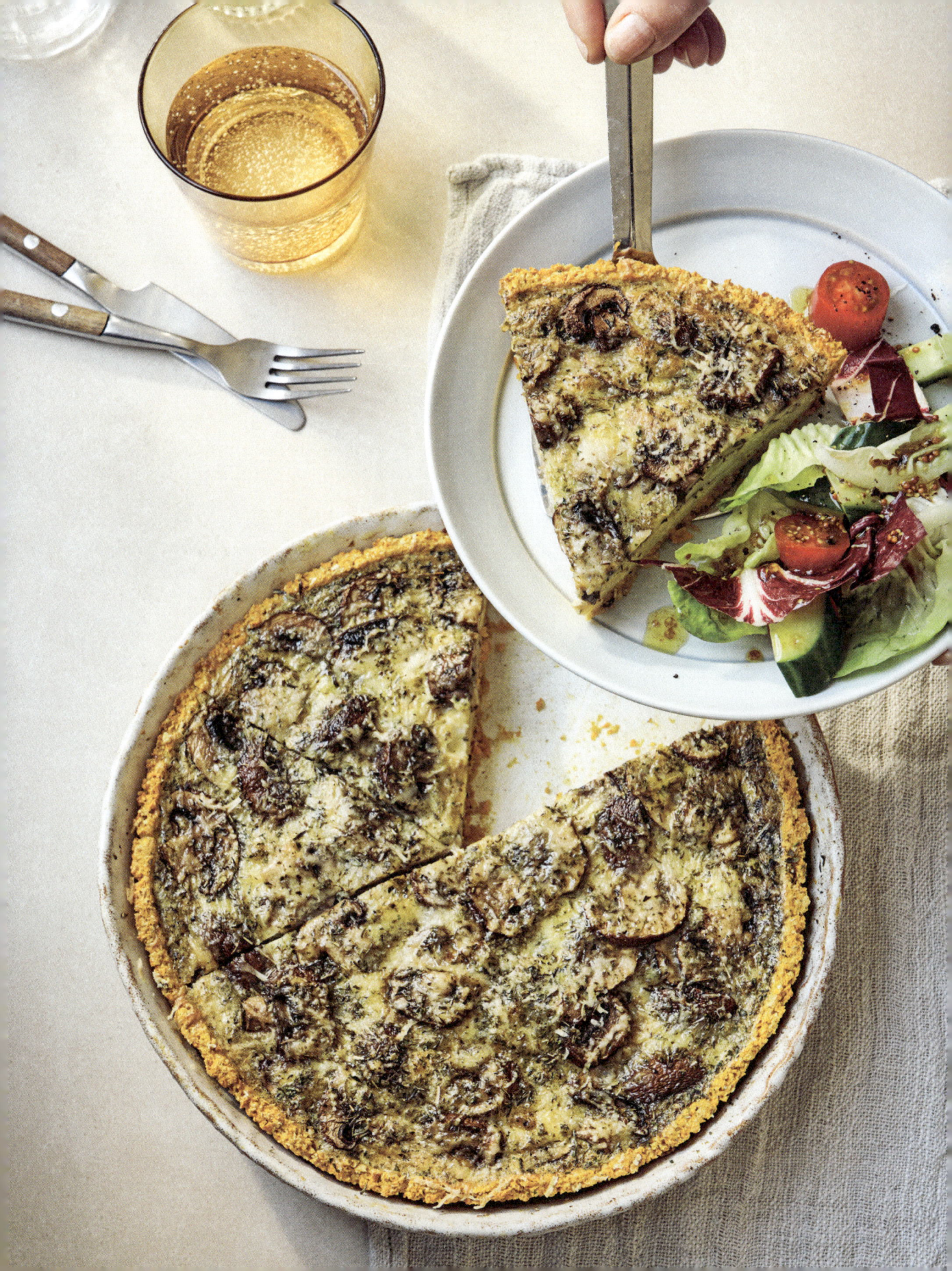

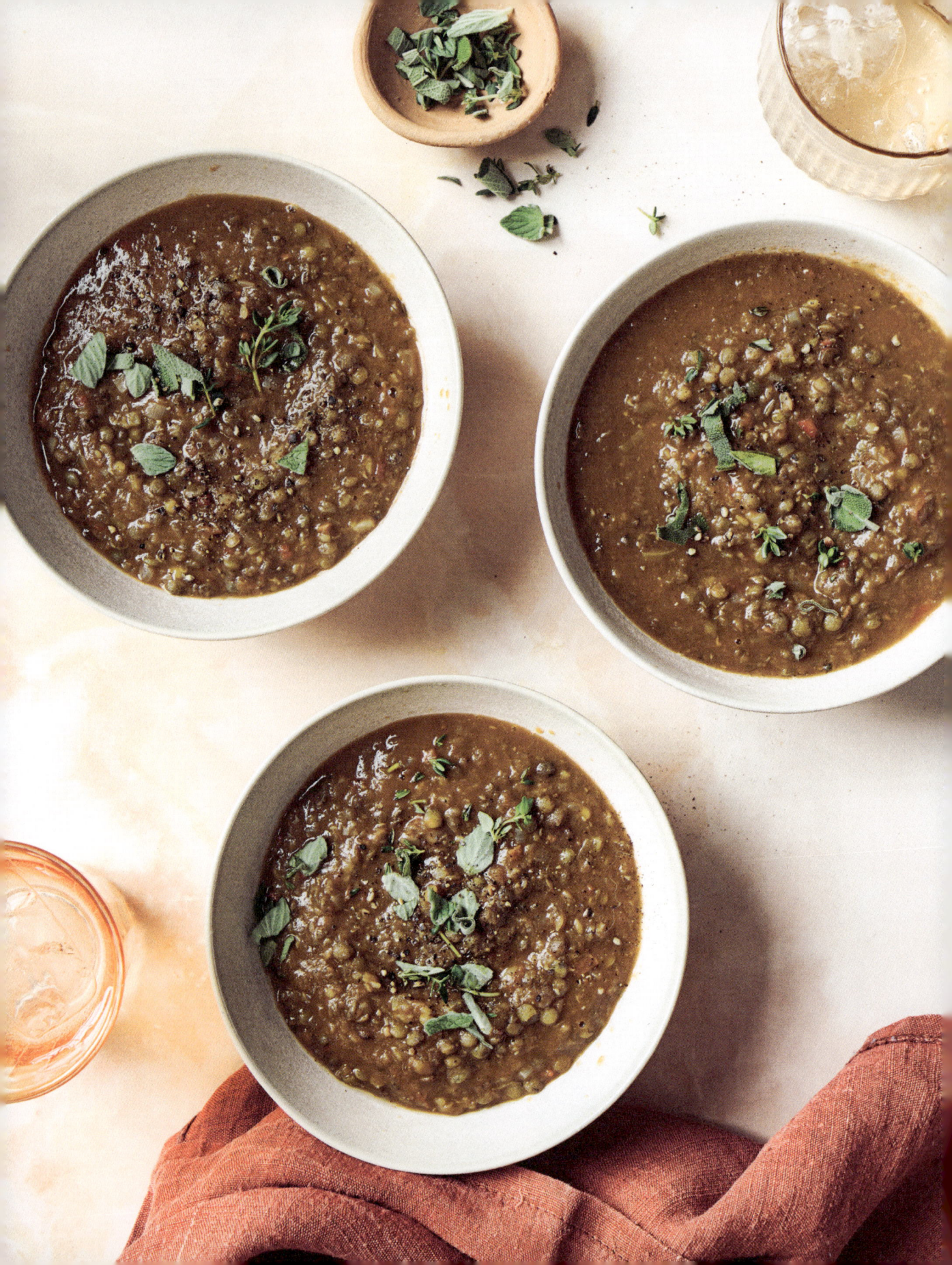

LENTIL, CHORIZO & RED CHILLI SOUP

SERVES 6
PREP TIME 10 minutes
COOK TIME 55 minutes

50g (1¾oz) chorizo, finely chopped

2 onions, finely chopped

2 leeks, trimmed, cleaned and finely chopped (see page 197)

1 red chilli, deseeded and finely chopped

2 garlic cloves, crushed

400g (14oz) can of chopped tomatoes

300g (10½oz) dried Puy lentils, or green lentils

1.5 litres (2½ pints) hot chicken stock

salt and pepper

any herbs you have: parsley, basil, oregano, sage or coriander would all work, to serve

A hearty lentil soup goes a long way: it's nourishing, filling and delicious. Just a small section of chorizo is enough to add great flavour to this recipe. Make a big batch to feed you easy lunches and dinners for days, adding bread on the side for extra filling-power, if you like.

1 Put the chorizo pieces into a large pan, which has a lid, and start to gently fry them over a medium heat. I use a shallow flameproof casserole dish here and I don't use additional oil as I find the chorizo releases enough to fry the vegetables.

2 Add the onions, leeks and chilli to the pan and stir-fry for 10 minutes.

3 Stir through the crushed garlic, then the chopped tomatoes.

4 Add the lentils, pour in the hot stock, stir thoroughly, then pop a lid on the pan and simmer gently for 45 minutes. Stir a couple of times while it is simmering, to ensure nothing sticks to the base of the pan.

5 After 45 minutes, try a lentil to check that they are soft and cooked through. Season to taste with salt and pepper.

6 Use a stick blender, either to partially blend the soup and give it a nice thick consistency, or to blend it completely smooth, if you prefer it that way. Scatter with herbs and serve in warmed bowls.

NOTE

Dried lentils are much more budget-friendly than canned and pre-cooked, though those are great for convenience and quicker meals. I really love Puy lentils, and if you can get hold of them (I buy them at my local health food shop), I think they make the nicest soup. Green lentils are still great though, if that's what you can find.

PER SERVING

CALORIES	FAT	SAT FAT	CARBS	SUGARS	FIBRE	PROTEIN	SALT
263	4.8G	1.5G	32G	9.1G	12G	16G	1.8G

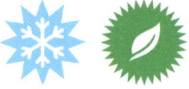

BATCH-COOKED JACKET POTATOES

MAKES 8
PREP TIME 5 minutes
COOK TIME 30–80 minutes, depending on method, plus reheating

8 baking potatoes
spray oil
coarse salt

These are a game-changer! I love the flavour of an oven-cooked jacket potato, but they usually take too long to make. These, on the other hand, make a convenient choice at lunchtime, because you can just quickly reheat them every time you fancy one, rather than waiting for them to fully cook. The best time to make a batch of these is when you have the oven going anyway; you can just pop in a tray of potatoes to make the most of it! The jackets will keep for five to seven days in the refrigerator and you might be surprised to know that you can also freeze them, once they have fully cooled: just seal into airtight freezer bags.

The calorie content will vary depending on the size of your potato, but a medium jacket potato without toppings is around **200 kcal**.

TO COOK

Oven method

1   Preheat the oven to 220°C/200°C fan (425°F), Gas Mark 7.

2   Use a sharp knife to make a cross in the top of each potato. Place them on a roasting tin, spray with oil and sprinkle with salt.

3   Bake for 20 minutes, then reduce the oven temperature to 190°C/170°C fan (375°F), Gas Mark 5 and bake for another 45–60 minutes, depending on how big your potatoes are. Check for doneness by inserting a sharp knife: after piercing the skin, it should easily slide through without resistance.

Microwave/oven combo method

1   Use a sharp knife to make a cross in the top of each potato. Put them into a large, microwave-safe bowl and cover with 2 layers of clingfilm. Microwave on high for 15 minutes (this does depend a bit on size; huge potatoes might need longer).

2   Preheat the oven to 220°C/200°C fan (425°F), Gas Mark 7.

3   Remove the bowl from the microwave, carefully peel back the clingfilm (the steam will be incredibly hot) and poke a sharp knife into one of the potatoes: it should go through easily, you want the insides to be fully cooked before oven-baking.

PER POTATO (WITHOUT TOPPINGS)

CALORIES	FAT	SAT FAT	CARBS	SUGARS	FIBRE	PROTEIN	SALT
205	1G	0.2G	41G	2.8G	5.2G	5G	0.14G

4 Tip the potatoes into a roasting tin, spray with oil, sprinkle with salt, then bake for 15 minutes.

5 Check them, give them a shake and return to the oven for another 5 minutes if needed: you want to crisp up the skin and give them that oven-baked taste.

Air-fryer method

1 Preheat the air fryer to 200°C (400°F) for a few minutes.

2 Use a sharp knife to make a cross in the top of each potato. Spray them with oil and sprinkle with salt. Place the potatoes in the air-fryer basket, making sure they are not overcrowded and have space between them for even cooking.

3 Cook for 40–50 minutes, depending on size. Check for doneness by inserting a fork into the centre of the largest potato; it should glide in easily with no resistance.

ONCE COOKED

Leave to fully cool before transferring to an airtight container to keep in the refrigerator, or freeze (see recipe introduction).

TO REHEAT

If your jacket potatoes are frozen, defrost thoroughly before reheating.

Oven method

1 Preheat the oven to 195°C/175°C fan (380°F), Gas Mark 5½.

2 Place the jacket potatoes on a baking tray, or in a roasting tin.

3 Bake for 15–20 minutes, or until heated through.

Microwave method

1 Place the jacket potatoes on a microwave-safe plate.

2 Microwave on high for 2–3 minutes per potato, depending on its size and the power of your microwave.

3 Check for doneness by inserting a fork into the centre of each potato; it should be hot all the way through. If necessary, continue microwaving in 1-minute increments until heated through.

4 Once heated, let the potatoes rest for a minute or so before serving.

Air-fryer method

1 Place the jacket potatoes in the air-fryer basket.

2 Cook for 5–8 minutes, depending on the size of the potatoes and the desired level of crispiness.

3 Check the potatoes halfway through cooking and shake the basket for even heating.

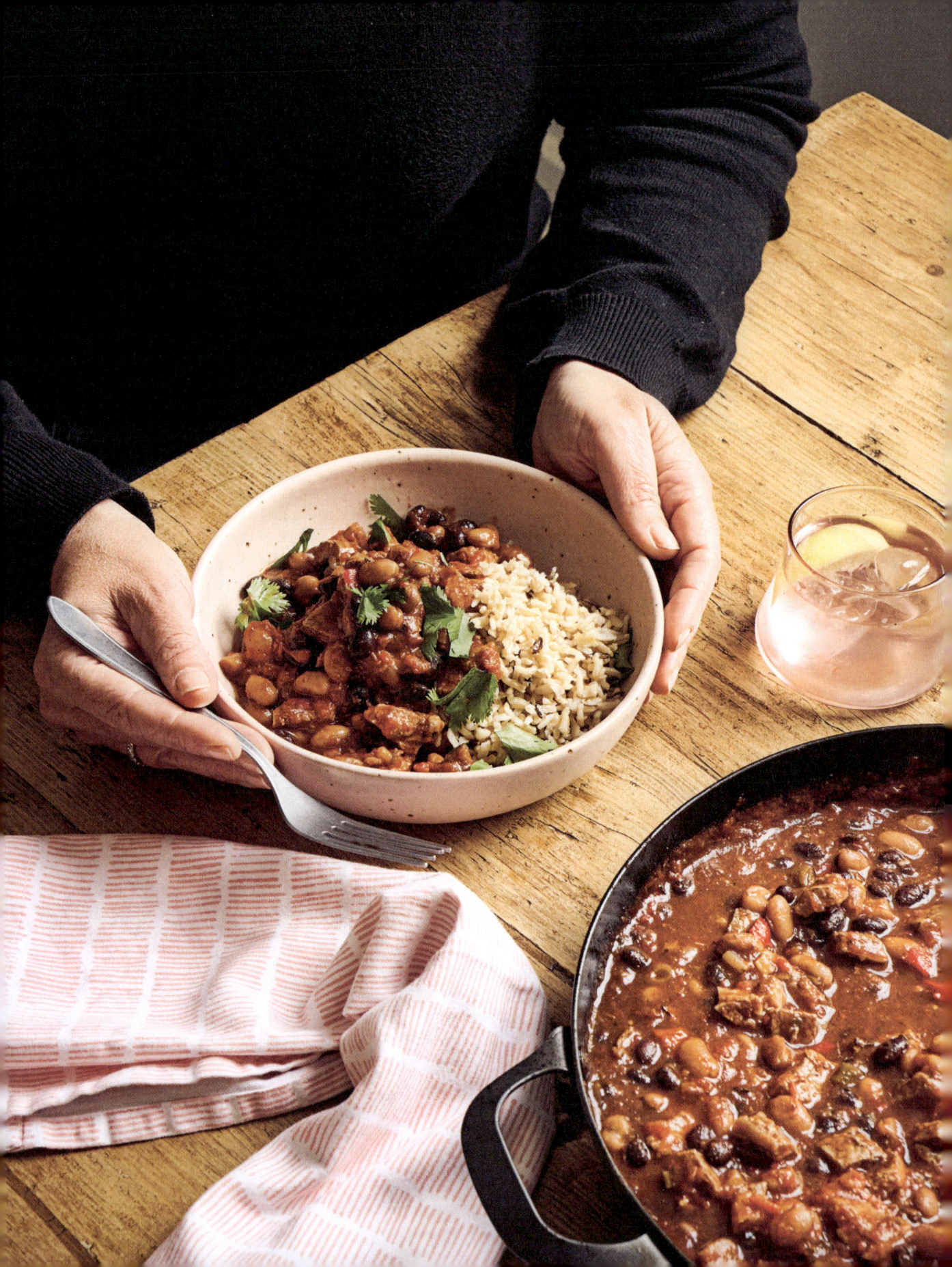

15-MINUTE CHILLI CON CARNE

SERVES 4
PREP TIME 10 minutes
COOK TIME 15 minutes

spray oil

2 frying steaks (total weight about 300g/10½oz), excess fat trimmed away

5 spring onions, sliced

1 red pepper, deseeded and finely chopped

400g (14oz) can of black beans, drained and rinsed

400g (14oz) can of pinto beans, drained and rinsed

2 tablespoons tomato purée

1 teaspoon ground cumin

1 teaspoon smoked paprika

1 teaspoon dried oregano

juice of 1 lime

salt and pepper

handful of chopped coriander leaves, to serve

FOR THE SAUCE

400g (14oz) can of chopped tomatoes

1 tablespoon finely chopped pickled jalapeños

3 garlic cloves

1 beef stock cube

1 red chilli, deseeded (optional)

Chilli con carne is a classic partner for rice or a jacket potato, but it's not usually quick, as a good chilli usually involves a slow simmer (you can find my more traditional recipe on page 183). This tasty version has a couple of little twists, which allow you to whip it up in no time at all: there's very little chopping, as the sauce is blended; and we're using frying steak, which is cheap, naturally lean, cooks fast and I think tastes better than minced meat in a limited time frame.

This recipe gives you enough to top a jacket potato, with leftovers to freeze or save for lunch another day.

1   Spray a sauté pan with oil and bring up to a high heat. Place the steaks into the pan and fry for 1–2 minutes on each side (for rare), or 3–4 minutes on each side (for medium/well). Remove from the pan and set aside on a plate.

2   Now spray a little more oil into the steak pan, add the spring onions and red pepper and set them to gently fry over a low heat for a couple of minutes while you prepare the sauce.

3   To make the sauce, use a mini chopper or food processor to whizz all the ingredients, including the chilli if you like it spicy, into a smooth sauce.

4   Increase the heat under the pepper and spring onions, stir-fry them for another minute, then pour in the sauce and stir it through. Add the beans, tomato purée, cumin, paprika and oregano, season with salt and pepper and simmer for 8 minutes.

5   Meanwhile, use a sharp knife to chop the steaks into very small pieces. After the sauce has simmered for 8 minutes, add the steaks and any juices back to the pan, stir through the lime juice, then try a little of the sauce to check the seasoning. Serve scattered with the chopped coriander.

NOTE

Red kidney beans are traditionally used in chilli, but personally I much prefer the smaller and softer black beans and pinto beans. Having a couple of different varieties of beans makes chilli more interesting, too, but feel free to substitute your preferred bean. I use canned beans for convenience, but it is cheaper to use dried.

PER SERVING

CALORIES	FAT	SAT FAT	CARBS	SUGARS	FIBRE	PROTEIN	SALT
300	6.3G	2.1G	24G	11G	12G	29G	0.87G

LIP SMACKIN' CHEESY BACON BEANS

SERVES 2
PREP TIME 5 minutes
COOK TIME 12 minutes

spray oil

1 red onion, finely chopped

4 smoked bacon medallions, finely chopped

400g (14oz) can of baked beans

1 roasted red pepper (from a jar), finely chopped

2 teaspoons Worcestershire sauce

½ teaspoon mild chilli powder

60g (2¼oz) Cheddar cheese, grated

freshly ground black pepper

chilli flakes, to garnish (optional)

I am a big advocate of a classic jacket potato with baked beans and cheese, but if you want to ramp it up to the next level, this simple jacket topping only takes a few more minutes to prepare and is unbelievably good! It is also great on toast, with mashed potato, or served up with a couple of fried eggs.

1   Spray a frying pan with oil and place over a medium-high heat. Stir-fry the onion and bacon pieces for 8 minutes.

2   Add the baked beans, red pepper, Worcestershire sauce and chilli powder and simmer gently for a few minutes to warm the beans through and allow them to soften a little.

3   Stir the cheese through until it's fully melted. Serve as you like (see recipe introduction), topped with some black pepper and chilli flakes, if you like.

NOTE

You could substitute the bacon here for roughly the same amount of finely chopped chorizo. Or, for a vegetarian option, replace the bacon with button mushrooms, add ½ teaspoon smoked paprika and use Henderson's relish instead of Worcestershire sauce.

PER SERVING

CALORIES	FAT	SAT FAT	CARBS	SUGARS	FIBRE	PROTEIN	SALT
460	16G	7.4G	40G	19G	12G	34G	2.85G

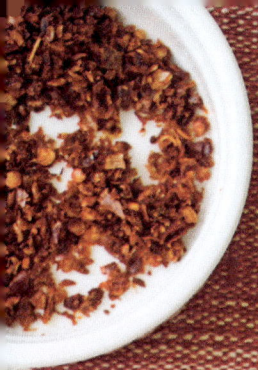

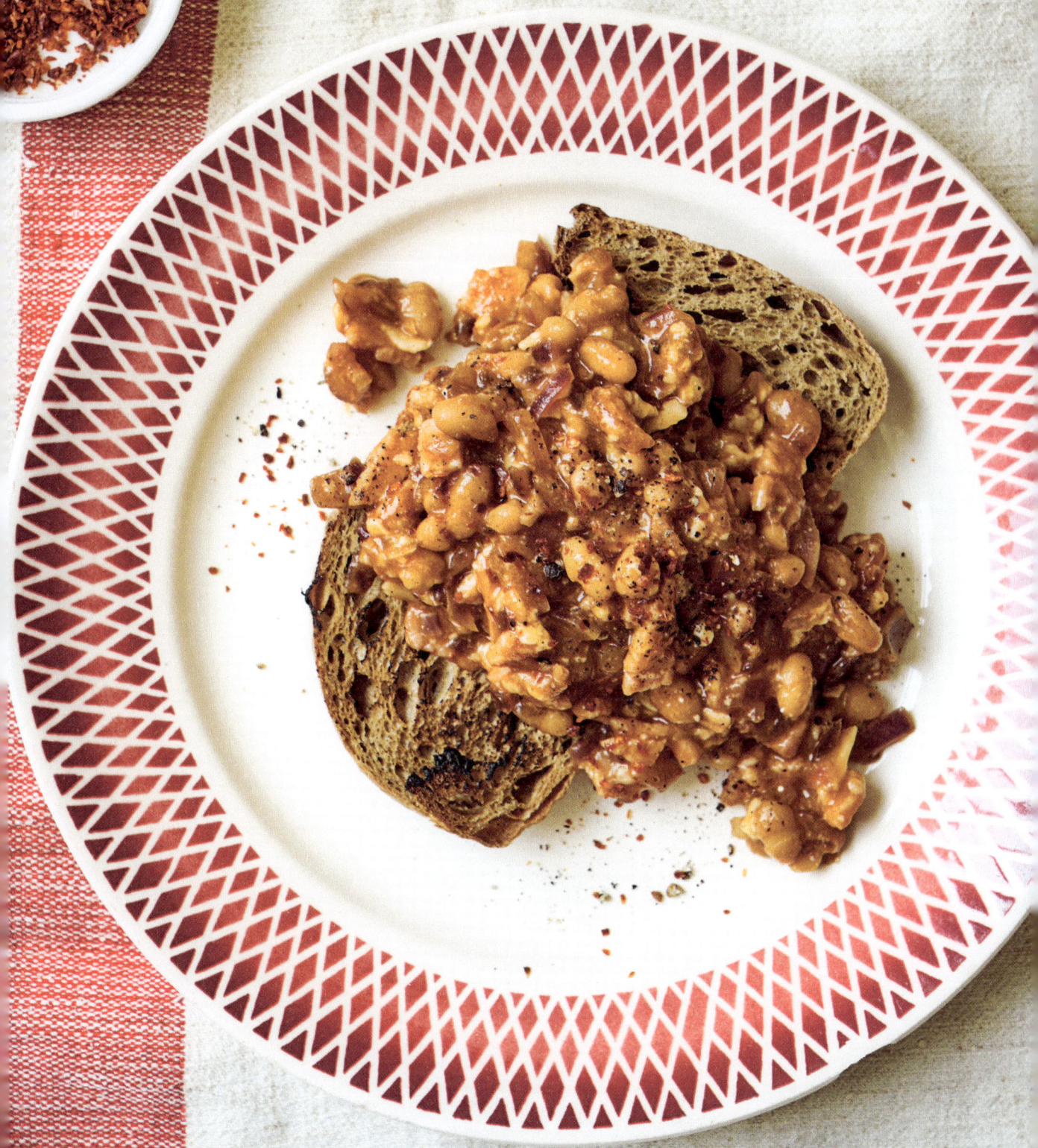

SPLIT PEA & HAM SOUP

SERVES 4
PREP TIME 10 minutes
COOK TIME 1 hour 8 minutes
(see note)

spray oil

1 onion, finely chopped

1 carrot, peeled and finely
 chopped

250g (9oz) yellow split peas,
 soaked and rinsed (see note)

1.5 litres (2½ pints) hot chicken
 stock made with 1 stock cube
 or pot

2 unsmoked gammon steaks (total
 weight about 300g/10½oz), fat
 trimmed away, finely chopped

freshly ground black pepper

This was a childhood favourite of mine, which my Mum would
make in a slow-cooker with a knuckle of ham from the butcher.
I was a fussy eater, but the comforting, wholesome taste of the
yellow split peas – delicately earthy with a slight sweetness and
a creamy texture – complemented by salty, savoury ham just hit
the spot, and my own children have always enjoyed this, too.
I have updated the recipe to make it a stove-top soup, using
readily available gammon steaks, and it's still a family favourite
for us. This is also a great way to use up leftover cooked ham,
simply add it for the last 10 minutes of the cooking time.

1 Spray a large saucepan with oil, place over a medium-low heat and fry
 the onion and carrot for 8 minutes, or until the onion has softened.

2 Add the split peas and pour over the hot stock. Bring to the boil, then
 reduce the heat and simmer for 40 minutes, stirring occasionally.

3 If you want a smooth base to your soup, use a stick blender to blend it
 now –if you choose to do this, you may just want to add some extra hot
 water as the gammon simmers, to ensure the soup does not get too dry.

4 Either way, add the gammon and simmer for a further 20 minutes; if
 you have chosen to leave it unblended, you will see that the peas have
 started to break down. Check the peas are tender before seasoning with
 pepper and serving in warmed bowls.

NOTE

Split peas can vary hugely in how long they take to cook, so you will need
to check yourself and decide if they need longer. You can shorten the
cooking time by soaking them overnight – or even just for a few hours
– before using them. If you have soaked them, you should find they are
tender in 30–45 minutes, as in the recipe above. If you have not pre-soaked
them, they are likely to take around 1 hour to reach the right consistency,
even a little longer. Just make sure you taste them to check they aren't still
hard. Occasionally, old split peas won't soften at all, so make sure yours
are in date before cooking them.

PER SERVING

CALORIES	FAT	SAT FAT	CARBS	SUGARS	FIBRE	PROTEIN	SALT
346	7.8G	2.3G	37G	5.5G	8.3G	27G	2.07G

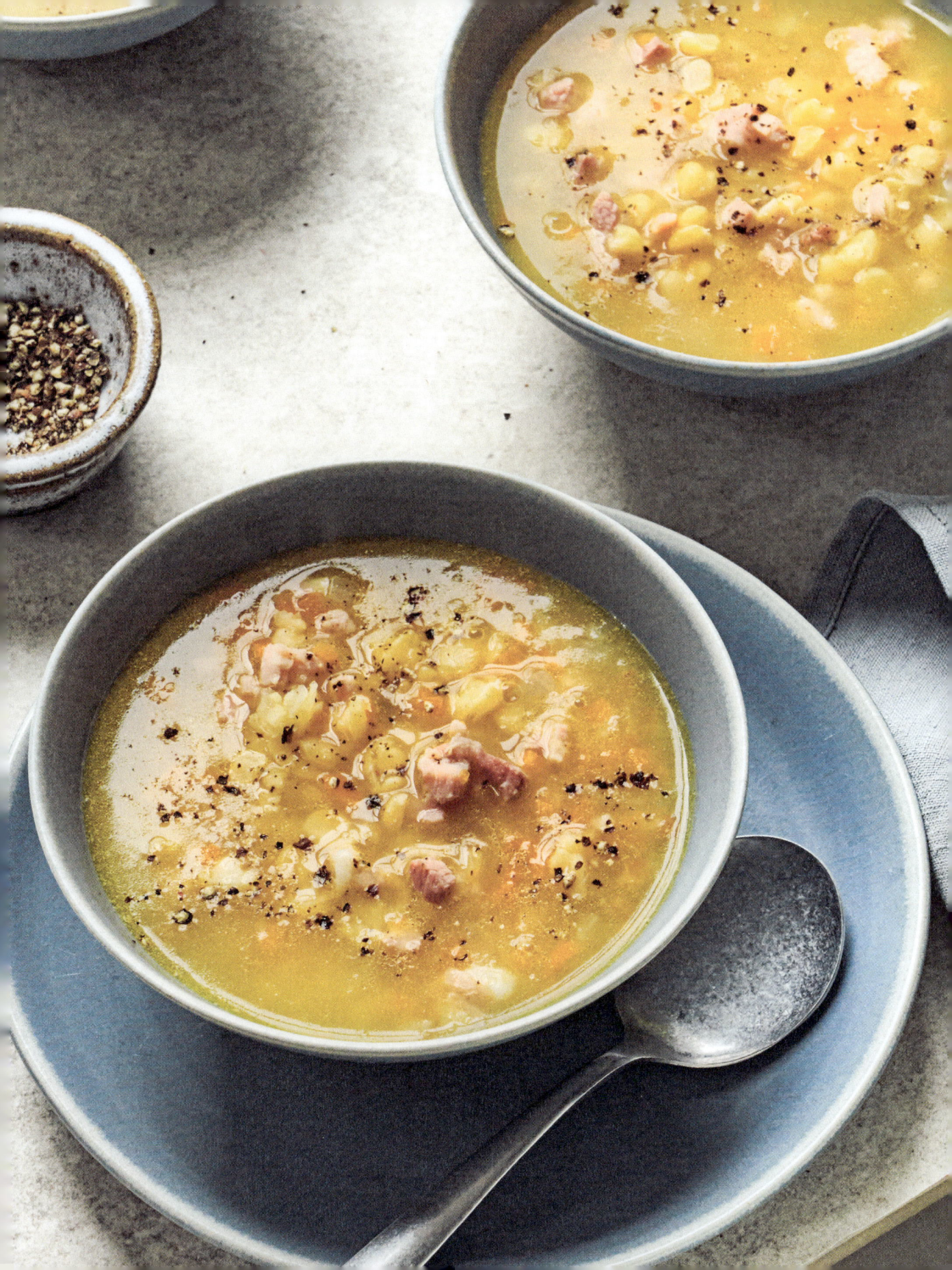

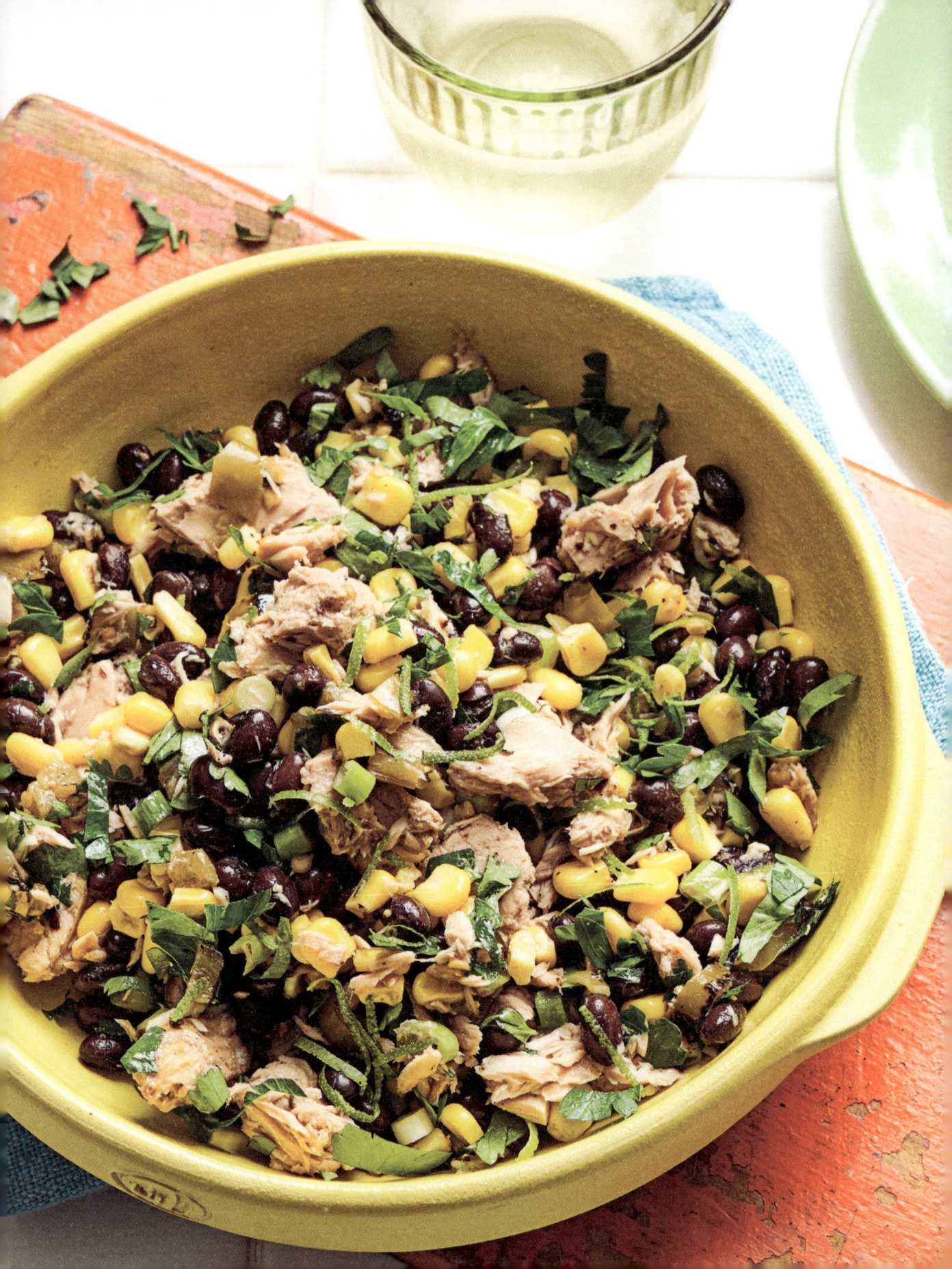

MEXICAN-INSPIRED TUNA & BEAN SALAD

SERVES 4
PREP TIME 10 minutes
COOK TIME none

This simple salad is so quick and easy to throw together – there's no cooking involved – and it tastes great over jacket potatoes, or just on its own.

145g (5¼oz) can of tuna in spring water or brine, drained

400g (14oz) can of black beans, drained and rinsed

160g (5¾oz) can of sweetcorn, drained

3 spring onions, finely sliced

2 tablespoons finely chopped pickled jalapeños

leaves from a few parsley sprigs, finely chopped

salt and pepper

FOR THE DRESSING

finely grated zest and juice of 1 lime

1 tablespoon honey

1 garlic clove, crushed or grated

1 tablespoon white wine vinegar

1   Put all the salad ingredients into a salad bowl and season to taste with salt and pepper.

2   Mix together the dressing ingredients in a small bowl, season this to taste, too, then add to the salad.

3   Stir everything together gently but thoroughly and serve.

NOTE

This salad is a great vehicle for all sorts of fresh vegetables, as well as a good way to use up bits and pieces from the refrigerator. Try adding salad leaves, chopped sweet peppers, tomatoes, avocado, cucumber, finely sliced radishes, sugar snap peas or chopped fine green beans.

PER SERVING

CALORIES	FAT	SAT FAT	CARBS	SUGARS	FIBRE	PROTEIN	SALT
152	1.2G	0.2G	17G	9.5G	6.7G	15G	0.7G

BASIC QUESADILLA

SERVES 1
PREP TIME 2 minutes
COOK TIME 5 minutes

2 mini tortilla wraps
30g (1oz) Cheddar cheese, grated

This is an incredibly simple recipe, and if it's not something you are already familiar with, you will find it so useful for fantastic quick lunches or accompaniments to soup. My youngest daughter loves these and, now she's 12, has learned to make them herself. I make them with mini tortilla wraps for the kids (I try to buy those which contain wholemeal flour, if I can), but you can use any size. Sometimes I make them for me and my husband to go alongside soup, in which case I'll use two medium-sized low-calorie wraps and we have half each.

1   Heat a frying pan over a medium heat. Put 1 wrap into the pan, scatter the cheese evenly over the top, then place the second tortilla on top. Cook for 2–3 minutes, until the bottom wrap is golden brown, toasted and crispy and the cheese has mostly melted.

2   Use a spatula to flip the quesadilla and cook for 2–3 minutes on the other side.

3   Once both sides are crisp, transfer to a plate and cut into quarters.

NOTE

I make a variation of this which, in our family, we call a 'pizzadilla'. You spread 1 teaspoon tomato purée or passata on the bottom wrap, sprinkle it with a few pinches of dried oregano or mixed herbs, then add the cheese. I've always found this a nice easy lunch to prepare when my girls have friends over and we need something quick that everybody likes!

PER SERVING

CALORIES	FAT	SAT FAT	CARBS	SUGARS	FIBRE	PROTEIN	SALT
296	14G	8G	30G	1.2G	2.2G	12G	1.5G

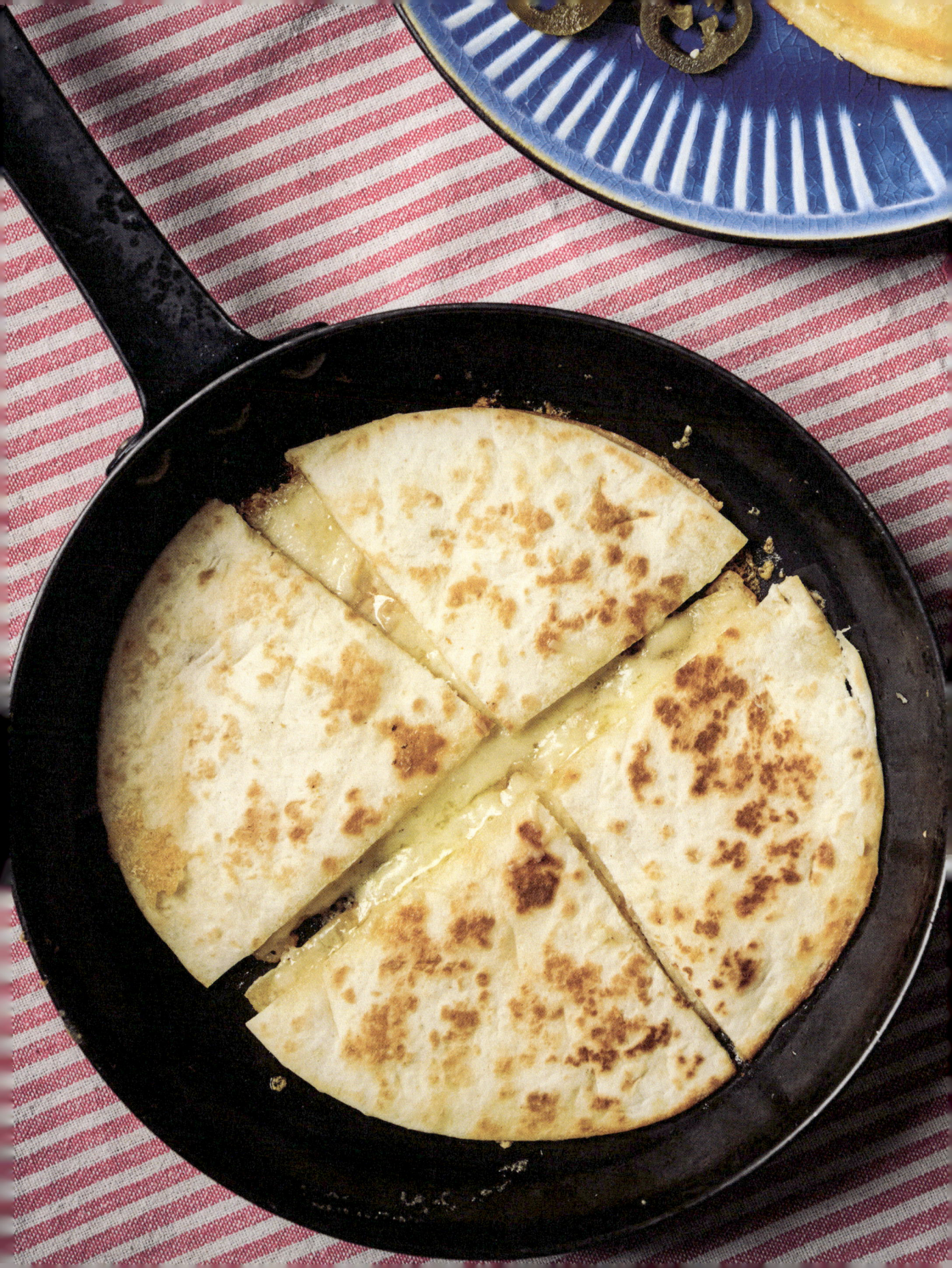

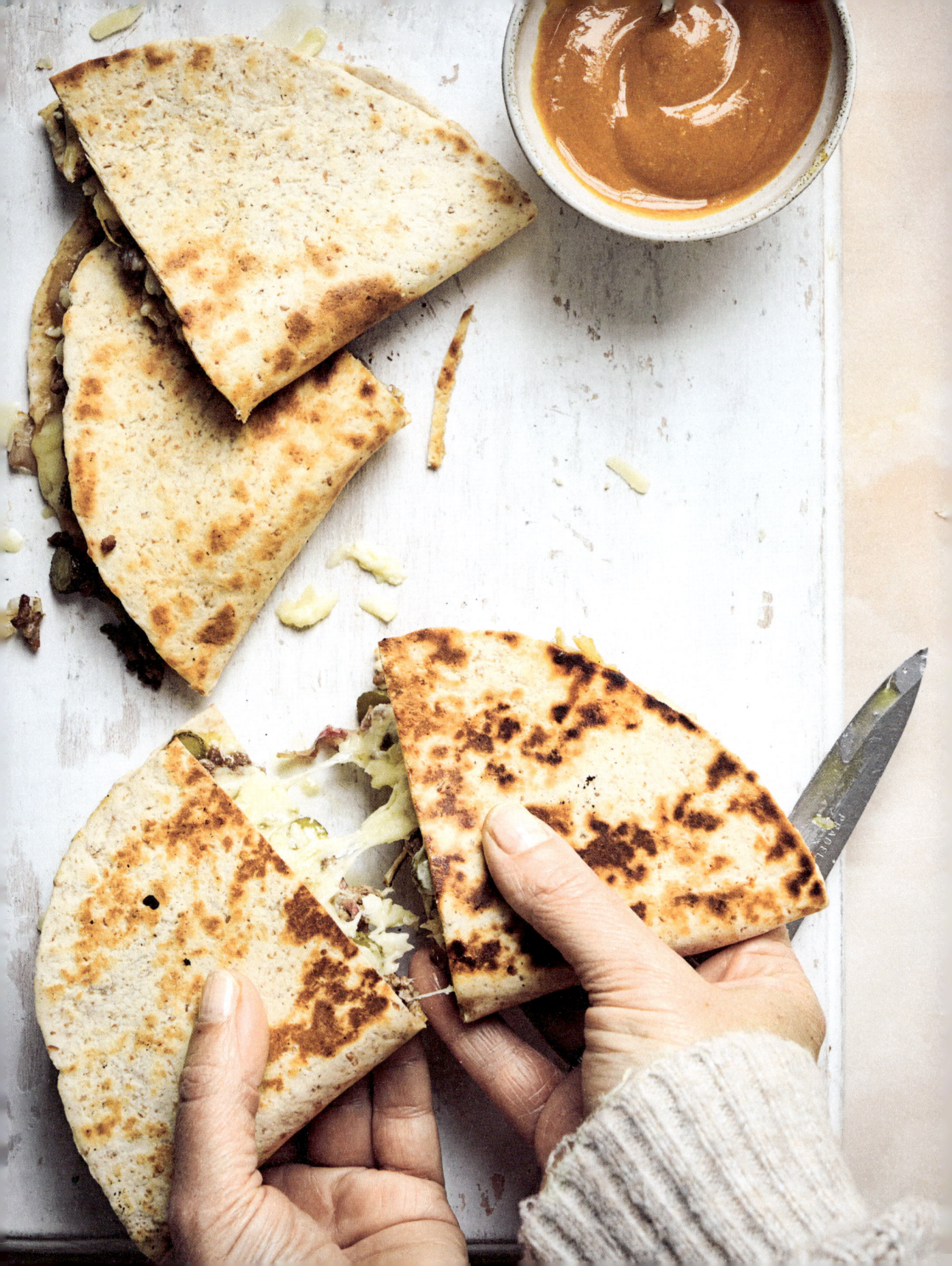

CHEESEBURGER QUESADILLA

SERVES 2
PREP TIME 5 minutes
COOK TIME 15 minutes

spray oil
1 small onion, finely sliced into
    half moons
150g (5½oz) lean minced beef
    (less than 5 per cent fat)
1 tablespoon American mustard
1 tablespoon tomato ketchup
1 tablespoon Worcestershire
    sauce
2 medium-sized low-calorie
    tortilla wraps
90g (3¼oz) Cheddar cheese,
    grated
2 cornichons, finely sliced
salt and pepper

All the flavours of a great cheeseburger come through in this quick lunch, a delicious treat, with a satisfying crisp on the outside. You don't need any extras, as the quesadillas themselves are filling, but you could serve them with a side salad, or if you are feeling cheeky, some homemade fries.

1   Spray a frying pan with oil and fry the onion and beef for 10 minutes, until the beef has browned and the onion has softened.

2   Add the mustard, ketchup and Worcestershire sauce, season with salt and pepper and stir thoroughly. Spoon into a bowl and clean the pan.

3   Put a tortilla wrap in the frying pan. Over one half of it (you are going to be folding it in half) sprinkle on about one-quarter of the cheese, half the beef mixture, then half the cornichons. Add another one-quarter of the cheese and fold the tortilla over the filling to create a half-moon shape. Press down gently but firmly with a spatula to help compress and start to bind the fillings. Repeat this with the other tortilla, so that the 2 are neatly back-to-back in the pan.

4   Cook over a medium heat for 2–3 minutes, until the bases are golden brown and the cheese is melty.

5   Use a spatula to carefully flip over each quesadilla (I do this by sliding the spatula underneath, laying a hand on top, then quickly flipping it over). If some filling does spill out, just push it back inside.

6   Fry on the other side for another 2–3 minutes until this side, too is golden brown and slightly crisp. The cooking time can vary depending on the pan and heat you are using, so if you begin to smell burning, flip the tortilla to prevent ending up with one over-charred side. Use a sharp knife to cut each quesadilla in half, then serve.

NOTE
You can really dress this up however you like in terms of extra fillings. Some of my favourite additions are fried mushrooms, pickled jalapeños, salsa, chopped avocado, hot sauce or herb leaves. You can also swap out the Cheddar for mozzarella.

PER SERVING

CALORIES	FAT	SAT FAT	CARBS	SUGARS	FIBRE	PROTEIN	SALT
438	20G	12G	29G	9.2G	3.8G	32G	2.1G

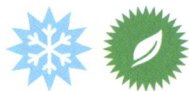

WHITE BEAN SOUP

SERVES 4
PREP TIME 5 minutes
COOK TIME 16 minutes

spray oil
1 onion, finely chopped
2 garlic cloves, sliced
1 green chilli, deseeded and finely
    chopped
500ml (18fl oz) hot vegetable
    stock
3 x 400g (14oz) cans of cannellini
    beans, drained and rinsed
1 teaspoon dried oregano
½ teaspoon ground cumin
½ teaspoon smoked paprika
1 teaspoon coarse salt
finely grated zest and juice
    of 1 lime
1 tablespoon finely chopped
    pickled jalapeños
3 spring onions, finely sliced
pepper, to serve

Using canned beans is a great way to make quick, easy and filling soup. This recipe, with its Mexican-inspired flavours, can be on the table in less than 20 minutes! If I'm feeling extra hungry, I serve it with a Basic Quesadilla on the side (see page 28).

1   Spray a saucepan with oil and fry the onion for 5 minutes, then add the garlic and chilli and stir-fry for another minute.

2   Add the hot stock, beans, oregano, cumin, paprika, salt and lime zest and simmer for 10 minutes.

3   Use a stick blender to purée the mixture into a smooth soup, then stir in the lime juice.

4   Ladle into warmed bowls, scatter with the jalapeños and spring onions and grind over some pepper to serve.

NOTE
You can add extra toppings to this, such as chopped avocado, coriander sprigs or a drizzle of chilli sauce.

PER SERVING

CALORIES	FAT	SAT FAT	CARBS	SUGARS	FIBRE	PROTEIN	SALT
238	3.4G	0.7G	30G	3.7G	13G	50G	1.5G

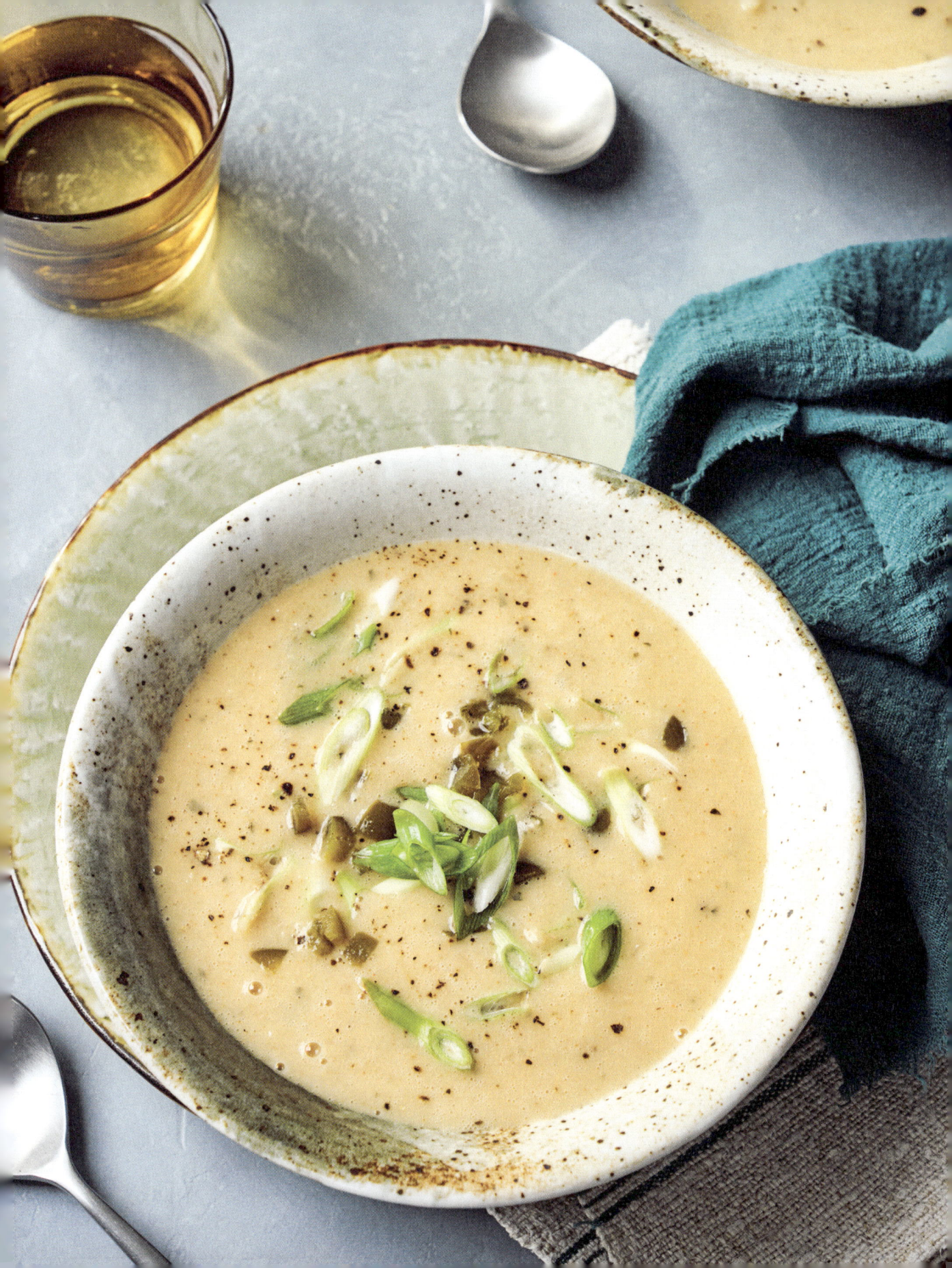

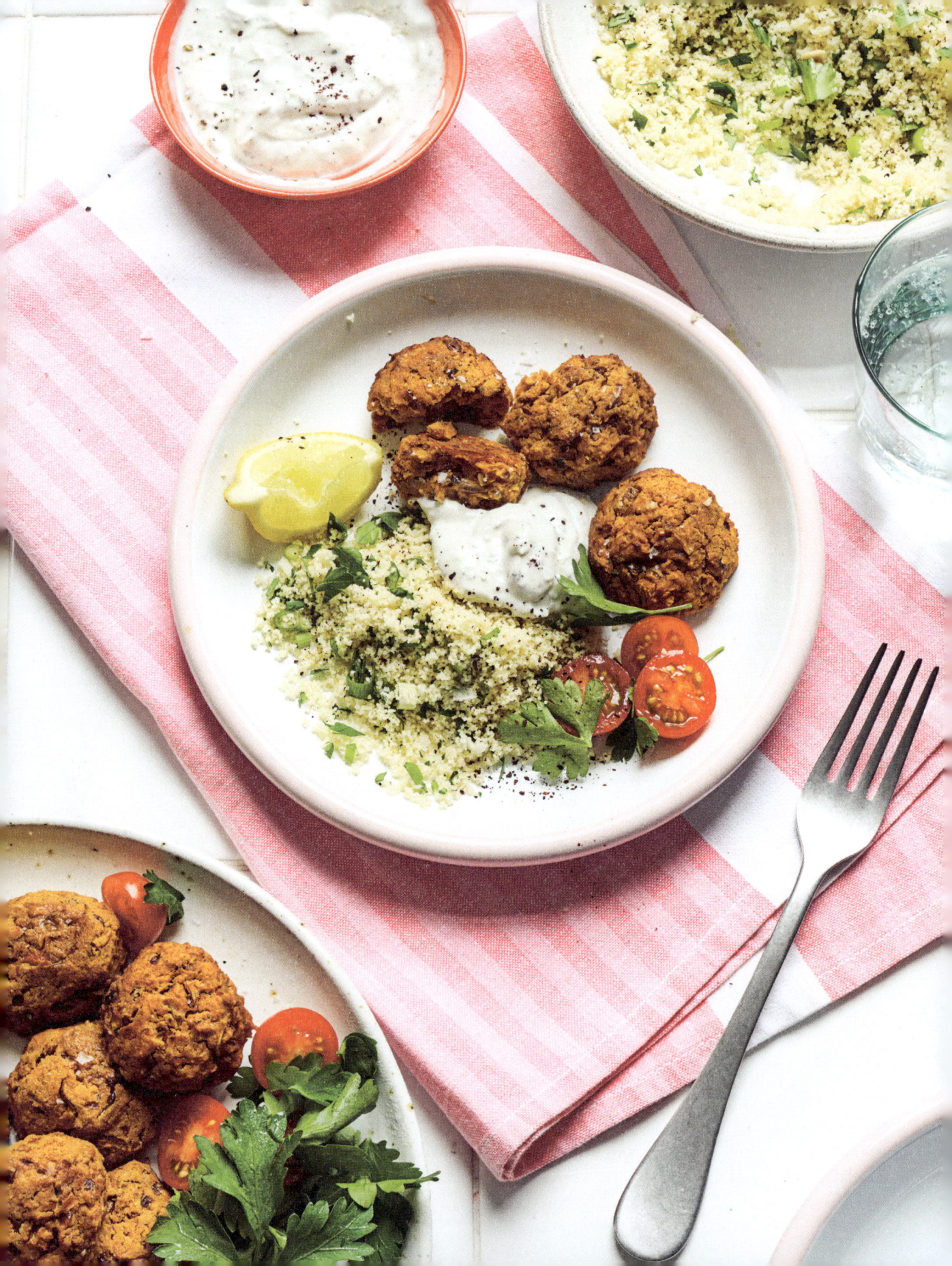

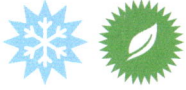

OVEN-BAKED FALAFELS

MAKES 18
PREP TIME 15 minutes
COOK TIME 30 minutes

spray oil
1 large red onion, finely chopped
2 large garlic cloves, crushed
1 teaspoon ground cumin
1 teaspoon ground coriander
1 teaspoon sweet (unsmoked)
    paprika
400g (14oz) can of chickpeas,
    drained and rinsed
400g (14oz) can of mixed beans,
    drained and rinsed
finely grated zest of 1 lime
1 tablespoon harissa paste
2 tablespoons plain flour
1 egg
1 teaspoon coarse salt
¼ teaspoon freshly ground
    black pepper

Making a batch of falafels in advance is a great way to take the hassle out of easy lunches and snacks, as you get lots of flavour in a tasty little package. They are so versatile: serve them in pitta bread, with a grain salad or salad leaves, or alongside some Greek yogurt and crisp fresh vegetables, such as cucumber and baby tomatoes.

1   Spray a frying pan with oil and fry the onion until it's soft (around 8 minutes), then add the garlic, cumin, coriander and paprika. Stir-fry for 2 minutes, then transfer to a mixing bowl to cool down while you prepare the other ingredients.

2   Put the chickpeas, mixed beans, lime zest, harissa, flour, egg, salt and pepper into a food processor and blend until smooth.

3   Transfer into the bowl containing the onions, then mix everything thoroughly together.

4   Preheat the oven to 210°C/190°C fan (410°F), Gas Mark 6½.

5   Line a baking tray with nonstick baking paper and shape the mixture into about 18 balls with your hands (if you wet your hands first, it helps prevent the mixture from sticking). Place them on the prepared tray as you shape them, leaving space between each, so they are able to crisp on the outside. You may need a second baking tray.

6   Spray the falafels with oil, then bake for 20 minutes. Allow them to cool for at least 10 minutes before removing from the tray.

NOTE

If you are going to eat these in pitta bread, or with a grain salad, you might want this quick and easy yogurt dip to go with them. Simply mix together 6 tablespoons of fat-free Greek yogurt, 1 finely grated garlic clove, the juice of the zested lime and 2 teaspoons Italian dried herbs, or za'atar or a mix of other dried herbs, such as oregano, thyme, basil or rosemary).

PER FALAFEL

CALORIES	FAT	SAT FAT	CARBS	SUGARS	FIBRE	PROTEIN	SALT
53	1.1G	0.14G	6.8G	0.83G	1.9G	2.9G	0.29G

BACON & SWEETCORN CHOWDER

SERVES 2
PREP TIME 5 minutes
COOK TIME 18 minutes

spray oil

3 smoked bacon medallions, chopped

1 onion, finely chopped

1 large potato (about 180g/6oz), peeled and chopped into 5mm (¼ inch) cubes

250ml (9fl oz) hot chicken stock

250ml (9fl oz) semi-skimmed milk

200g (7oz) sweetcorn, frozen or canned

salt and pepper

chopped chives, to serve

Quick, filling and full of flavour, this is an easy lunch to whip up in a pinch and it is great for taking to work in a soup container.

1   Spray a saucepan with oil, then fry the bacon, onion and potato for 8 minutes, stirring regularly.

2   Pour in the hot stock and milk and simmer for 5 minutes.

3   Now add the sweetcorn and simmer for another 5 minutes.

4   Season (you may not need much salt as the bacon is salty), divide between 2 warmed bowls and sprinkle with chopped chives.

NOTE

Stir through some grated Cheddar before serving, for extra flavour and (of course) cheesiness!

PER SERVING

CALORIES	FAT	SAT FAT	CARBS	SUGARS	FIBRE	PROTEIN	SALT
372	6.9G	2.2G	53G	18G	5.7G	22G	2.5G

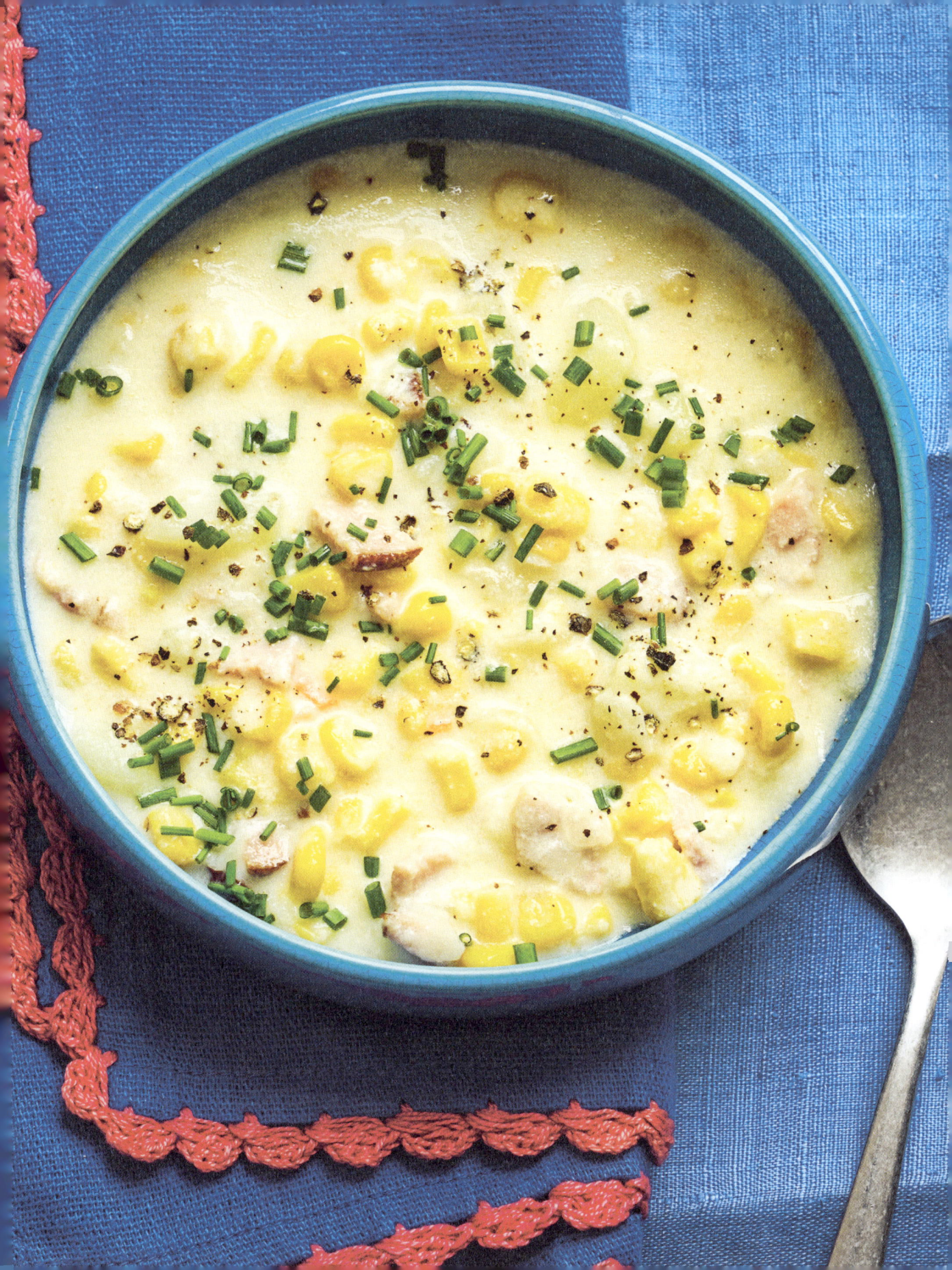

BRIGHT & BREEZY

2

TANDOORI CHICKEN TENDERS

SERVES 4
PREP TIME 5 minutes,
plus 30 minutes marinating
COOK TIME 10 minutes

2 tablespoons fat-free Greek
   yogurt
1½ tablespoons shop-bought
   tandoori spice mix
2 garlic cloves, crushed
juice of 1 lemon
½ teaspoon coarse salt
4 skinless chicken breasts, each
   cut into 5 strips lengthways

I always keep a pot of tandoori spice mix in the cupboard, both because tandoori-style chicken is one of my children's favourite foods and because it is such a quick and easy meal: this marinade can be put together in minutes. It's a recipe that's perfect for both barbecuing and grilling and easy to scale up or down, depending how many you are feeding. The tenders are delicious hot, or make perfect picnic food and easy lunches when cold, too.

1 Make up the marinade by combining the yogurt, spice mix, garlic, lemon juice and salt in a mixing bowl, then stir in the chicken strips. Cover and allow to marinate for at least 30 minutes (or longer if you prefer, overnight in the refrigerator is fine).

2 Preheat the grill to high and lay the chicken pieces on the grill rack, or a rack over a baking tray. Grill for 4–5 minutes on each side, or until cooked, depending on how thick your chicken pieces are.

3 When the chicken is cooked, it should be a rich golden-orange colour with some browning on the edges. You can cut the thickest chicken piece in half to check that it is cooked through and not pink in the middle, or use a meat thermometer to check it has reached a safe temperature (75°C/167°F for chicken).

NOTE

Some serving suggestions:

Wraps Fill warmed tortillas with the cooked tandoori chicken, lettuce, sliced tomatoes, cucumber and a dollop of minty yogurt sauce (combine chopped fresh mint leaves with fat-free yogurt).

Salad Slice the cooked chicken and toss with mixed salad leaves, cherry tomatoes, sliced red onions and cucumber. Drizzle with a simple dressing made with lemon juice, a dash of olive oil and a pinch of tandoori spice mix.

Skewers Thread the uncooked marinated chicken strips on to skewers with chunks of sweet pepper, onion wedges and cherry tomatoes. Grill until the chicken is cooked through and serve with a side of basmati rice, with mango chutney or aubergine pickle.

Tandoori platter Arrange the grilled chicken on a platter alongside basmati rice, warmed mini naans and steamed green veg, such as broccoli, green beans or asparagus.

Bounty bowl Build a bowl with a base of cooked quinoa or brown rice, topped with sliced avocado, steamed broccoli, shredded carrots and sliced tandoori chicken tenders. Drizzle with a minty yogurt sauce (see Wraps, above).

PER SERVING

CALORIES	FAT	SAT FAT	CARBS	SUGARS	FIBRE	PROTEIN	SALT
203	2.2G	0.6G	1.6G	0.8G	0.8G	44G	0.93G

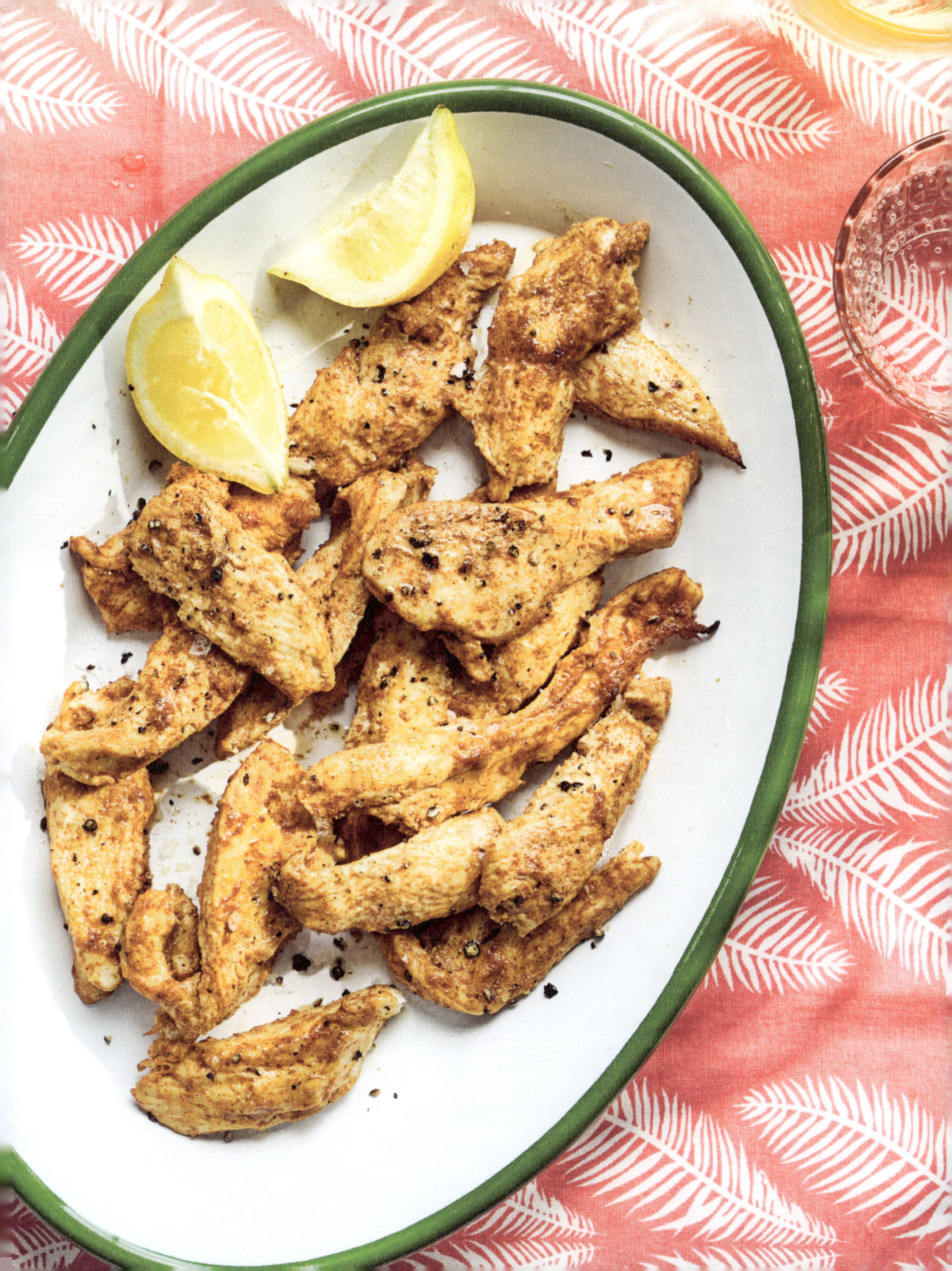

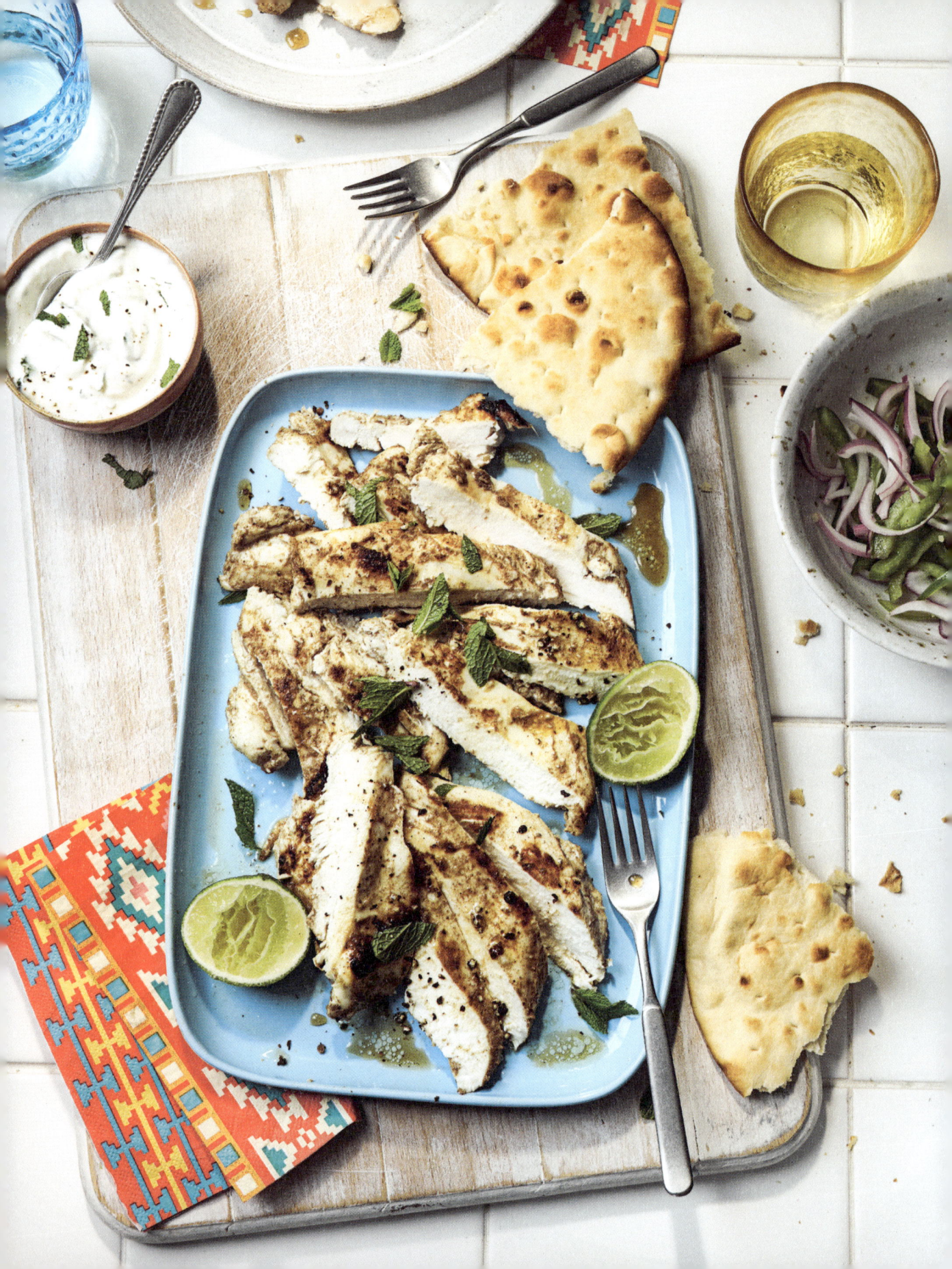

CHICKEN SHAWARMA WITH GARLIC SAUCE

SERVES 4
PREP TIME 20 minutes
(plus marinating)
COOK TIME 15 minutes

FOR THE CHICKEN & MARINADE
4 skinless chicken breasts
4 garlic cloves, crushed
juice of 2 limes
1 teaspoon ground allspice
1 teaspoon ground cinnamon
1 teaspoon ground cumin
1 teaspoon ground coriander
1 teaspoon freshly ground black pepper
1 teaspoon coarse salt

FOR THE CREAMY GARLIC SAUCE
125g (4½oz) fat-free Greek yogurt
2 garlic cloves, crushed
juice of ½ lemon
¼ teaspoon salt
10 mint leaves, finely chopped

FOR THE SALAD
½ red onion, very finely sliced
1 green pepper, very finely sliced

TO SERVE
4 white flatbreads, or wholemeal pitta breads
lime wedges

This recipe is not in any way an authentic shawarma (in the Middle East, the meat would traditionally be cooked on a vertical rotisserie), but the results are still delicious. This chicken would taste even better cooked on a barbecue, but a regular oven grill will do just fine. You can decide whether you pair this with wholemeal pitta, or a white flatbread, though the calorie count will be different. Serve this with a salad or some homemade fries for an extra element.

1   Place the chicken breasts, 1 at a time, between 2 sheets of clingfilm, and gently beat with a rolling pin, or the underside of a saucepan, to flatten.

2   Mix the marinade ingredients in a bowl and spread it evenly over each flattened chicken breast (I pile them up in a bowl with the marinade between each).

3   Set the chicken aside while you prepare the other ingredients, and allow to marinate for at least 10 minutes. If you want, you can cover and marinate in the refrigerator for a few hours, or overnight, for extra flavour.

4   Make the garlic sauce by mixing together all the ingredients in a bowl.

5   Preheat the grill to high and grill the chicken for 15 minutes, turning halfway. It should be cooked through after this time, but double-check by slicing into the thickest part.

6   Set the chicken aside while you heat up your flatbreads or pittas. You can do this under the grill or in the toaster, depending on their size.

7   I put everything into the middle of the table so everyone can construct their own meal to taste. Slice the chicken breasts into strips, mix the red onion and green pepper together in a bowl and place everything on the table with the warm flatbreads, garlic sauce and lime wedges.

NOTE

If you are cooking the chicken on a barbecue, you will need to cook each breast for about 10 minutes, turning halfway through. If you are going to be having a barbecue anyway, it's really worth just making some of this chicken for some delicious lunches later in the week.

PER SERVING (WITH WHITE FLATBREAD)

CALORIES	FAT	SAT FAT	CARBS	SUGARS	FIBRE	PROTEIN	SALT
487	6.9G	1.1G	48G	6.9G	6.1G	53G	2.4G

PENNE SICILIANA

SERVES 4
PREP TIME 10 minutes
COOK TIME 40 minutes

2 large aubergines

1 tablespoon olive oil

400g (14oz) can of chopped or plum tomatoes

4 garlic cloves

½ teaspoon dried oregano

½ teaspoon salt, plus more for the aubergines

300g (10½oz) penne

200g (7oz) mozzarella balls, torn into small pieces

45g (1¾oz) finely grated Parmesan-style vegetarian cheese

freshly ground black pepper

When I worked in Covent Garden in London, I became completely addicted to two dishes from an amazing restaurant called Pasta Brown. They made an unrivalled penne arrabbiata, or, my other favourite from the menu, penne Siciliana. It's a combination of super-soft, silky-textured aubergine with rich tomato, garlic and herb sauce and gooey, melty mozzarella; probably my favourite way to enjoy aubergine, which is both readily available and good value in summer in the UK. This is my easy but still absolutely delicious version.

1   Preheat the oven to 240°C/220°C fan (475°F), Gas Mark 9.

2   Prepare the aubergines. Trim away the stalks at the top, then slice the aubergines lengthways at 3cm (1¼ inch) intervals. Once you have the slices, cut each into quarters.

3   Place the aubergine pieces into a bowl, drizzle over the 1 tablespoon of olive oil and stir well to coat the pieces as much as possible. Season with salt and pepper. Lay them on a baking tray in a single layer and roast for 20 minutes, then flip them over and roast for another 10 minutes.

4   Meanwhile, prepare the sauce. Simply put the canned tomatoes, whole garlic cloves, oregano and ½ teaspoon salt in a mini chopper and blend into a smooth sauce.

5   Cook the penne according to the packet instructions, drain, then set aside until the aubergine is ready.

6   Remove the aubergine from the oven and reduce the oven temperature to 200°C/180°C fan (400°F), Gas Mark 6. In an ovenproof dish, mix the cooked pasta, tomato sauce and roasted aubergine. Add the torn mozzarella and half the grated Parmesan and mix the cheeses through. Top with the remaining Parmesan and freshly ground black pepper.

7   Put the baking dish into the oven and bake for 10 minutes, by which time the cheeses should be deliciously gooey.

NOTE

Add some extra vegetables to the sauce, if you like: peppers, courgette and cherry tomatoes all work well. Or whizz a pinch of chilli flakes, or a fresh chilli into the tomato sauce, for a spicy kick.

Roast the aubergine ahead of time, if you have the oven on, and store it in the refrigerator until ready to use. This allows you to assemble the dish quickly on busy weeknights.

PER SERVING

CALORIES	FAT	SAT FAT	CARBS	SUGARS	FIBRE	PROTEIN	SALT
520	19G	9.8G	59G	8.5G	6.7G	25G	2.1G

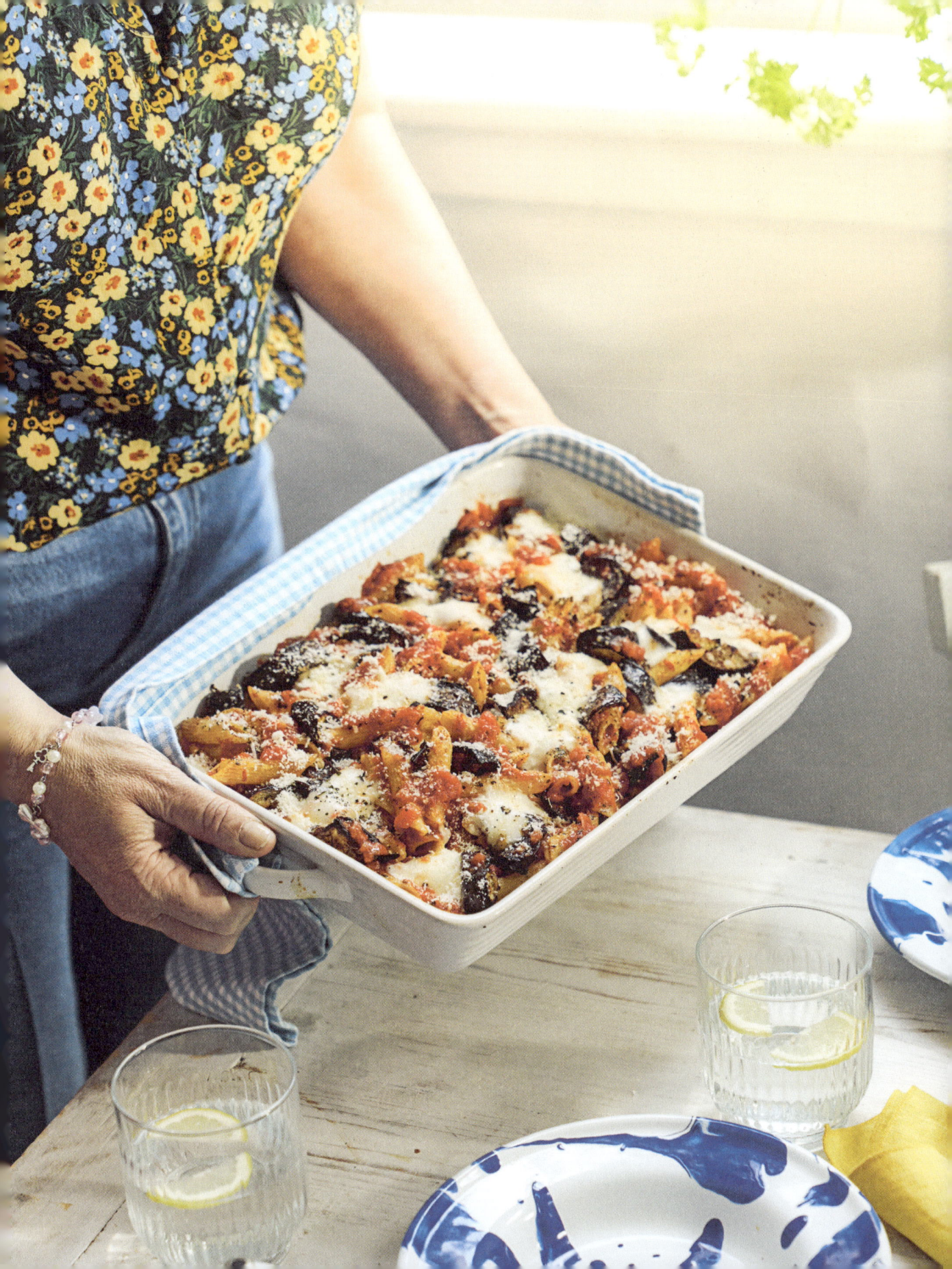

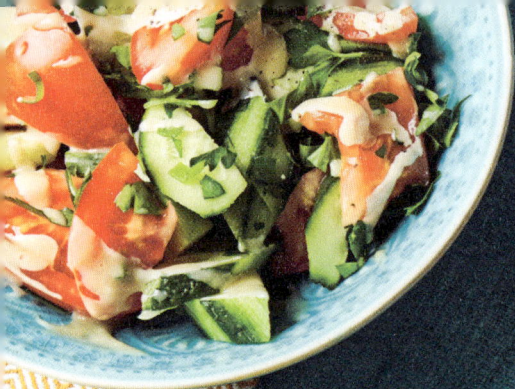

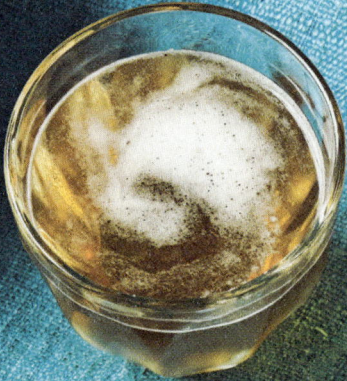

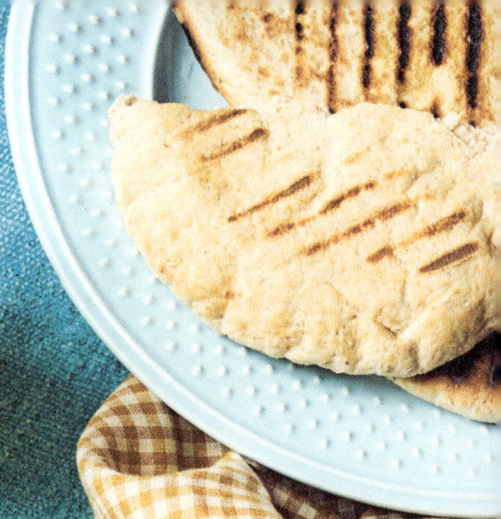

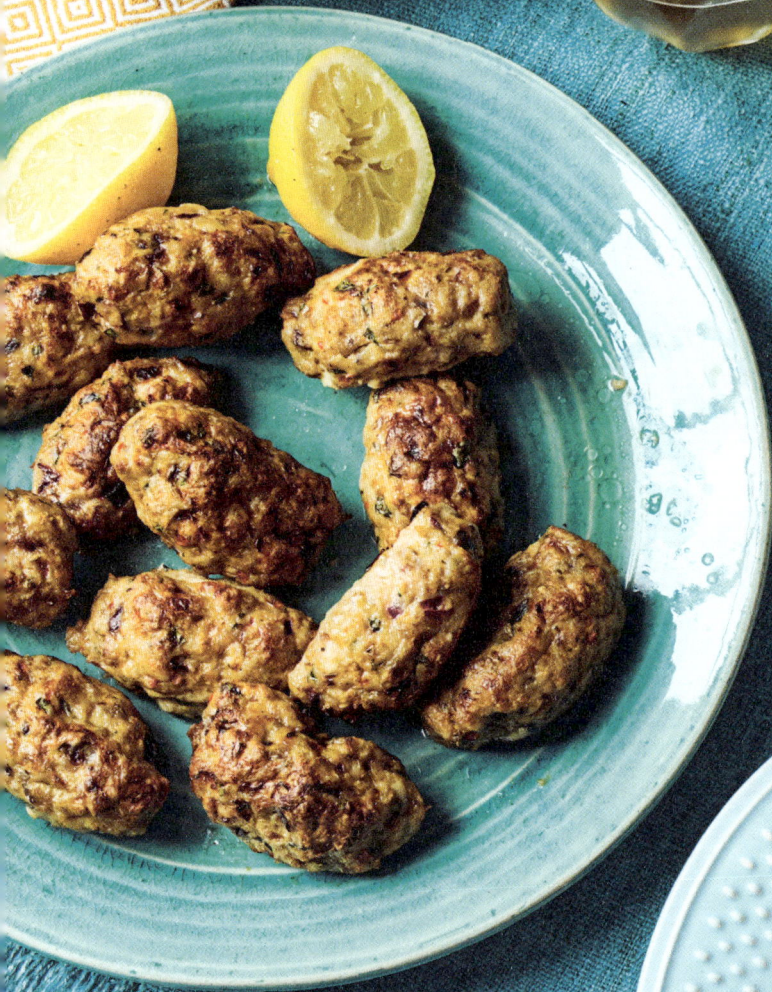

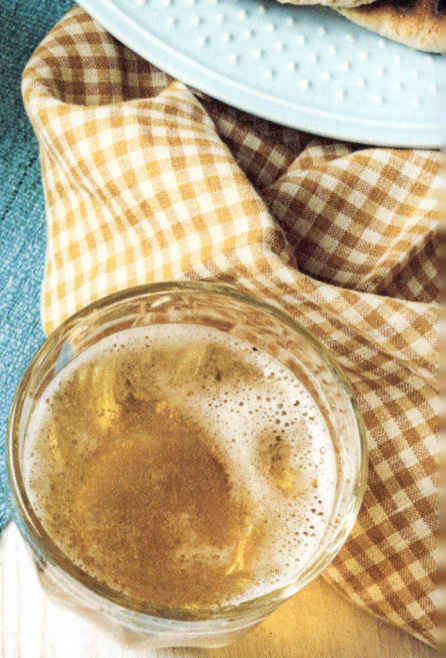

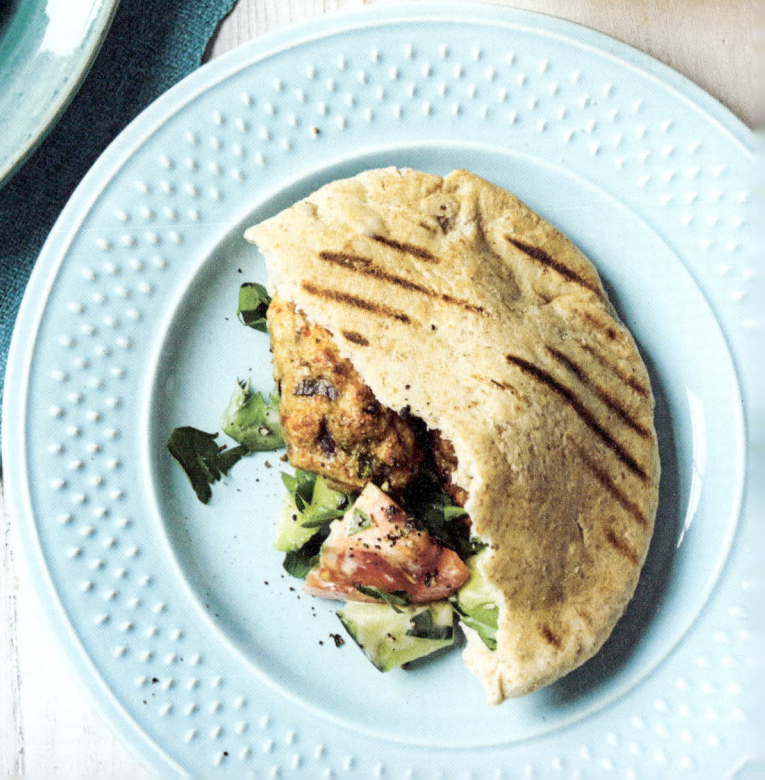

CHICKEN KOFTA & SUMMER SALAD

SERVES 4
PREP TIME 15 minutes
COOK TIME 16 minutes

Packed with flavour and great cooked on the barbecue or under the grill, serve these kofta up with a simple tahini-dressed salad and toasted pitta. Any leftovers are great in lunchboxes.

1 wholemeal pitta bread
50ml (1¾fl oz) water
500g (1lb 2oz) minced chicken
1 red onion, finely chopped
1 red chilli, deseeded and finely chopped
1 garlic clove, crushed
1 egg, lightly beaten
1 tablespoon baharat spice mix (see note)
1 teaspoon coarse salt
handful of parsley leaves, finely chopped
handful of mint leaves, finely chopped
spray oil

FOR THE SALAD
6 salad tomatoes, chopped
1 cucumber, chopped into 1cm (½ inch) pieces
handful of parsley leaves, finely chopped

FOR THE DRESSING
1 tablespoon tahini, well stirred
juice of 1 lemon
1 tablespoon honey
½ teaspoon salt

1   Pop the pitta bread in the toaster and toast it until golden brown. Allow it to cool enough to handle, then tear it into small pieces into a large mixing bowl and add the measured water. Leave this for a few minutes (I do this before I chop my onion and chilli, so I have something to do while I am waiting).

2   Add the minced chicken, onion, chilli, garlic, egg, baharat spice, salt and herbs to the mixing bowl, then use your hands to thoroughly combine all the ingredients, breaking up any larger pieces of pitta bread with your fingers as you go.

3   Preheat the grill to high and line the grill pan with foil. With wet hands, to stop the mixture sticking, shape the chicken mixture into 12 sausage-shaped patties, 4–5cm (1½–2 inches) in length. Place these on the prepared grill pan as you make them and spray with oil.

4   Grill for about 8 minutes on each side, until the kofta are fully cooked through and nicely golden brown on the outside. You can use a meat thermometer to check that the internal temperature of the kofta has reached 75°C (167°F) if you aren't sure.

5   Meanwhile, mix the salad ingredients in a mixing bowl. Stir the dressing ingredients in a small bowl until thoroughly combined.

6   Serve up the kofta, divide the salad between the plates and drizzle the dressing over the salad.

NOTE

You can find baharat spice blend in some supermarkets, but if you can't get hold of it, you can make a simplified version using 1 teaspoon ground cumin, 1 teaspoon ground coriander, 1 teaspoon sweet paprika and ½ teaspoon ground cinnamon. See also my recipe on page 202.

PER SERVING

CALORIES	FAT	SAT FAT	CARBS	SUGARS	FIBRE	PROTEIN	SALT
347	11G	2.6G	22G	12G	4.6G	36G	1.7G

LEMON ORZO WITH RAS EL HANOUT LAMB

SERVES 4
PREP TIME 15 minutes
COOK TIME 20 minutes

Zesty lemon orzo makes a light base for lamb in a rich and flavoursome ras el hanout sauce. For extra flavour, barbecue the lamb leg steaks rather than grilling: you can then wrap them in foil to rest while you prepare the orzo.

300g (10½oz) lamb leg steaks

1 red onion, sliced into half moons

200g (7oz) cherry tomatoes, halved

250g (9oz) chestnut mushrooms, sliced

1 tablespoon ras el hanout

2 tablespoons tomato purée

1 tablespoon honey

juice of 1 lemon

salt and pepper

handful of chopped parsley leaves, to serve

FOR THE ORZO

spray oil

2 garlic cloves, crushed

300g (10½oz) orzo

1 litre (1¾ pints) hot chicken stock

finely grated zest and juice of 1 lemon

1   Preheat the grill to high. Season the lamb steaks and put them under the grill to cook for 6–8 minutes on each side. Have a timer going so you remember to turn them. When the lamb is ready, just leave it to rest on a warm plate: it's best if it has a few minutes to rest.

2   For the orzo, spray a saucepan with a little oil and fry the garlic for 1 minute. Stir in the orzo, then pour in three-quarters of the hot stock. Bring up to a gentle simmer and cook for 10–12 minutes until the orzo is tender, topping up with the remaining stock if it starts to dry out. Give it a stir now and again to ensure it is not sticking to the pan.

3   Spray a sauté pan or frying pan with oil and fry the onion for 5 minutes. Add the cherry tomatoes and mushrooms and fry for another 5 minutes. Stir through the ras el hanout for 1 minute, then add the tomato purée, honey and lemon juice, then season with salt and pepper. Leave to cook over a low heat, stirring occasionally, until everything else is ready.

4   Once the orzo is cooked, stir through the lemon zest and juice and season with salt and pepper.

5   Thinly slice the lamb steaks, discarding any fatty bits, and stir the strips through the tomato sauce. You can add a little hot water if you need to loosen it up a bit.

6   Divide the orzo between 4 warmed pasta bowls and top with the lamb sauce. Sprinkle over the chopped parsley and serve.

NOTE

Cooking lamb Cook until the meat reaches an internal temperature of 63–70°C (145–158°F) on a meat thermometer for medium to well-done. Depending on the thickness of the steak, this takes roughly 6–8 minutes under a domestic grill on each side. If you are barbecuing the lamb, it will cook more quickly as the temperature will be higher, usually about 3 minutes on each side.

PER SERVING

CALORIES	FAT	SAT FAT	CARBS	SUGARS	FIBRE	PROTEIN	SALT
508	12G	5G	69G	15G	6.2G	27G	1.2G

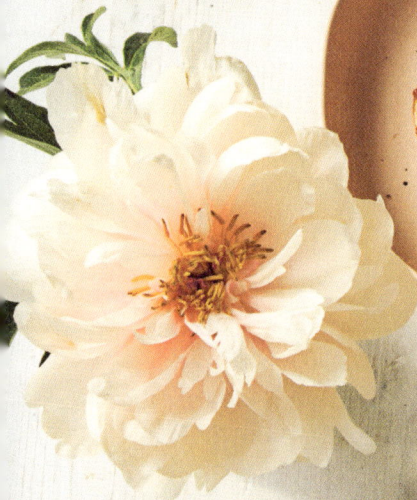

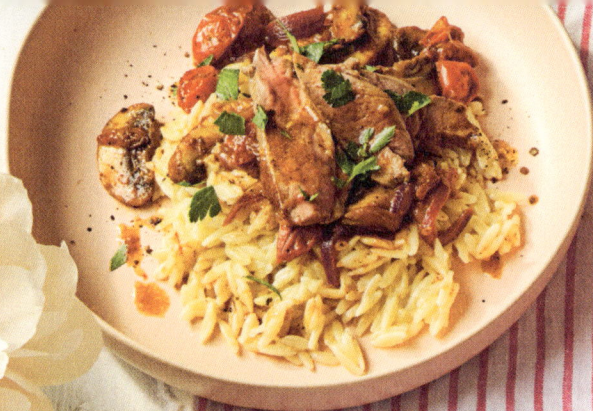

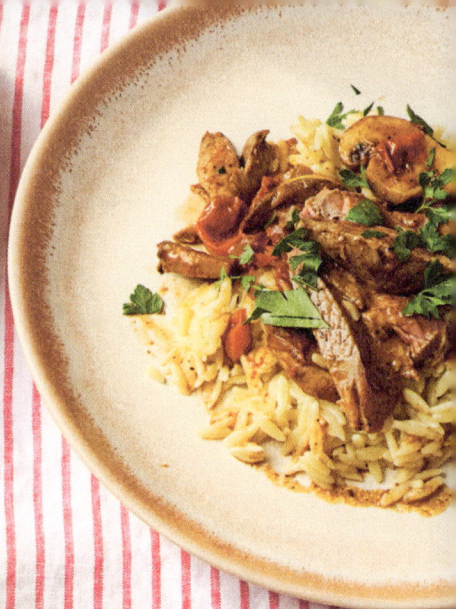

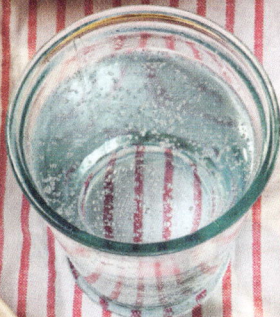

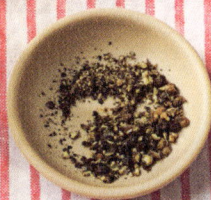

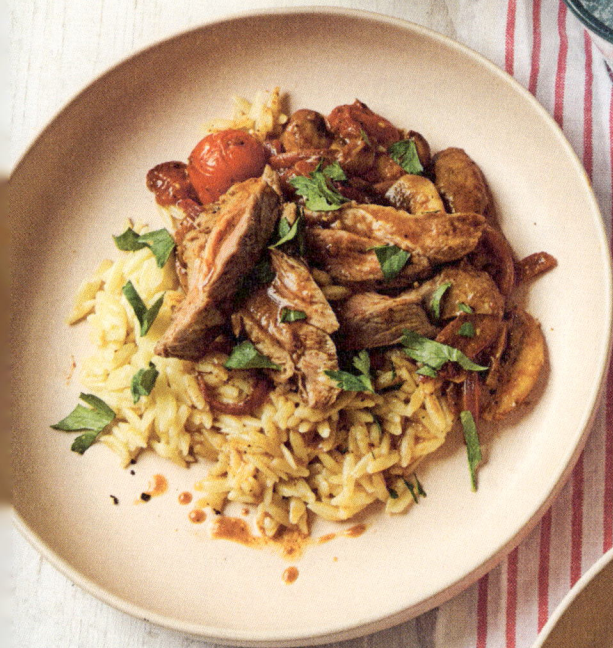

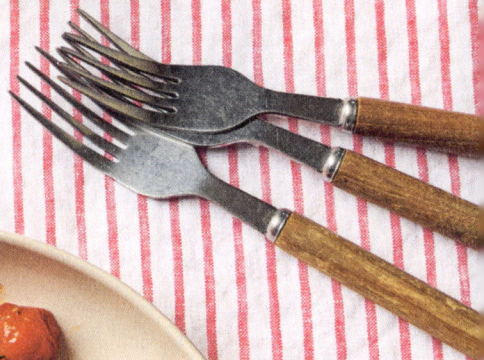

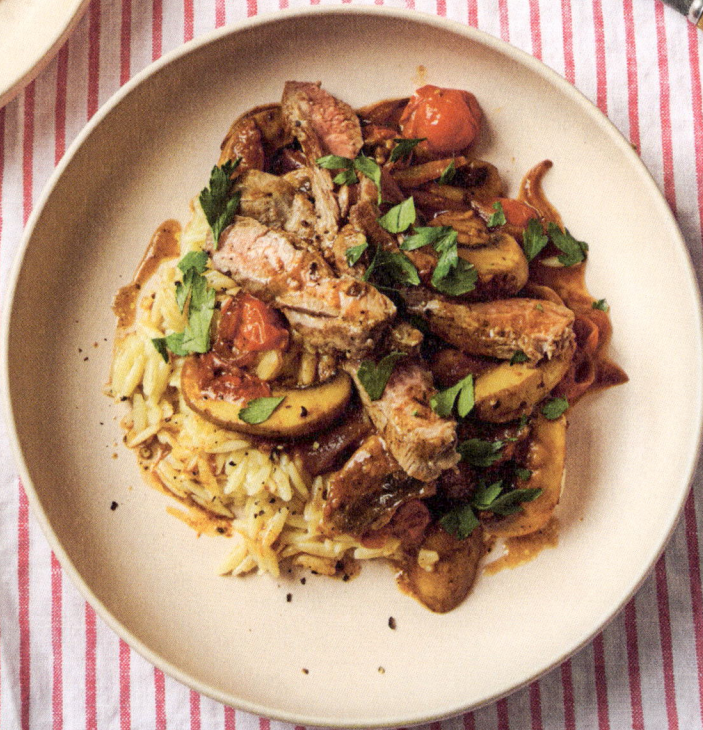

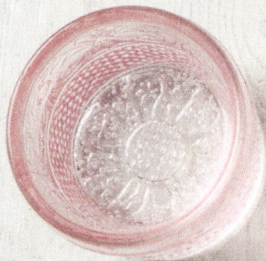

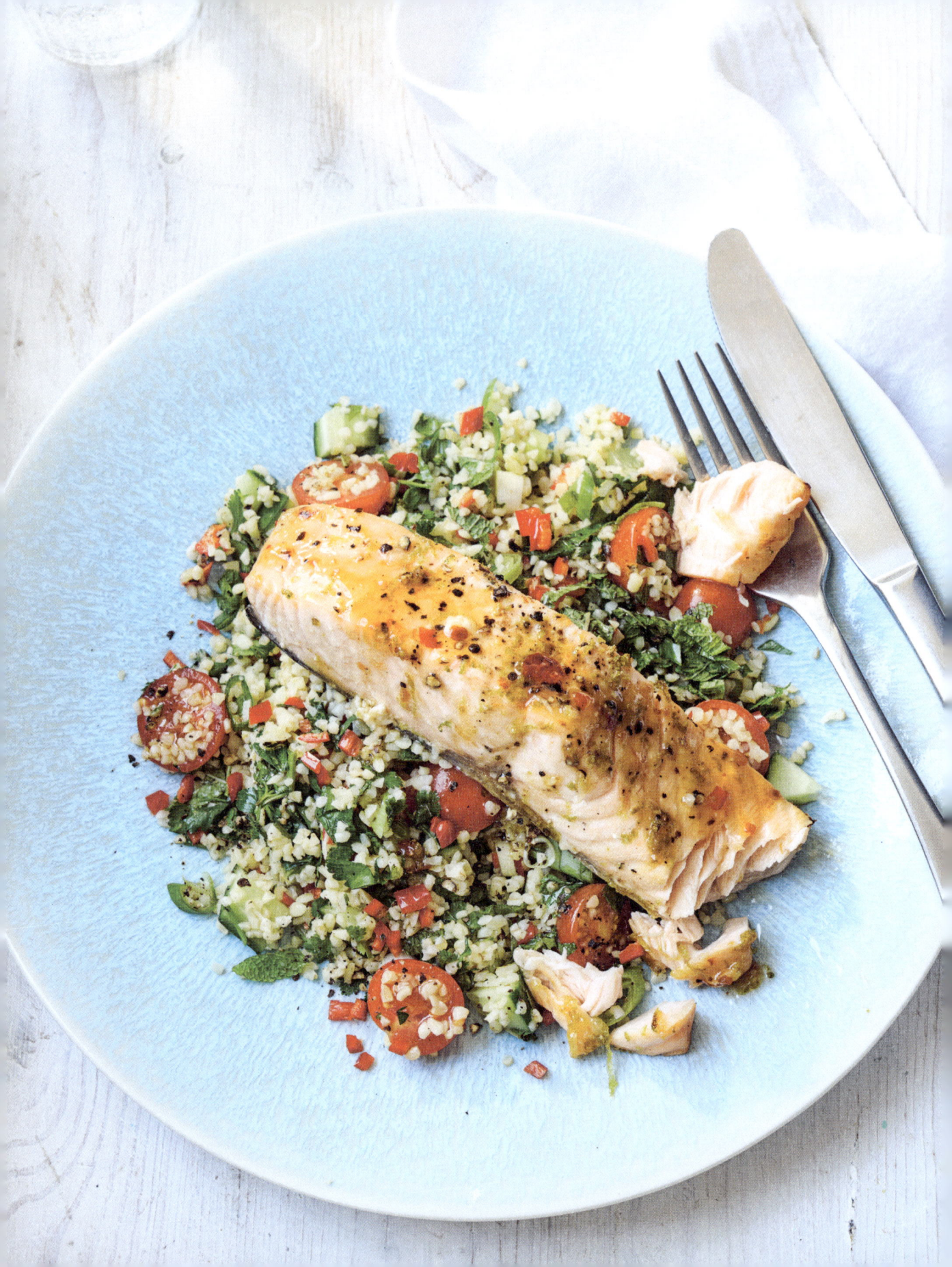

SWEET CHILLI SALMON WITH THAI-STYLE GRAIN SALAD

SERVES 2
PREP TIME 10 minutes
COOK TIME 20 minutes

Succulent salmon fillets glazed with sweet chilli sauce and zesty lime, with a refreshing salad with aromatic Thai-inspired flavours. A lovely light and refreshing meal.

100g (3½oz) bulgur wheat
2 salmon fillets
1 tablespoon sweet chilli sauce
50g (1¾oz) cucumber, finely chopped
10 cherry tomatoes, halved
2 spring onions, finely sliced
large handful of coriander
large handful of mint leaves
finely grated zest of 1 lime, to serve

FOR THE SALAD DRESSING
1 tablespoon fish sauce
½ tablespoon honey
juice of 1 lime
¼ teaspoon coarse salt
1 garlic clove, crushed
½ red chilli, finely chopped

1   Cook the bulgur wheat according to the packet instructions, tip into a sieve, then rinse with cold water to cool it rapidly. Leave to drain well.

2   Preheat the grill to high, line the grill pan with foil and lay the salmon on skin side down. Spread ½ tablespoon sweet chilli sauce over each salmon fillet, then grill for 6–8 minutes until just cooked through.

3   Meanwhile, mix up the dressing ingredients in a small bowl, making sure they are well combined (be sure to zest the lime before juicing it, setting the zest aside to serve).

4   In a separate mixing bowl, combine all the salad ingredients.

5   Stir the dressing through the bulgur wheat salad, then divide between 2 plates.

6   Top each portion with a cooked salmon fillet (you may wish to remove the skin first), then sprinkle over the lime zest and serve.

NOTE

Sometimes at special occasions, such as Christmas and Easter, supermarkets sell whole sides of salmon. If you can get hold of one, it is a more cost-effective way of buying salmon fillets. Simply cut it down into fillets, then freeze (I place 2 in each freezer bag), so you have it in for quick and easy meals.

PER SERVING

CALORIES	FAT	SAT FAT	CARBS	SUGARS	FIBRE	PROTEIN	SALT
457	22.3G	4.1G	23.9G	14.1G	4.3G	33.8G	2.6G

ONE-DISH FRAGRANT CHICKEN, CHICKPEA & COUSCOUS BAKE

SERVES 6
PREP TIME 15 minutes
COOK TIME 35 minutes

2 x 400g (14oz) cans of chickpeas, drained and rinsed

2 tablespoons chermoula spice blend, bought or homemade (see page 205), or Moroccan spice mix

500g (1lb 2oz) tomato passata

1 large red onion, finely chopped

2 celery sticks, finely chopped

3 garlic cloves, crushed

finely grated zest and juice of 1 lemon

1 red chilli, deseeded and finely chopped

250g (9oz) wholewheat couscous

400ml (14fl oz) hot chicken stock

6 skinless chicken thigh fillets

spray oil

salt and pepper

TO SERVE

8 tablespoons fat-free Greek yogurt

leaves from a couple of mint sprigs, chopped

lemon wedges

A satisfying one-dish meal which is easy to prepare and perfect for busy weeknights. You can use my homemade Chermoula Spice Blend (see page 205), or just find a Moroccan-style spice blend in the supermarket.

1 Preheat the oven to 220°C/200°C fan (425°F), Gas Mark 7.

2 Tip the chickpeas into a large baking dish with 1½ tablespoons of the chermoula or Moroccan spice mix, the passata, onion, celery, garlic, lemon zest and juice, chilli, couscous and hot stock.

3 Stir everything together, then place the chicken thigh pieces on top, sprinkle the remaining ½ tablespoon of chermoula over the chicken, season with salt and pepper, then spray everything with spray oil.

4 Bake on the middle shelf of the oven for 35 minutes. Meanwhile, mix together the yogurt and mint in a bowl, and season with salt and pepper.

5 Serve the chicken and couscous with a dollop of minty yogurt on top and lemon wedges on the side.

NOTE

I have used 1 chicken thigh per person here, as there are so many other elements to this dish. If you think that your family will eat more chicken, you can easily add some extra thighs. Sometimes I will cut each chicken thigh fillet into 6 before I bake this, to make the chicken go further.

You can add additional ingredients to make this even tastier, try pitted olives, cherry tomatoes, roasted peppers, feta cut into cubes or fresh herbs, such as parsley and mint. Pine nuts, sunflower seeds or flaked almonds sprinkled over the top for the final 10 minutes of cooking adds a nice crunch.

PER SERVING

CALORIES	FAT	SAT FAT	CARBS	SUGARS	FIBRE	PROTEIN	SALT
382	6.7G	1.3G	36G	10G	10G	38G	0.87G

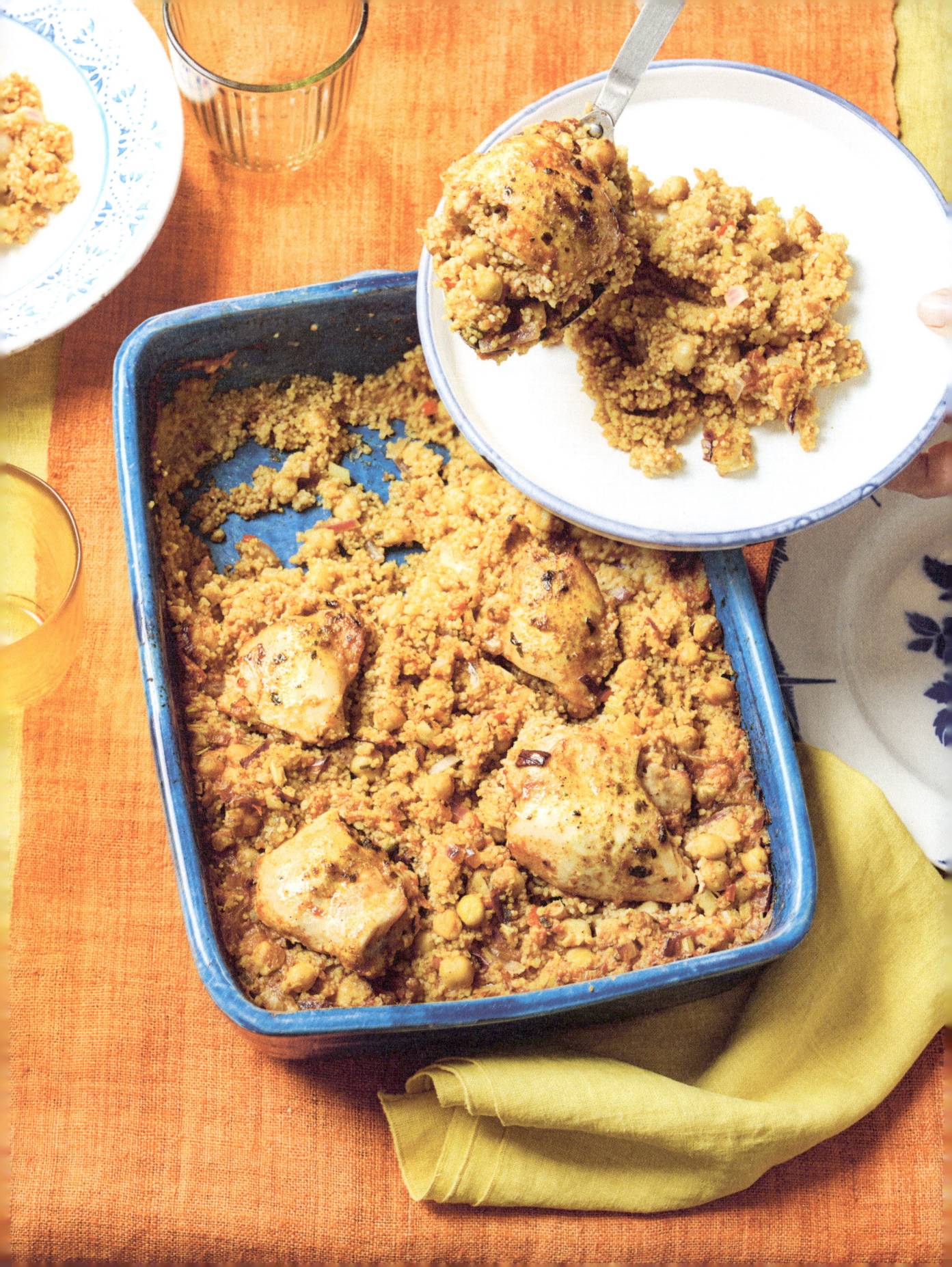

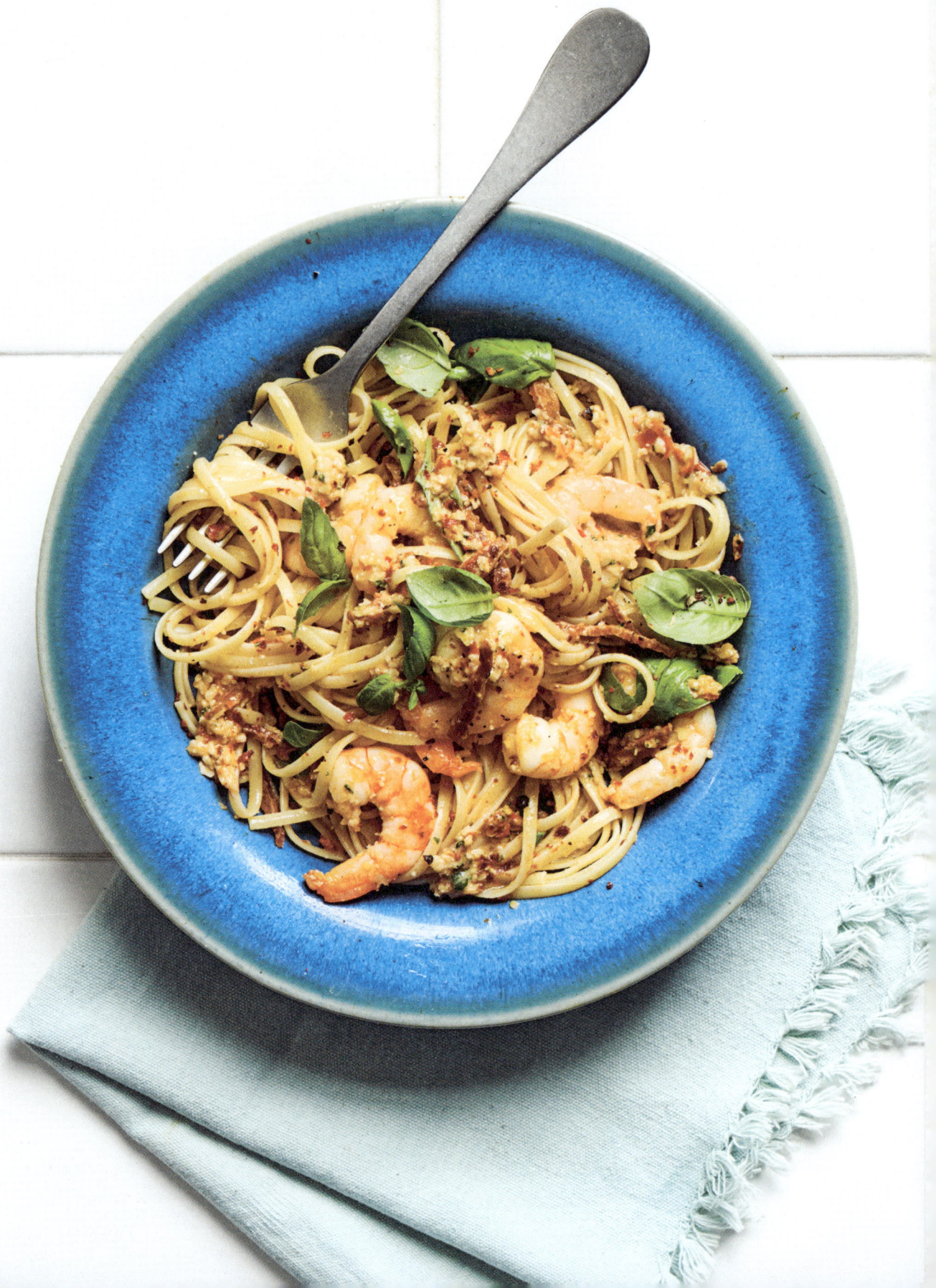

CHORIZO & PRAWN TOMATO PESTO LINGUINE

SERVES 4
PREP TIME 5 minutes
COOK TIME 11 minutes

This pesto is the perfect easy, light summer pasta sauce, with just a few simple ingredients – and no cheese – it still has so much flavour and you can pair it with any pasta shape. This is lovely served with a rocket salad.

FOR THE PESTO

50g (1¾oz) flaked almonds
250g (9oz) cherry tomatoes
large handful of basil leaves
1 garlic clove
1 teaspoon red wine vinegar
¼ teaspoon chilli flakes
¾ teaspoon coarse salt
1 teaspoon olive oil

FOR THE LINGUINE

300g (10½oz) linguine
40g (1½oz) thin chorizo slices, sliced into thin strips
250g (9oz) cooked king prawns

TO SERVE (OPTIONAL)

grated Parmesan cheese
freshly ground black pepper
torn basil leaves

1 Make the pesto. Start by dry-frying the almonds for a couple of minutes to lightly toast them. Put the almonds into a mini chopper or small food processor bowl along with all the other pesto ingredients. Blend into a smooth sauce.

2 Put the linguine on to cook according to the packet instructions (usually 9–11 minutes).

3 Meanwhile, in a frying pan, gently fry the chorizo for 3 minutes, then add the prawns and fry for another 2 minutes. Remove from the heat, but keep in the pan until the pasta is ready.

4 Drain the linguine, add it to the pan with the chorizo and prawns and spoon on the pesto. Mix well to coat the linguine in sauce and distribute the prawns and chorizo evenly.

5 Serve with grated Parmesan, freshly ground black pepper and torn basil leaves.

NOTE

This also makes a great vegetarian summer dish if you omit the chorizo and prawns for fried mushrooms and/or chopped raw courgettes and swap the Parmesan for a vegetarian alternative.

PER SERVING

CALORIES	FAT	SAT FAT	CARBS	SUGARS	FIBRE	PROTEIN	SALT
473	15G	3.2G	55G	5.3G	5.8G	2.6G	2.4G

SUMMERY CHICKEN STEW

SERVES 4
PREP TIME 15 minutes
COOK TIME 38 minutes

Stews can work for summer, too! This one uses seasonal new potatoes and vegetables, with a light gravy flavoured with mint and rosemary.

spray oil

2 smoked bacon medallions, finely chopped

leaves from 2 rosemary sprigs, finely chopped

1 onion, finely chopped

3 skinless chicken breasts, chopped

500ml (18fl oz) hot chicken stock

500g (1lb 2oz) new potatoes, halved or cut into bite-sized pieces, depending on size

2 carrots, peeled and sliced

400g (14oz) can of cannellini beans, drained and rinsed

1 courgette, cut into bite-sized chunks

bunch of asparagus spears, trimmed and cut into 3cm (1¼ inch) pieces

½ head of broccoli, cut into florets

2 tablespoons mint sauce

salt and pepper

1   Spray a flameproof casserole dish or large sauté pan, which has a lid, with oil, then fry the bacon, rosemary and onion for 10 minutes, stirring regularly.

2   Add the chicken and stir-fry for about 3 minutes, just to lightly cook it on the outside.

3   Now pour in the hot stock, add the potatoes and carrots, pop a lid on and leave to simmer gently for 20 minutes.

4   Tip in the cannellini beans, courgette, asparagus and broccoli, put the lid back on and simmer for 5 minutes, until the vegetables are al dente (if you prefer them softer, just cook for a few minutes longer).

5   Season with salt and pepper, stir through the mint sauce and serve.

NOTE

This is the perfect dish in which to use the freshest seasonal vegetables, depending on the time of year. You could substitute the courgette, broccoli and asparagus for green beans, runner beans, broad beans, sugar snap peas, sliced spring greens, or baby spinach. Or, for a more year-round option, you could even use frozen sweetcorn and peas.

PER SERVING

CALORIES	FAT	SAT FAT	CARBS	SUGARS	FIBRE	PROTEIN	SALT
403	4.2G	1G	38G	14G	11G	48G	1.8G

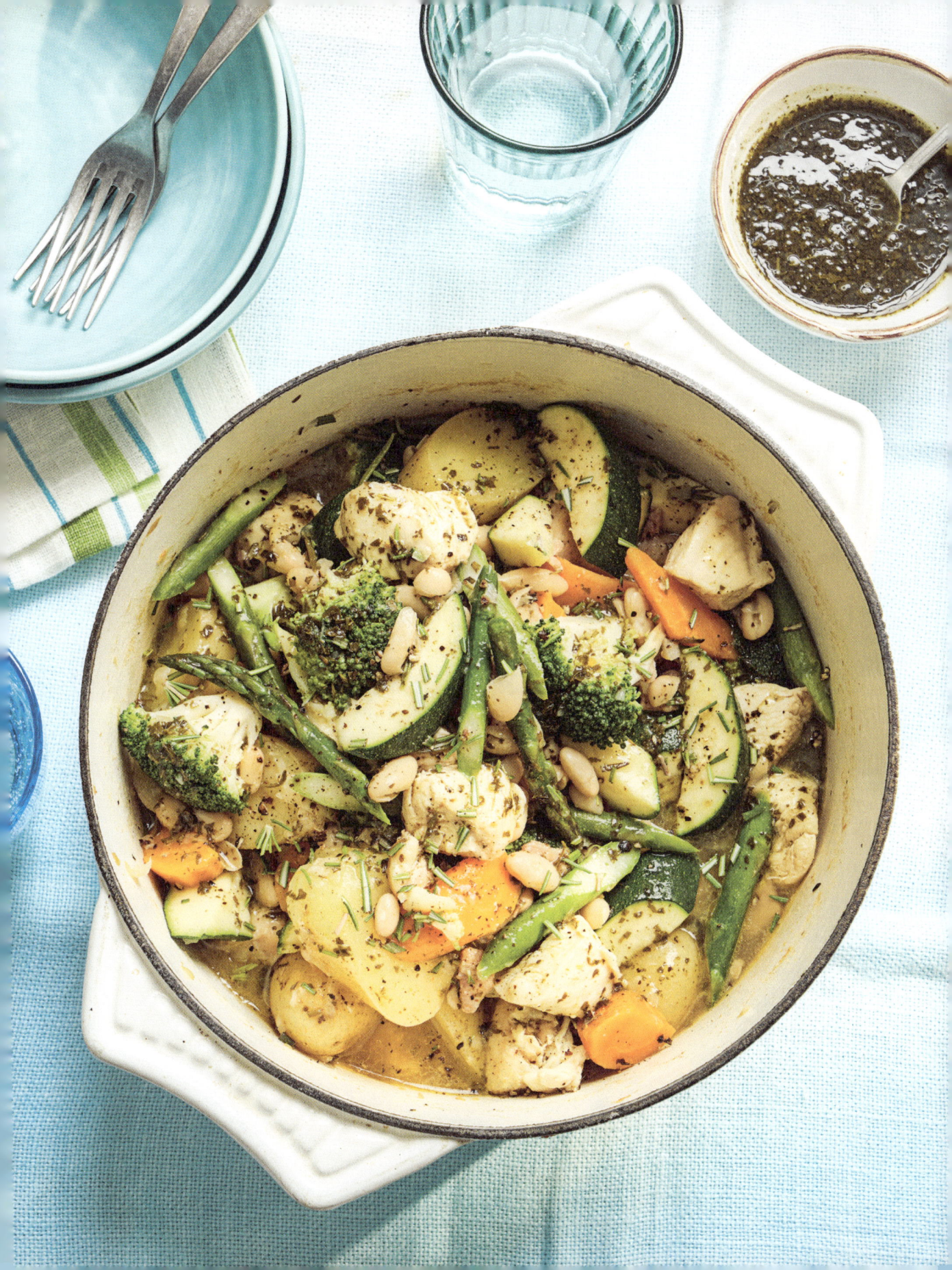

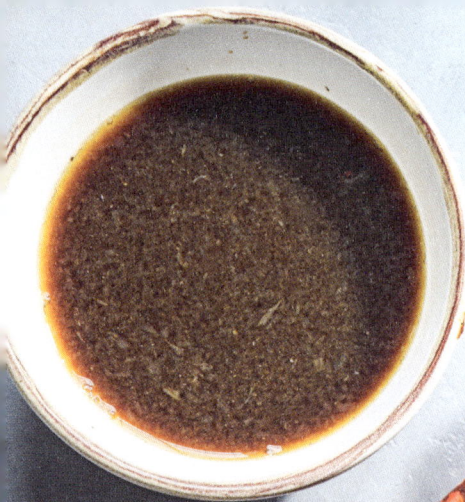

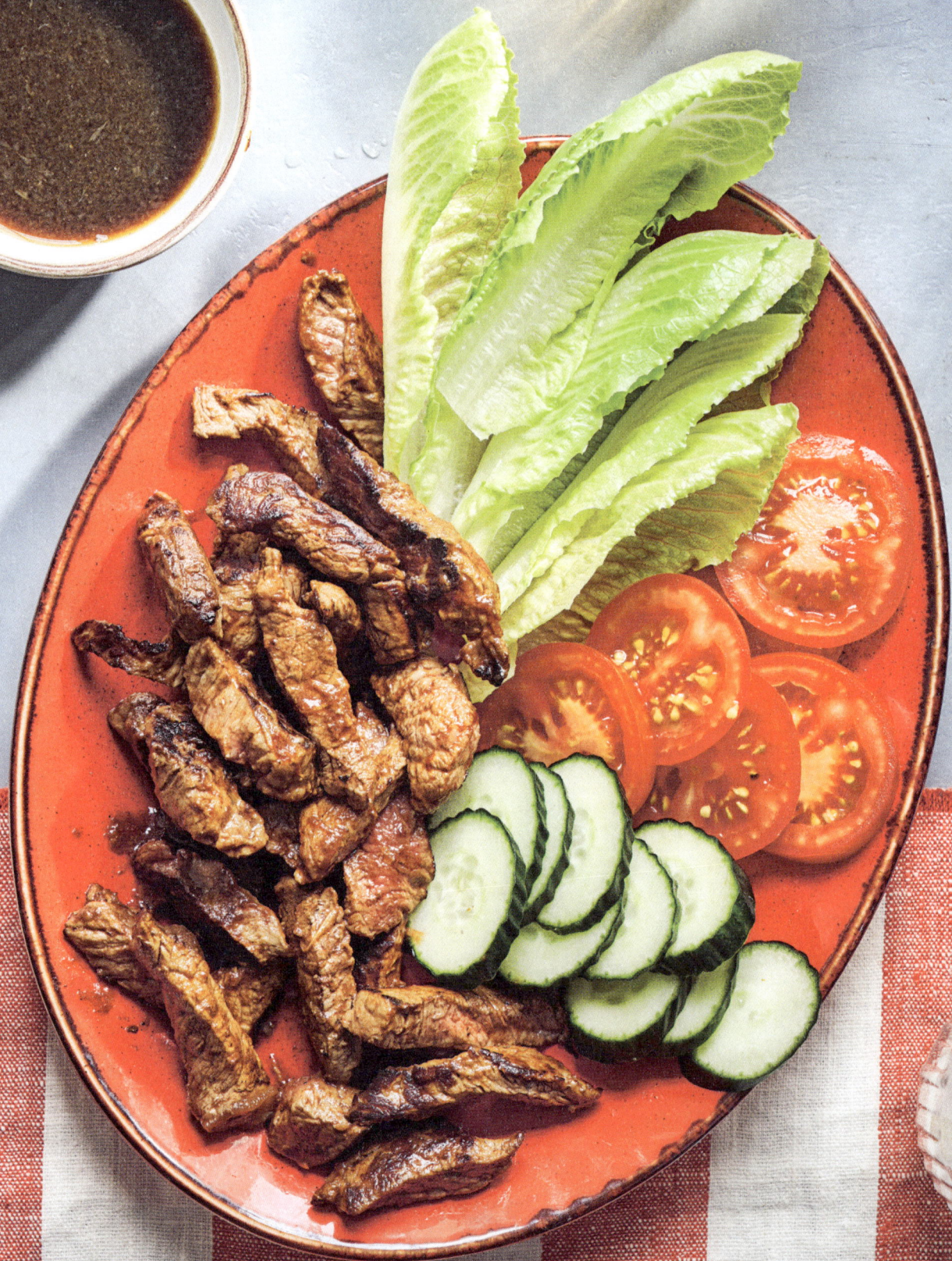

LOK LAK

SERVES 4
PREP TIME 15 minutes
COOK TIME 12 minutes

1 tablespoon vegetable oil

2 tablespoons dark soy sauce

1 tablespoon oyster sauce

1 tablespoon tomato purée

2 garlic cloves, crushed

600g (1lb 5oz) rump or sirloin steak, fat trimmed away, chopped into small bite-sized pieces

FOR THE DIPPING SAUCE

juice of 2 limes

4 tablespoons cold water

2 teaspoons brown sugar

2 teaspoons fish sauce

1 teaspoon freshly ground black pepper

FOR THE SALAD

2 small crisp lettuces, such as Little Gem, leaves separated

4 salad tomatoes, sliced

½ cucumber, sliced

TO SERVE

200g (7oz) basmati rice, cooked

sliced spring onions or chives

1 lime, cut into wedges

Lok lak is a Cambodian dish of tender marinated beef with a peppery, tangy dipping sauce, served with rice and contrasting crunchy-fresh vegetables. For my simplified version, I use rump or sirloin steak. You can use the lettuce leaves as a 'wrap' and layer in the rice, meat and a drizzle of dipping sauce.

1   Mix the oil, soy sauce, oyster sauce, tomato purée and crushed garlic in a bowl, add the beef and stir to thoroughly coat.

2   Make up the dipping sauce by mixing the ingredients in a bowl, then divide between 4 dipping bowls or ramekins ready to serve. Make sure the sugar and black pepper have been well dispersed.

3   Put the rice on to cook according to the packet instructions (usually around 12 minutes).

4   Mix all the salad ingredients in a bowl. Get 4 plates out ready and arrange the salad between the plates.

5   When the rice has about 5 minutes remaining, heat up a sauté pan over a high heat, add the beef and marinade and stir-fry for 4 minutes, keeping the heat high: it should be sizzling the whole time. You want the beef to be tender on the inside and slightly charred on the outside, so be careful not to overcook, or it could be chewy! Remove the beef from the heat and share it out between the plates.

6   Drain the rice and divide between the plates. Scatter with sliced spring onions or chives and serve with the dipping sauce on the side and a lime wedge on every plate.

NOTE

Traditionally, lok lak uses Kampot peppercorns; I have used regular black pepper here, as it's easily available in the UK, but if you fancy trying it with Kampot peppercorns for a more authentic experience, you can find them online.

PER SERVING

CALORIES	FAT	SAT FAT	CARBS	SUGARS	FIBRE	PROTEIN	SALT
472	11G	3.5G	48G	9.4G	2.8G	42G	2.5G

PRAWN, COURGETTE & MINT SALAD

SERVES 2
PREP TIME 5 minutes
COOK TIME none

1 courgette (150g/5½oz), sliced into thin matchsticks

½ red pepper, deseeded and finely chopped

225g (8oz) cooked, peeled prawns

juice of 1 lemon

1 teaspoon olive oil

1 tablespoon chopped parsley leaves

8 mint leaves, shredded

salt and pepper

A light, fresh salad, with crisp vegetables, salty little prawns and a simple dressing, perfect for hot summer days as it's cool and refreshing. This recipe makes two modest portions ideal for a lunch or light supper, but you can easily toss in salad leaves to bulk it out, or serve it with toasted wholemeal pitta breads.

1   Put the vegetables and prawns into a mixing bowl and add the lemon juice, olive oil, parsley and mint. Season with salt and pepper and toss the salad to evenly distribute all the ingredients.

2   Serve immediately, or chill until ready to serve.

NOTE

You can change this salad by adding cherry tomatoes, cucumber slices or avocado chunks. It's also delicious with a sprinkling of crumbled or cubed feta cheese.

PER SERVING

CALORIES	FAT	SAT FAT	CARBS	SUGARS	FIBRE	PROTEIN	SALT
128	2.8G	0.5G	4.2G	3.9G	1.6G	2G	1.92G

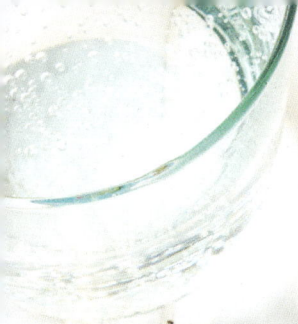

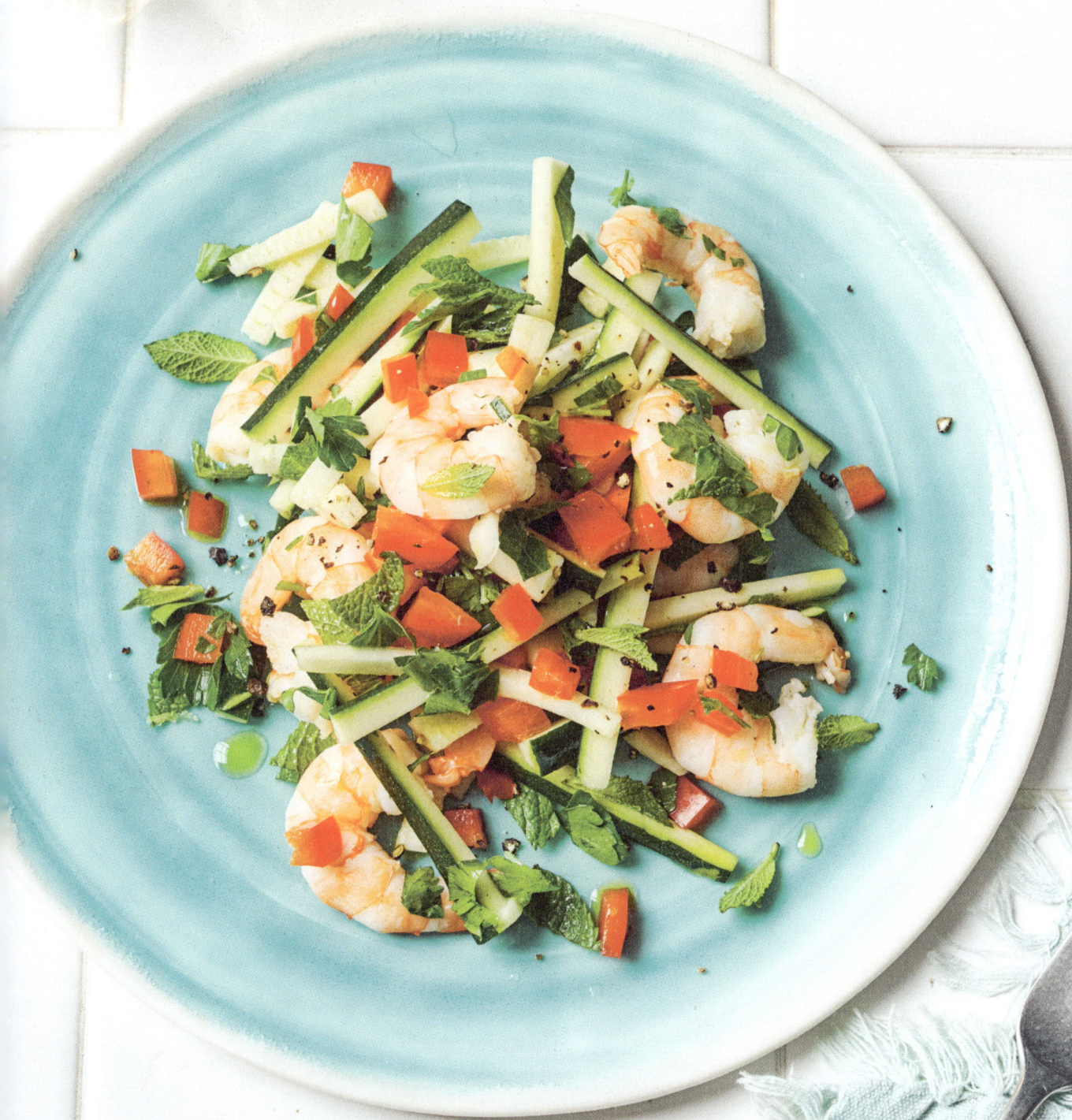

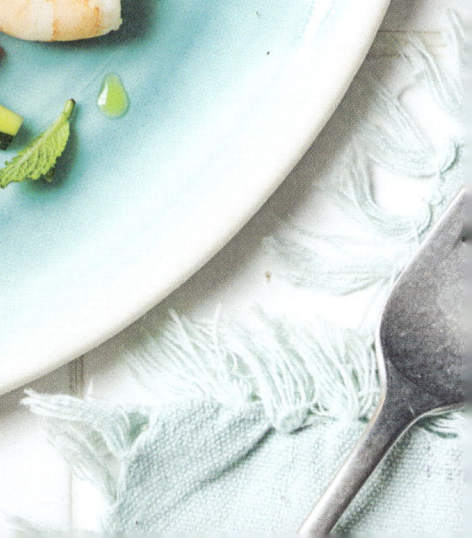

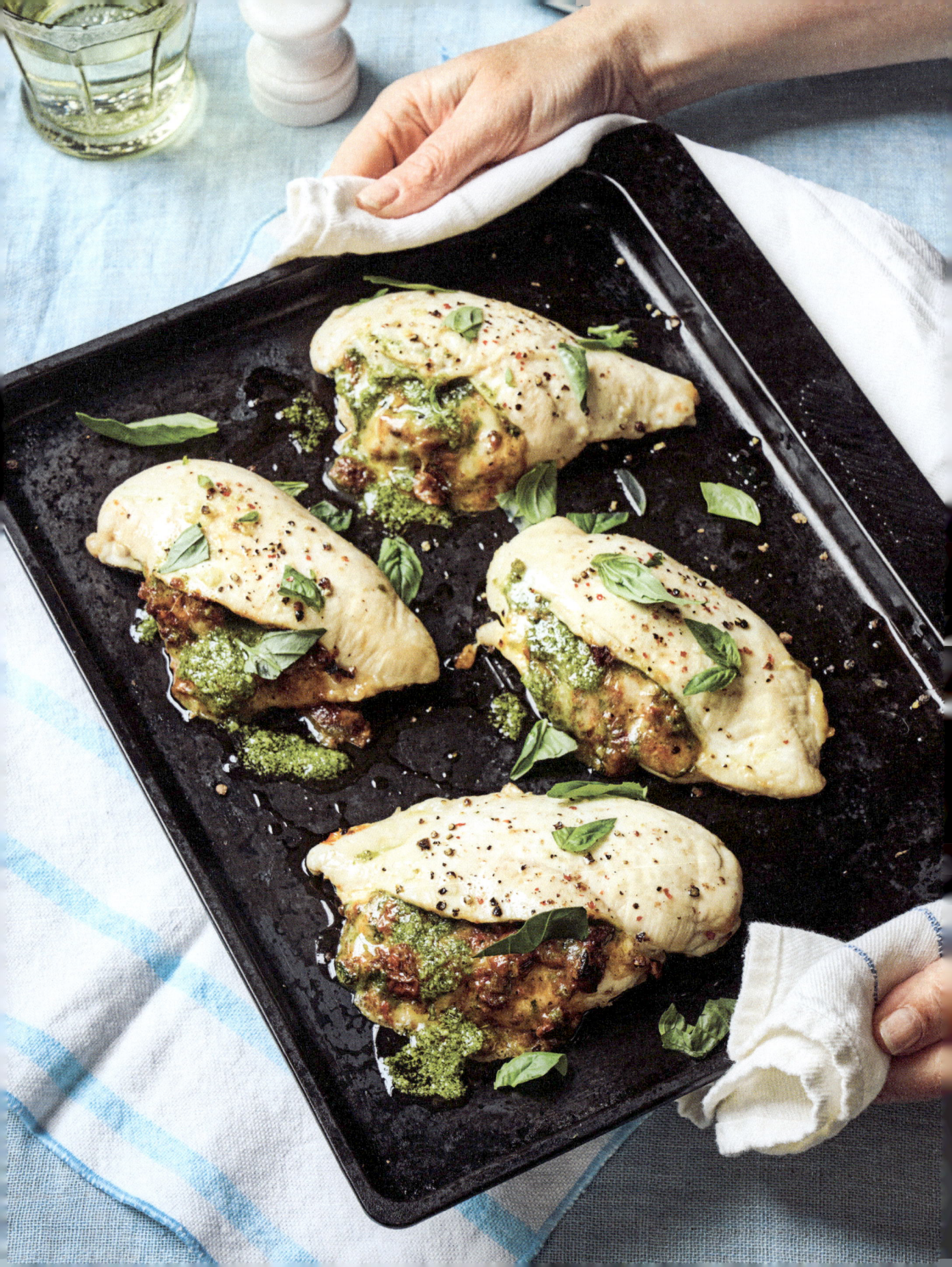

PESTO, SUNDRIED TOMATO & MOZZARELLA-STUFFED CHICKEN BREASTS

SERVES 4
PREP TIME 20 minutes
COOK TIME 25 minutes

4 chicken breasts

4 sundried tomatoes, drained and patted dry with kitchen paper, then finely chopped

125g (4½oz) ball of mozzarella, torn into pieces

1 tablespoon balsamic vinegar

handful of basil leaves, finely chopped

4 teaspoons basil pesto

spray oil

salt and pepper

Elevate chicken breasts with this simple stuffing for a tasty dish full of summery flavours. Serve alongside a rocket salad with balsamic vinegar dressing or glaze, or with mashed potato, roasted vegetables or Ratatouille, or Cannellini Bean Mash with Rosemary & Lemon (see pages 137 and 198).

1   Preheat the oven to 210°C/190°C fan (410°F), Gas Mark 6½.

2   Use a sharp knife to cut a pocket in each chicken breast: cut the side where the meat has a fold, rather than the smooth side, and do not cut all the way through, as you want to be able to push in the stuffing without it coming out the other side.

3   In a bowl, mix the sundried tomatoes, mozzarella, balsamic vinegar and basil, then season with salt and pepper and mix again.

4   Spread 1 teaspoon of pesto into the pocket of each chicken breast.

5   Divide the mozzarella mix evenly between the 4 chicken breasts, stuffing it into the pocket.

6   Line a baking tray with nonstick baking paper, lay each chicken breast on the baking paper, season and spray with oil.

7   Bake in the oven for 25 minutes. Check that the chicken is cooked through (you can use a meat thermometer for this, it should read 75°C/167°F), then serve.

NOTE

You can customize this recipe by adding ingredients to the stuffing, such as chopped spinach, roasted chopped red peppers or sliced black olives. For a crispier exterior, you can dredge the stuffed chicken breasts in crumbs, or finely grated Parmesan cheese, before baking.

PER SERVING

CALORIES	FAT	SAT FAT	CARBS	SUGARS	FIBRE	PROTEIN	SALT
325	13G	5.9G	2G	1.5G	0.9G	49G	1.1G

BUDGET
STARS

3

CHEESY MARMITE BAKED OATS

SERVES 2
PREP TIME 5 minutes
COOK TIME 25 minutes

80g (2¾oz) porridge oats
80g (2¾oz) fat-free cottage cheese
1 egg
2 teaspoons Marmite
30g (1oz) Cheddar cheese, grated
1 teaspoon baking powder
¼ teaspoon dried mixed herbs
¼ teaspoon pepper
spray oil

Baked oats have been a staple breakfast in my life for years, but savoury baked oats are a fairly new discovery to me. This recipe is brilliant for when you are craving a really filling, satisfying start to the day. Years ago, I used to love a cheese and Marmite toastie for breakfast, and these oats hit the spot in just the same way.

1 Preheat the oven to 200°C/180°C fan (400°F), Gas Mark 6.

2 In a bowl, mix all the ingredients, except the spray oil, until they are thoroughly combined.

3 Spray 2 ramekins or mini casserole dishes with oil, then divide the mixture evenly between the dishes.

4 Bake for 25 minutes. Serve hot.

NOTE

If you aren't a fan of Marmite, try playing around with different flavours for your savoury baked oats:

Pizza Add 1 teaspoon tomato purée, dried oregano and grated mozzarella cheese, perhaps even sprinkle a little finely chopped chorizo on top.

Sundried tomato & basil Add chopped sundried tomatoes and basil leaves.

Pesto & Parmesan Swirl in some pesto and sprinkle with grated Parmesan cheese.

Spinach & feta Fold in chopped spinach leaves and crumbled feta cheese.

Salsa & jalapeño Mix in tomato salsa and finely chopped pickled jalapeños.

Roasted red pepper & goat's cheese Stir in roasted red pepper strips and crumbled goat's cheese.

Mushroom & thyme Add sautéed mushrooms and thyme leaves.

Sriracha Add sriracha sauce for a spicy kick.

PER SERVING

CALORIES	FAT	SAT FAT	CARBS	SUGARS	FIBRE	PROTEIN	SALT
314	12G	4.6G	30G	1.4G	3.2G	19G	2.4G

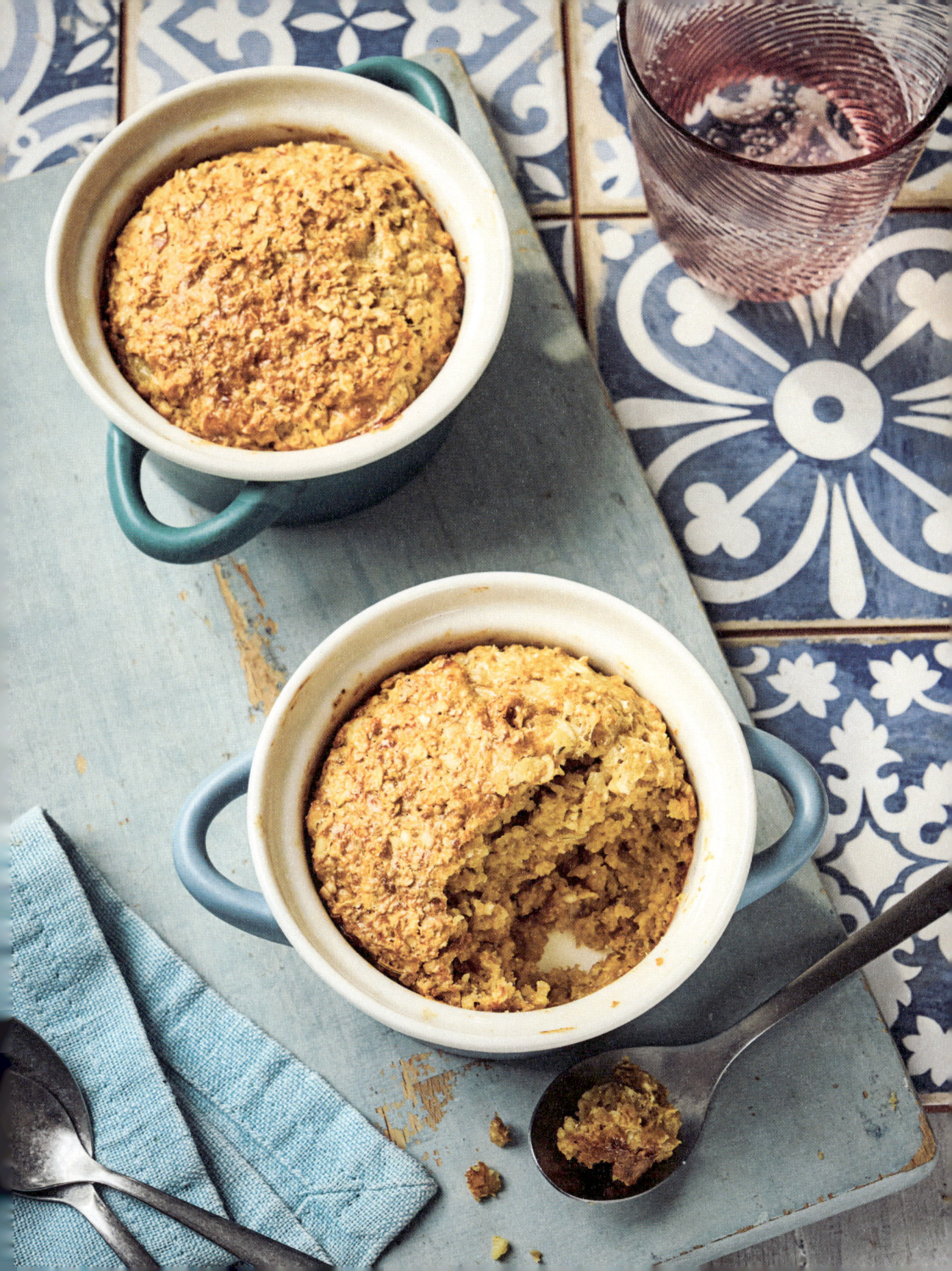

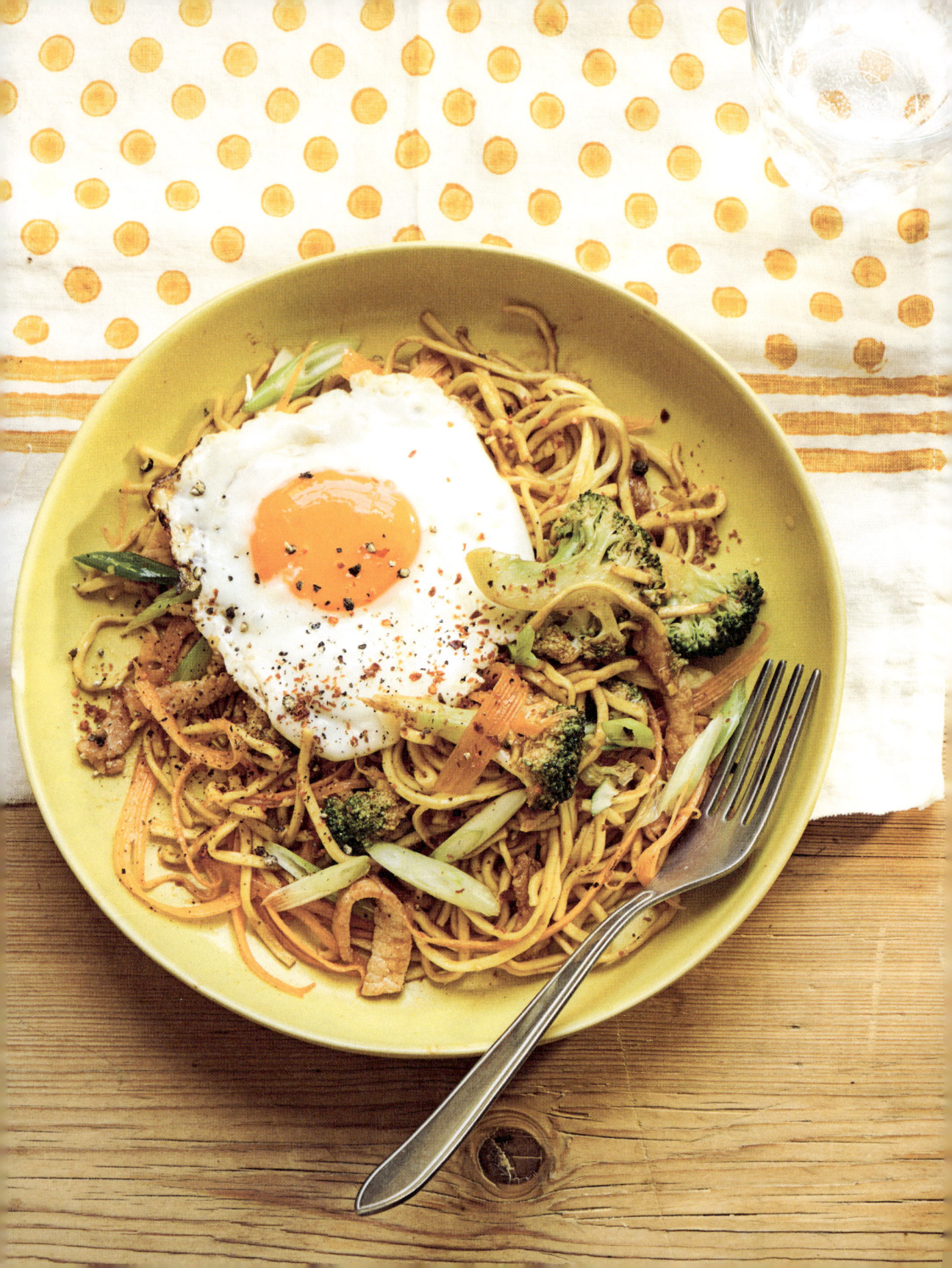

HAM & EGG HOISIN NOODLES

SERVES 4
PREP TIME 10 minutes
COOK TIME 10 minutes

Hoisin sauce is great for packing fast flavour into meals. This simple noodle dish is filling, tasty and satisfying, plus it's a great way to get two gammon steaks to stretch between four people.

4 nests of medium egg noodles (250g/9oz)

spray oil

2 unsmoked gammon steaks (300g/10½oz), very finely sliced

4 spring onions, sliced

½ head of broccoli, cut into small bite-sized florets

4 eggs

1 garlic clove, crushed

1 large carrot, sliced into thin ribbons with a vegetable peeler

6 tablespoons hoisin sauce

1 Put the noodles on to cook according to the packet instructions. When they are cooked, drain, rinse with cold water and set aside.

2 Spray a sauté pan or wok with oil and fry the gammon pieces for 3 minutes, then add the spring onions and broccoli florets and stir-fry for a further 5 minutes.

3 Meanwhile, spray a frying pan with spray oil and put the 4 eggs on to fry.

4 Add the garlic to the ham and broccoli, stir through, then tip in the drained noodles and carrot ribbons and add the hoisin sauce. Stir-fry to bring everything together and heat the noodles through.

5 Divide the noodles between 4 warmed bowls and top each with a fried egg.

NOTE

This is a great way to use up veg from the refrigerator, just add it during step 2 with the spring onions and broccoli. You could try sliced sweet peppers, mushrooms, shredded cabbage, baby corn, courgette batons or green beans. Any leafy greens, such as spinach, spring greens or bok choi, can go in at the same time as the carrot ribbons, in step 4.

PER SERVING

CALORIES	FAT	SAT FAT	CARBS	SUGARS	FIBRE	PROTEIN	SALT
481	12G	3.7G	56G	12G	5.9G	34G	3.1G

BUTTERNUT SQUASH MAC 'N' CHEESE

SERVES 4
PREP TIME 10 minutes
COOK TIME 20 minutes

spray oil
1 onion, finely chopped
400g (14oz) butternut squash, chopped
1 garlic clove, crushed
½ teaspoon sweet (unsmoked) paprika
½ teaspoon onion granules
½ teaspoon coarse salt
½ teaspoon pepper
300ml (½ pint) semi-skimmed milk
300g (10½oz) macaroni
1 chicken stock cube, crumbled
90g (3¼oz) mature Cheddar cheese, grated

TO GARNISH
handful of chopped parsley leaves
Parmesan cheese

Using butternut squash is a great way to achieve a beautiful, silky and creamy sauce for your mac 'n' cheese without having to go overboard with the cheese! This recipe is a great way to get vegetables into fussy eaters and it's good value, too! Serve it with green vegetables or salad.

1 Spray a flameproof casserole dish with oil and fry the onion for 5 minutes.

2 Stir in the butternut squash, then add the garlic, paprika, onion granules, salt and pepper, pour in the milk, cover and leave to simmer while you cook the pasta.

3 Cook the macaroni, with the crumbled chicken stock cube, in a large pan of simmering water according to the packet instructions (usually 10–12 minutes) until soft. Drain, reserving some of the pasta cooking water.

4 Check that the butternut squash is tender, then use a stick blender to blitz the butternut squash and milk into a smooth sauce. If you think it seems too thick, or it's hard to blend, add a ladleful of the pasta water.

5 Preheat the grill to high.

6 Stir the cooked macaroni and 60g (2¼oz) of the Cheddar into the squash sauce.

7 Transfer the mixture to an oven dish or pan suitable to go under the grill, top with the remaining 30g (1oz) Cheddar and grill for about 5 minutes, until the cheese is golden brown and bubbling. Serve with chopped parsley scattered over the top, with Parmesan for grating.

NOTE

How to prepare a butternut squash Slice off the stalk and root end with a sharp knife, then use a Y-shaped peeler to remove the skin. Cut the squash in half lengthways (you need a large, sharp knife for this) and use a dessertspoon to scrape out the seeds and fibrous parts around the seeds. Lay the squash halves down on their flat sides and use the large sharp knife to chop it.

Make it veggie Swap the chicken stock cube for vegetable and serve with a Parmesan-style vegetarian cheese.

Make it meaty Fry some chopped bacon or chorizo, add with the Cheddar.

PER SERVING

CALORIES	FAT	SAT FAT	CARBS	SUGARS	FIBRE	PROTEIN	SALT
521	16G	8.9G	66G	13G	6.7G	25G	2.4G

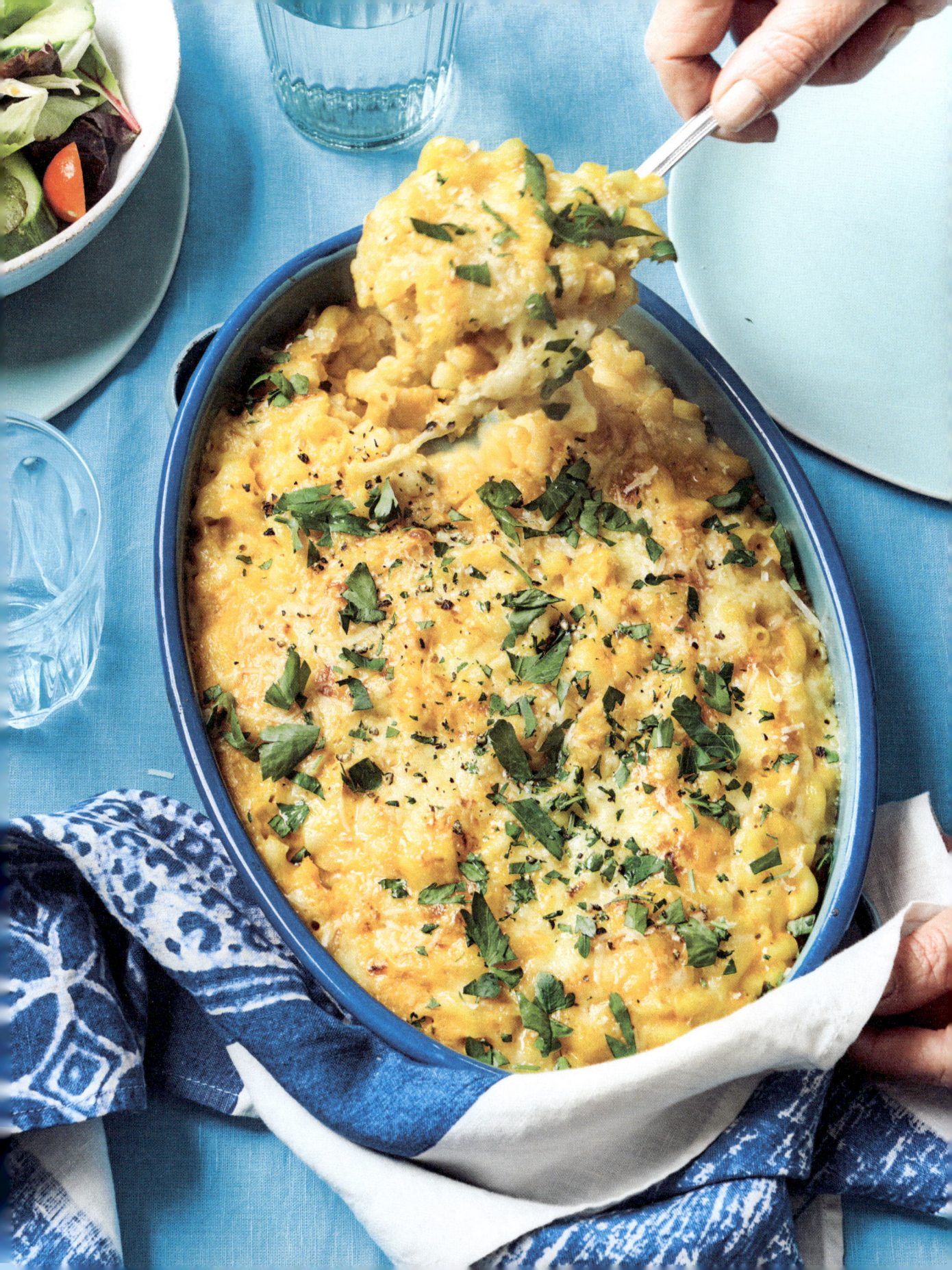

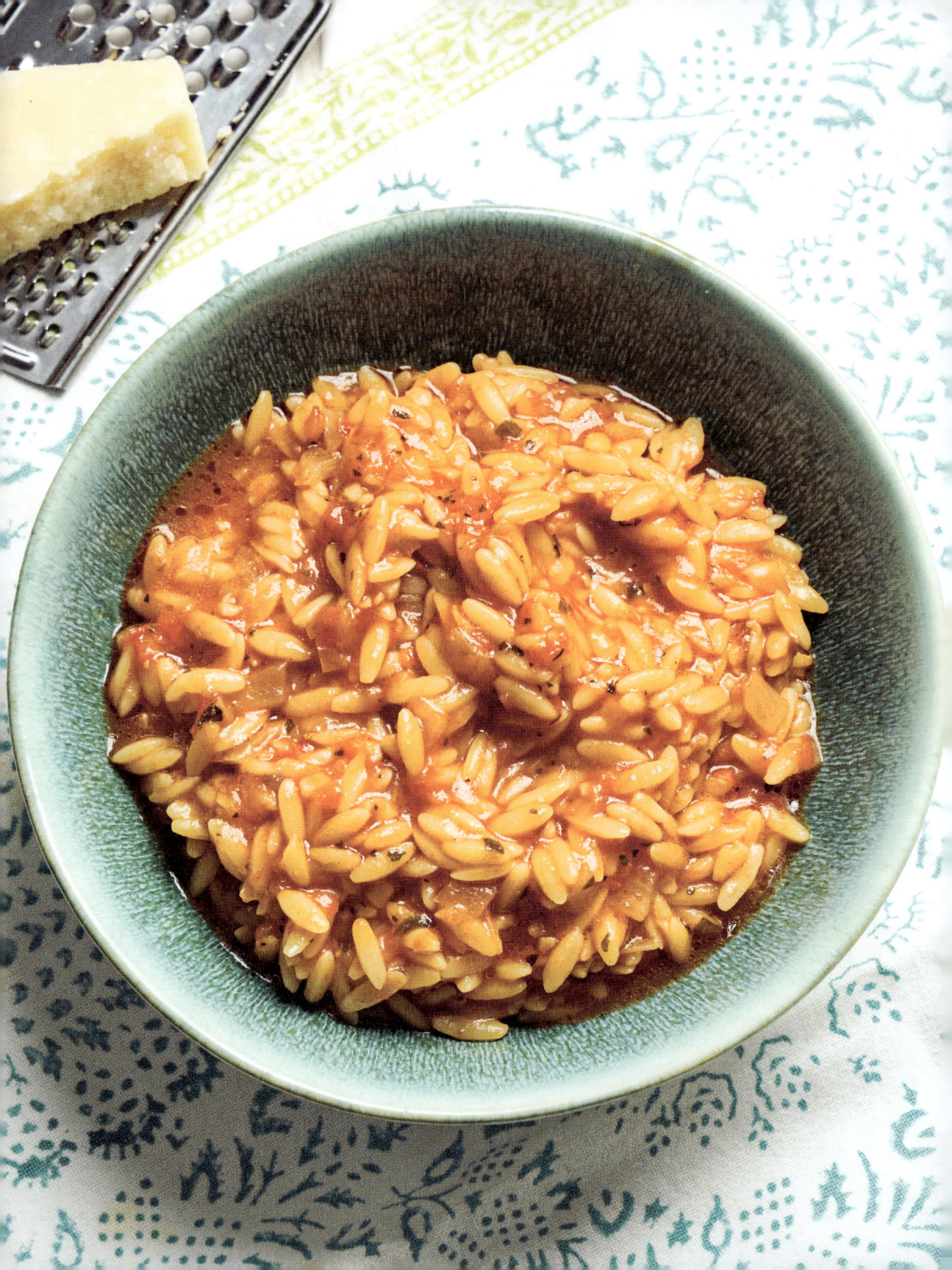

TOMATO ORZO

SERVES 4
PREP TIME 5 minutes
COOK TIME 26 minutes

spray oil

1 onion, finely chopped

3 garlic cloves, crushed

350g (12oz) orzo

400g (14oz) can of chopped
   tomatoes

1 litre (1¾ pints) hot vegetable
   stock

2 teaspoons dried mixed herbs

1 teaspoon sweet (unsmoked)
   paprika

60g (2¼oz) Parmesan-style
   vegetarian cheese

salt and pepper

A simple, budget-friendly and quick one-pot pasta dish for days
when you want to eat good, easy homemade food, but don't
have too much time.

1   Spray a saucepan or sauté pan with oil and fry the onion for 5 minutes.

2   Add the garlic and stir-fry for 1 minute.

3   Now add the orzo and tomatoes, then the hot stock, herbs and paprika
and simmer gently until the orzo is cooked, about 20 minutes.

4   Season with salt and pepper, stir in the Parmesan-style cheese and
serve in warmed bowls.

NOTE

There are plenty of ways that you can jazz this up, and it's a great way to
use leftovers. Vegetables, such as mushrooms, cherry tomatoes, leeks,
celery, sweet peppers, courgettes and aubergines will all work well fried
in with the onion (just fry the onion for a few minutes on its own first, then
add the extra veg and fry for a few more minutes). If you want to add
meat, try finely chopped bacon or chorizo fried at the same time as the
onion, or you can stir in leftover roast chicken, beef or pork for the last
5 minutes of cooking. Different cheeses also work well, try Cheddar,
mozzarella, Gruyère, Swiss, Boursin or cream cheese.

PER SERVING

CALORIES	FAT	SAT FAT	CARBS	SUGARS	FIBRE	PROTEIN	SALT
438	7.3G	3.4G	71G	10G	6.4G	18G	2.4G

SUPER-CREAMY SWEET POTATO & CHICKPEA CURRY

SERVES 4
PREP TIME 5 minutes
COOK TIME 30 minutes

1 large sweet potato (500g/
   1lb 2oz), chopped, or frozen
   sweet potato cubes, if you prefer
spray oil
1 onion, finely chopped
400ml (14fl oz) can of light
   (reduced-fat) coconut milk
1 tablespoon mild curry powder
½ teaspoon sweet (unsmoked)
   paprika
½ teaspoon ground ginger
½ teaspoon coarse salt
½ teaspoon cayenne pepper
150ml (¼ pint) hot vegetable stock
1 garlic clove, crushed
2 x 400g (14oz) cans of chickpeas,
   drained and rinsed
coriander or mint leaves, to serve
   (optional)

This has a thick and satisfying creamy sweet potato-based sauce which is mildly spiced and works perfectly with nutritious, cheap chickpeas. I serve it simply, with naan or a homemade flatbread on the side, or with basmati rice and a spoonful of mango chutney.

1. Place the sweet potato into a pan of boiling water and simmer for 12–15 minutes, or until tender.

2. Meanwhile, spray a saucepan with oil and fry the onion gently to soften and sweeten it, stirring every now and again to prevent it from catching and burning (see note).

3. Once the sweet potato is tender, put it into a food processor or blender with the coconut milk, curry powder, paprika, ground ginger, salt, cayenne pepper and hot stock, then blend it until you have a smooth and creamy sauce.

4. Add the garlic to the onions and fry gently for 1 minute, then tip in the creamy sauce.

5. Stir the chickpeas in and simmer gently for 15 minutes, then serve, scattered with herbs, if you have them.

NOTE

I just keep the onions frying gently until the sweet potato is cooked, but if you are only using a little oil, they can dry out. If they are looking a bit dry, add a big splash of boiling water and stir it through, to help them to soften up, rather than adding more oil.

Fancy packing some extra veggies into this? Fry chopped sweet peppers with the onions, add cauliflower or broccoli florets at the same time as the chickpeas, or stir baby spinach leaves through for the last couple of minutes of cooking.

PER SERVING

CALORIES	FAT	SAT FAT	CARBS	SUGARS	FIBRE	PROTEIN	SALT
386	12G	6.8G	50G	11G	14G	13G	0.8G

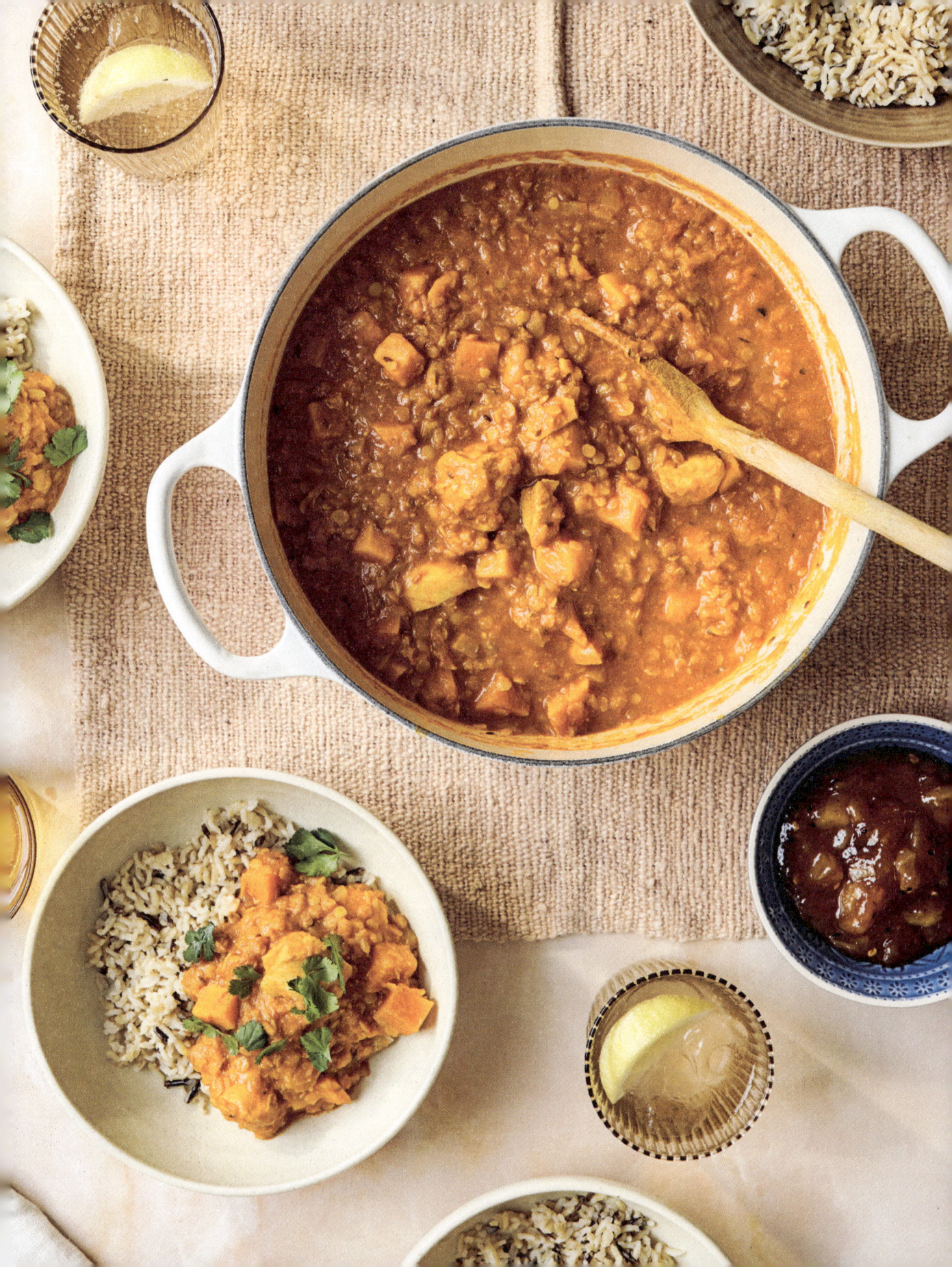

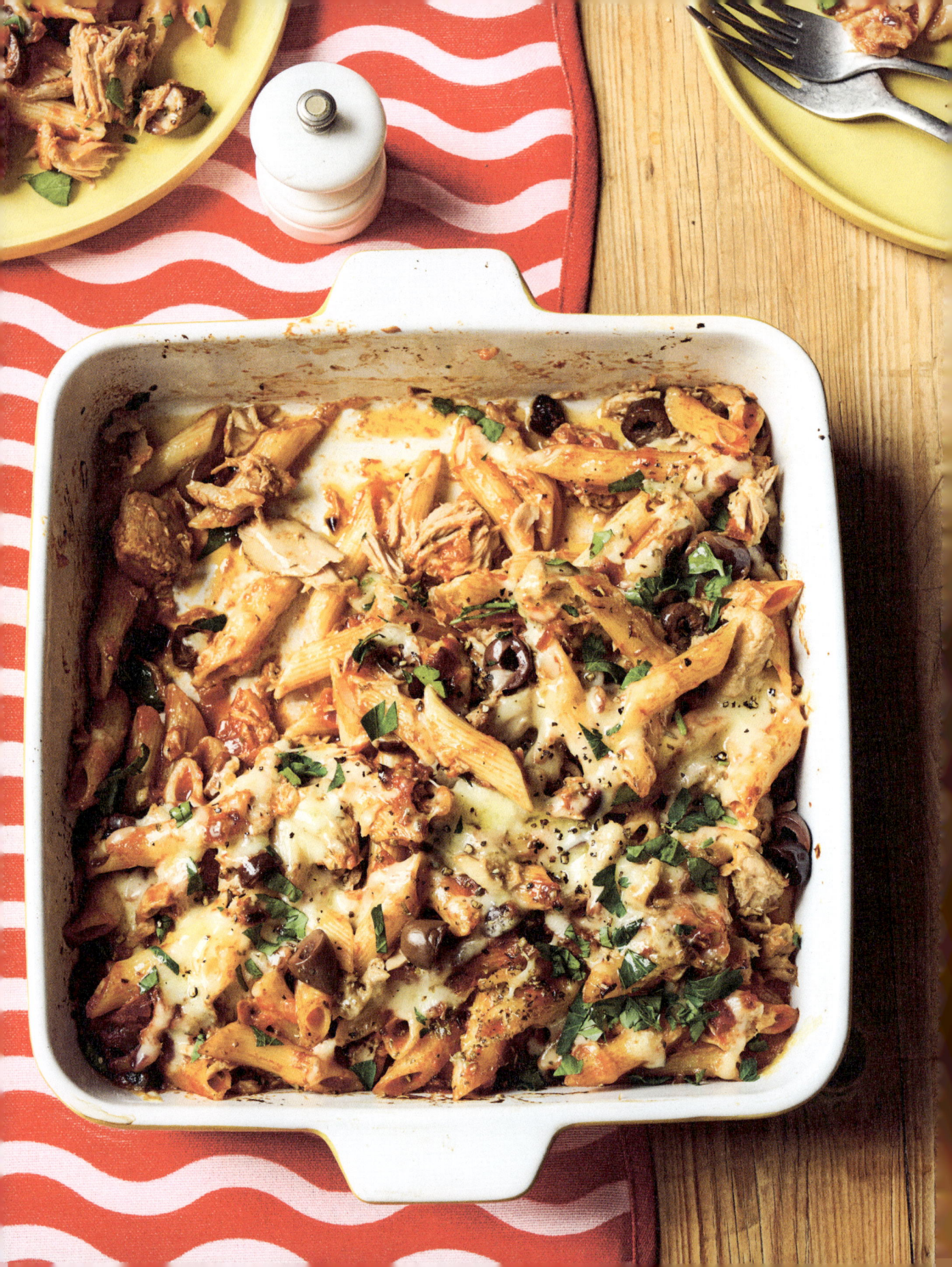

SPICY TUNA PASTA BAKE

SERVES 4
PREP TIME 5 minutes
COOK TIME 30 minutes

300g (10½oz) penne, or other short pasta shape

spray oil

1 onion, finely chopped

2 garlic cloves, crushed

500g (1lb 2oz) tomato passata

1 tablespoon dried Italian herbs

1 teaspoon coarse salt

1 teaspoon chilli flakes

75g (2¾oz) pitted black olives, sliced

2 x 145g (5¼oz) cans of tuna in spring water, drained

60g (2¼oz) Cheddar cheese, grated

parsley leaves, finely chopped, to serve

freshly ground black pepper

I think this is a really comforting dish. With the added elements of olives and chilli, this recipe is so tasty, but incredibly quick to throw together.

1 Preheat the oven to 200°C/180°C fan (400°F), Gas Mark 6.

2 Put the pasta on to cook in boiling water until al dente (usually 10–12 minutes), then drain, reserving some of the pasta cooking water.

3 Meanwhile, spray a frying pan with oil and fry the onion gently for 10 minutes until it is soft, adding the garlic for the final minute.

4 Add the passata, herbs, salt and chilli flakes, then simmer for a further 3 minutes.

5 Add the olives, tuna and drained pasta, adding some of the pasta cooking water if needed, then mix everything together.

6 Transfer into a baking dish, sprinkle with the cheese and bake for 15 minutes. Scatter with parsley and season with black pepper before serving.

NOTE

Grated mozzarella melted on top of this goes down a treat. If you want to increase the vegetable content, add chopped sweet peppers or mushrooms when you are frying the onion, or chopped spinach with the tomato passata, or try adding chopped courgette or halved cherry tomatoes into the mix at the same time as the olives.

PER SERVING

CALORIES	FAT	SAT FAT	CARBS	SUGARS	FIBRE	PROTEIN	SALT
477	9.8G	3.9G	62G	12G	7.4G	29G	2.2G

PEANUT MISO RAMEN

SERVES 2
PREP TIME 5 minutes
COOK TIME 10 minutes

spray oil

250g (9oz) closed-cup or chestnut mushrooms, sliced

2 garlic cloves, finely grated

¼ teaspoon chilli flakes

4 spring onions, sliced, plus more to serve

1 tablespoon peanut butter

1 tablespoon miso paste

500ml (18fl oz) hot water, plus more for the peanut paste

2 x 100g (3½oz) packets of instant noodles (set aside the seasoning packets)

100g (3½oz) pak choi, or sweetheart/hispi cabbage, finely sliced

1 tablespoon soy sauce

coriander leaves, to serve

So quick, but so flavoursome, this easy ramen recipe is always a winner!

1 Spray a saucepan with oil and fry the mushrooms for a few minutes, then stir through the garlic, chilli flakes and spring onions.

2 In a small bowl, mix together the peanut butter, miso paste and a little bit of hot water, just enough to loosen it up and allow it to mix.

3 Add the paste to the pan with the mushrooms, then pour in the hot water and bring to a simmer.

4 Add the noodles, submerge them in the liquid, tip in the cabbage, then simmer until the noodles are soft (instant noodles usually take 3–4 minutes).

5 Stir through the soy sauce, divide between 2 warmed bowls and scatter with coriander and spring onions to serve.

NOTE

You can add any extra quick-cooking vegetables you fancy and simply simmer them with the rest of the ingredients – try frozen sweetcorn, sugar snap peas, mange tout, fine green beans, broccoli florets, carrot matchsticks or beansprouts.

PER SERVING

CALORIES	FAT	SAT FAT	CARBS	SUGARS	FIBRE	PROTEIN	SALT
507	7.8G	1.6G	92G	5.5G	4.1G	15G	2.1G

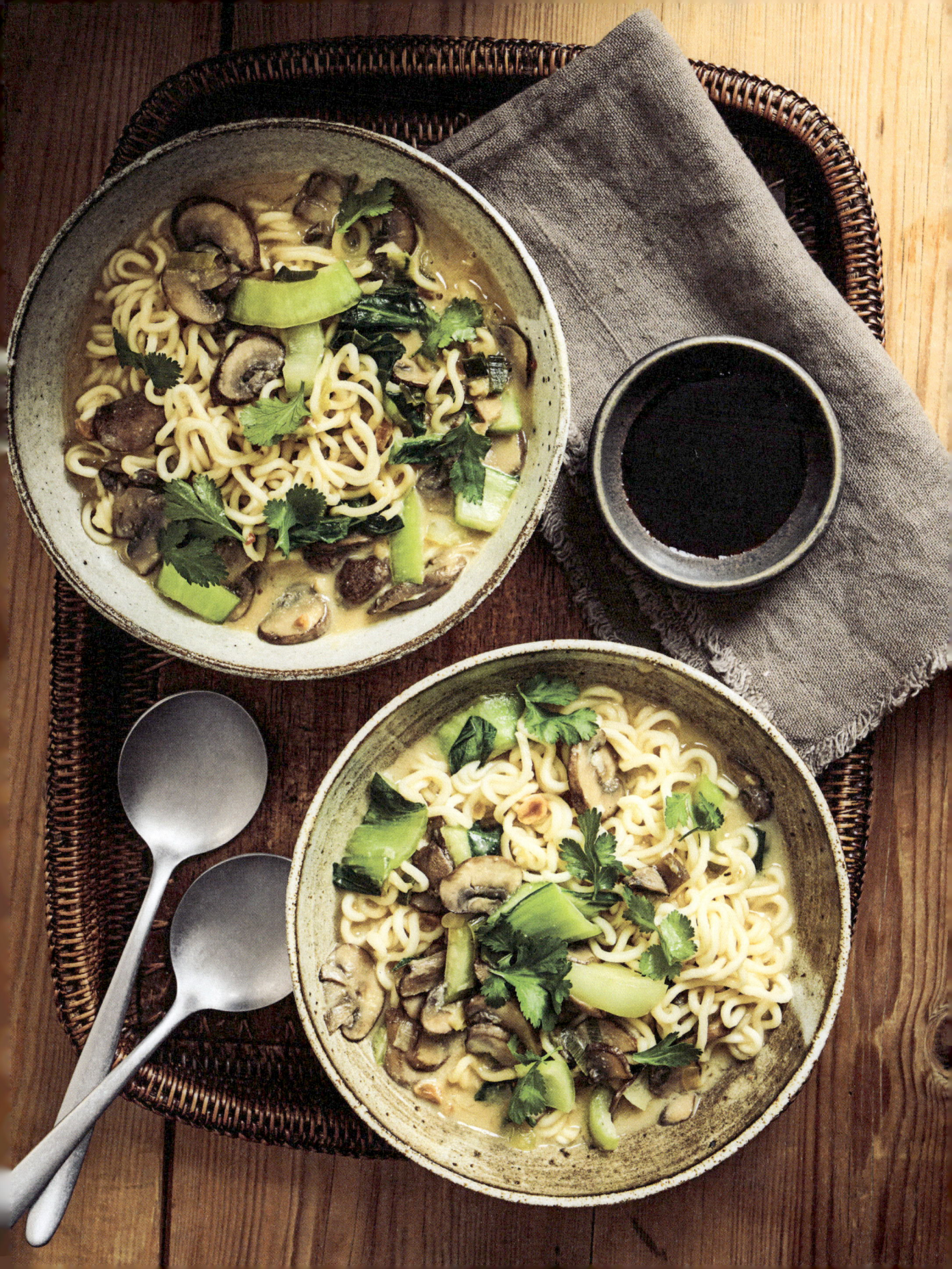

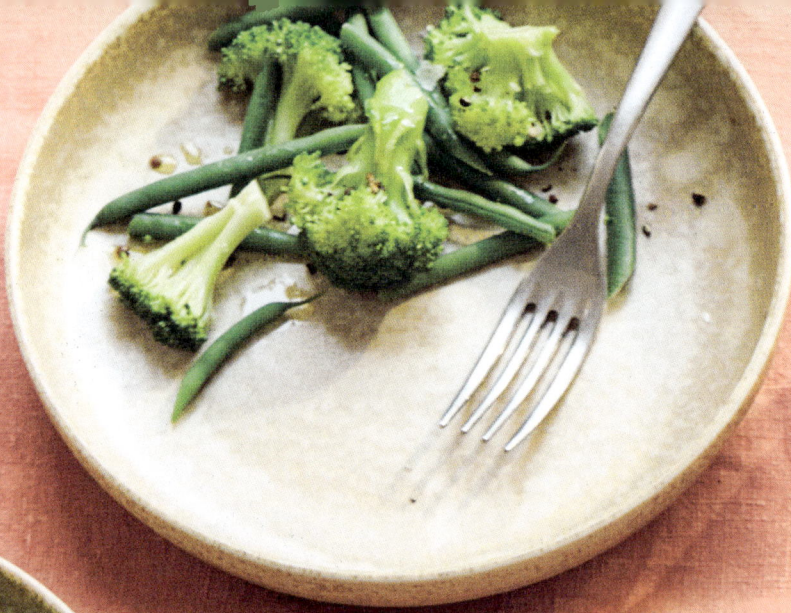

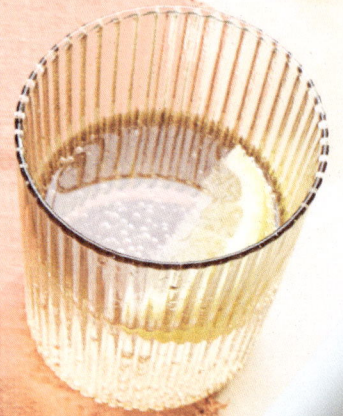

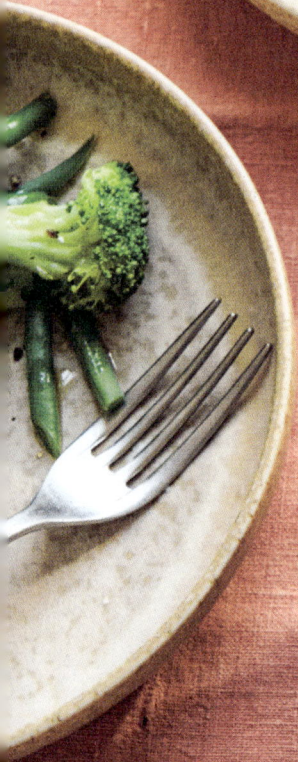

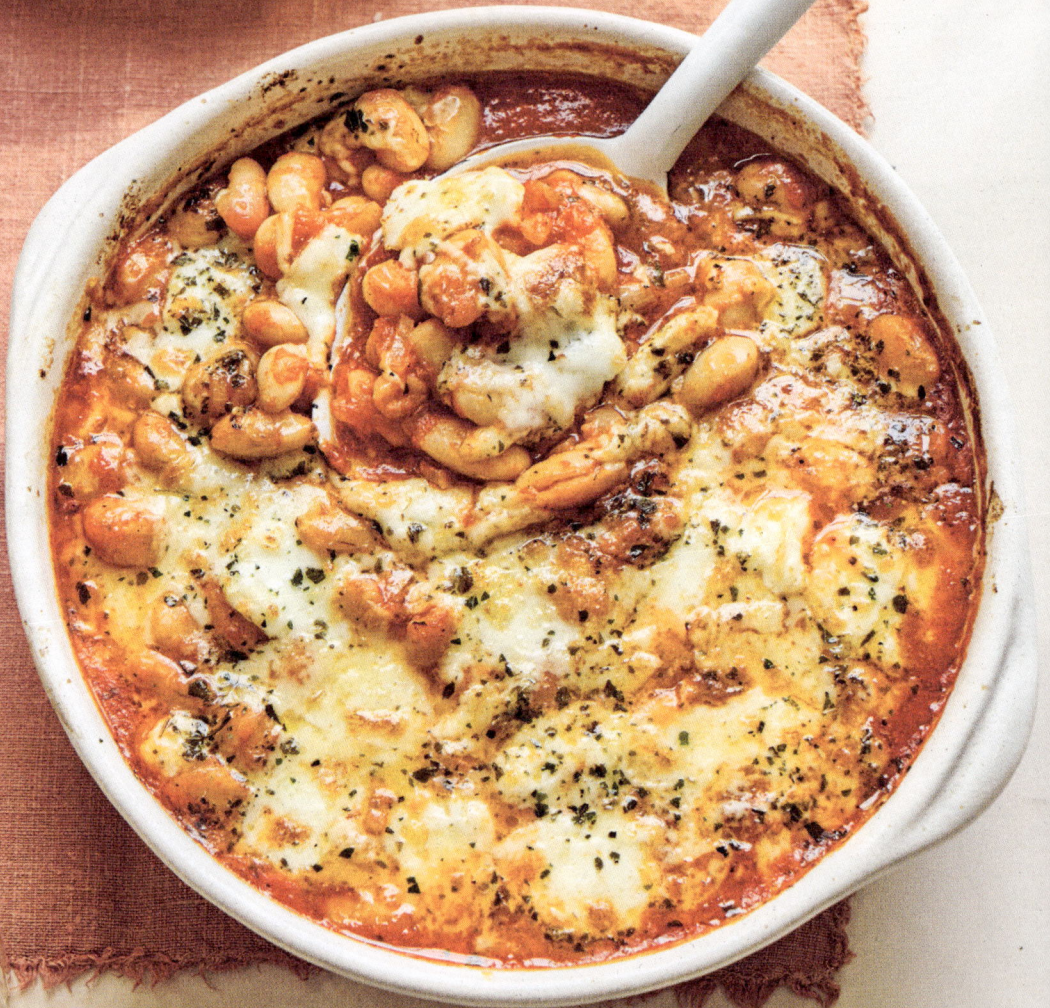

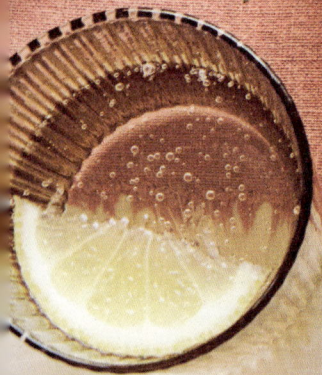

CHEESY MARINARA BUTTER BEAN BAKE

SERVES 4
PREP TIME 5 minutes
COOK TIME 25 minutes

spray oil

1 onion, finely chopped

2 garlic cloves, crushed

500g (1lb 2oz) tomato passata

100ml (3½fl oz) water

1 teaspoon dried oregano, plus more for the top

1 teaspoon dried basil

3 x 400g (14oz) cans of butter beans, drained and rinsed

125g (4½oz) ball of mozzarella, torn into pieces

45g (1½oz) Cheddar cheese, grated

salt and pepper

Butter beans encased in a thick marinara sauce with oozing, melted cheese: a simple comfort food dish which is filling and nutritious. I serve this up with a side of green vegetables, whatever I have in.

1   If you can use a hob-to-oven pan here, it will save on washing up. Spray a sauté pan with oil and fry the onion until soft, about 8 minutes. Preheat the grill to high.

2   Stir the garlic into the onion and stir-fry for 1 minute.

3   Add the passata and measured water, then the dried herbs. Stir in the butter beans, season with salt and pepper, then simmer for 10 minutes.

4   If you are using an ovenproof pan, then add the cheese to it directly; if not, transfer the beans to an oven dish first. Scatter the torn mozzarella over the top, then sprinkle on the Cheddar with a pinch of oregano.

5   Put the pan or dish under the hot grill for 4–5 minutes until the cheese is golden and bubbling. Serve with the vegetables of your choice.

NOTE

You can raid the refrigerator for extras to add to this if you wish – vegetables such as mushrooms, spinach, courgettes, cherry tomatoes and sweet peppers all work well, as does finely chopped chorizo, bacon or sausage, if you fry them for a few minutes with the onion. You could also add leftover cooked meat, such as chicken, lamb or beef, along with the butter beans. If you fancy a bit of crunch on the top, you could add breadcrumbs along with the cheese (spray with oil before grilling).

PER SERVING

CALORIES	FAT	SAT FAT	CARBS	SUGARS	FIBRE	PROTEIN	SALT
311	11G	6.9G	24G	11G	13G	19G	0.57G

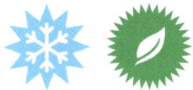

VEGGIE CURRIED 'SHEPHERD'S' PIE

SERVES 4 generously, this could easily feed 6
PREP TIME 15 minutes
COOK TIME 45 minutes

This tasty twist on shepherd's pie uses mainly store cupboard ingredients, swapping out the traditional minced lamb for curried lentils, chickpeas and vegetables, and regular potatoes for sweet potatoes. Serve with green vegetables.

600g (1lb 5oz) sweet potato, chopped, or frozen sweet potato chunks

spray oil

1 onion, finely chopped

3 garlic cloves, crushed

2.5cm (1 inch) piece of root ginger, peeled and finely grated

2 carrots, finely chopped

2 celery sticks, finely chopped

1 tablespoon garam masala

1 teaspoon chilli powder

500g (1lb 2oz) tomato passata

2 x 400g (14oz) cans of green lentils, drained and rinsed

400g (14oz) can of chickpeas, drained and rinsed

100g (3½oz) frozen peas

1 vegetable stock cube, crumbled

½ teaspoon coarse salt

2 tablespoons mango chutney

pepper

1. Preheat the oven to 200°C/180°C (400°F), Gas Mark 6.

2. Put the cubed sweet potato into a large saucepan of boiling water and simmer until tender. This should take around 15 minutes, but may take less time if you are using frozen sweet potato, so just follow the packet instructions.

3. Meanwhile, spray a sauté pan with oil and cook the onion for 5 minutes, then add the garlic, ginger, carrots and celery. Sauté these for 10 minutes, stirring regularly.

4. Add the garam masala and chilli powder to the sauté pan, cook for 1 minute, then tip in the passata, lentils, chickpeas, frozen peas, crumbled stock cube, salt and 1 tablespoon of the mango chutney. Stir well and leave to simmer for a few minutes while you prepare the potatoes.

5. Drain the sweet potatoes, allow them to steam for a couple of minutes in the colander, then pop them back into their pan (or a bowl). Add the remaining tablespoon of mango chutney and a few grinds of pepper, then mash them until there are no lumps remaining.

6. Transfer the lentil mixture to a baking dish (I use a 5cm-/2 inch-deep 24cm/9½ inch square oven dish) and spread it out evenly.

7. Spoon the sweet potato over the top of the lentil mixture – I space spoonfuls evenly over the top, which then helps when spreading it out. Use a fork to spread the sweet potato to fully cover the lentil mixture, then use the prongs to create a cross-hatch pattern. Spray with oil, then bake for 30 minutes. If you want a little more crispiness and colour on the top of the pie, leave it under a hot grill for a few minutes after baking.

NOTE

This is perfect for using up bits and pieces of leftover vegetables; you can add almost anything! Try mushrooms, spinach, sweet peppers, cauliflower, green beans, broccoli, spinach, leeks or sweetcorn. If you don't need it to be vegetarian, then adding leftover roast meats, such as lamb, beef, chicken or pork, or frying in some bacon, chorizo or sausage pieces with the carrots and celery also works really well.

PER SERVING

CALORIES	FAT	SAT FAT	CARBS	SUGARS	FIBRE	PROTEIN	SALT
472	4.4G	0.7G	76G	28G	21G	20G	1.7G

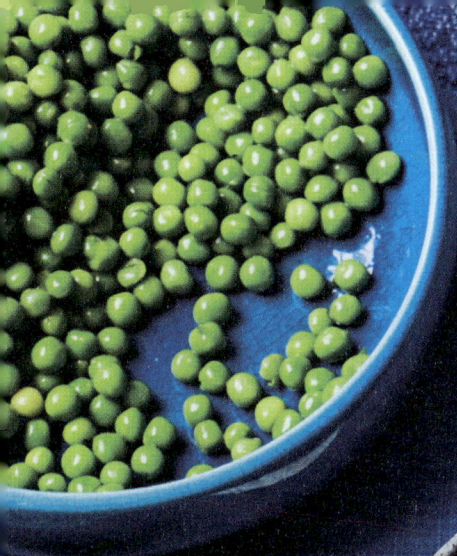

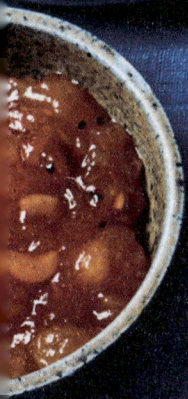

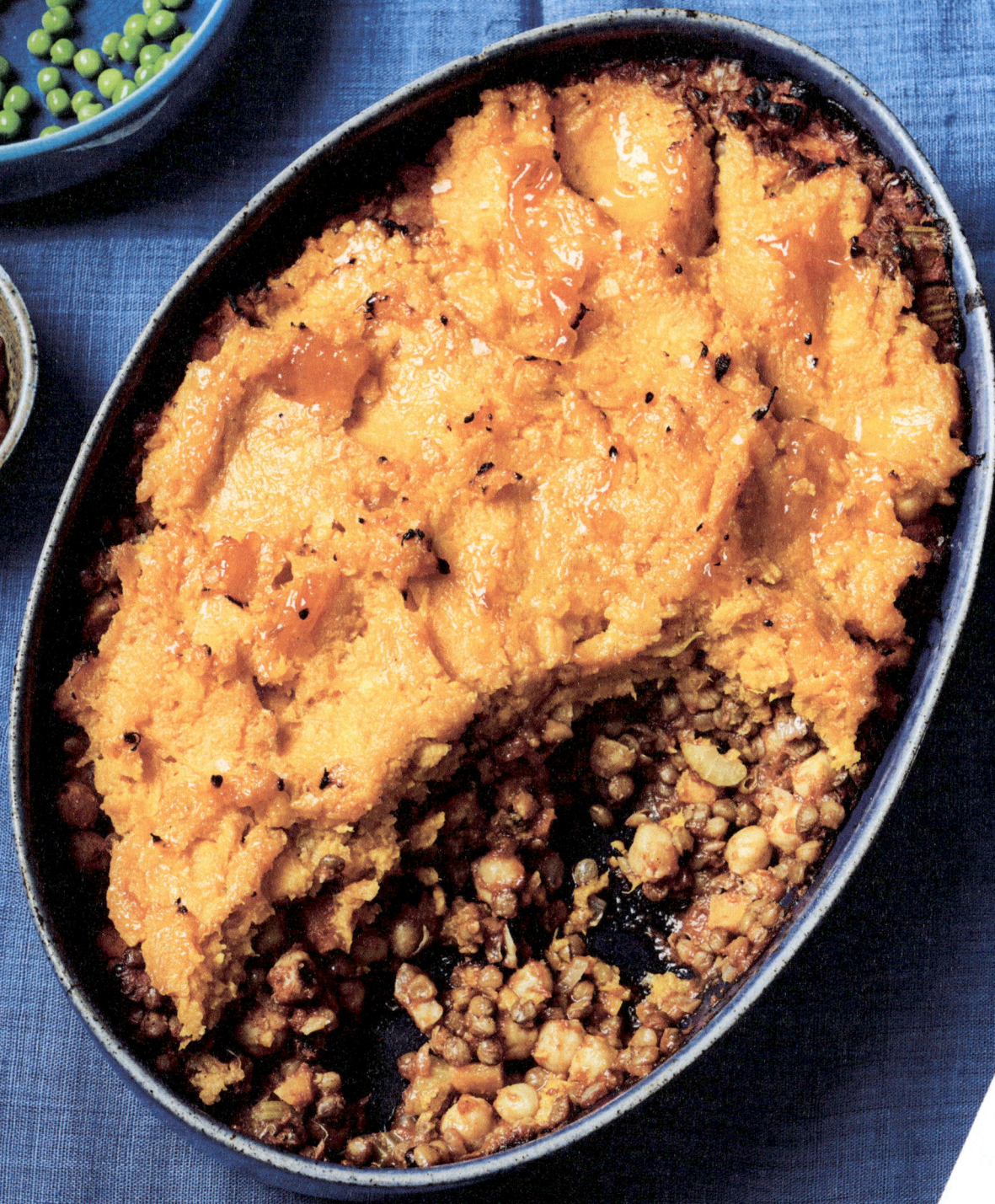

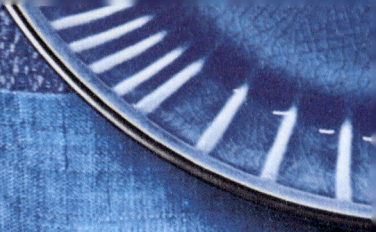

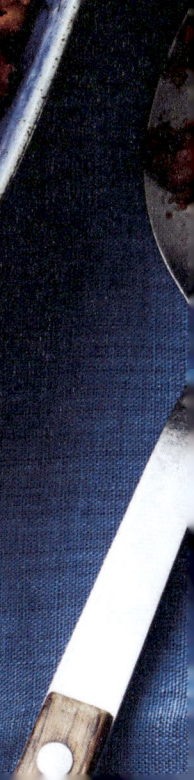

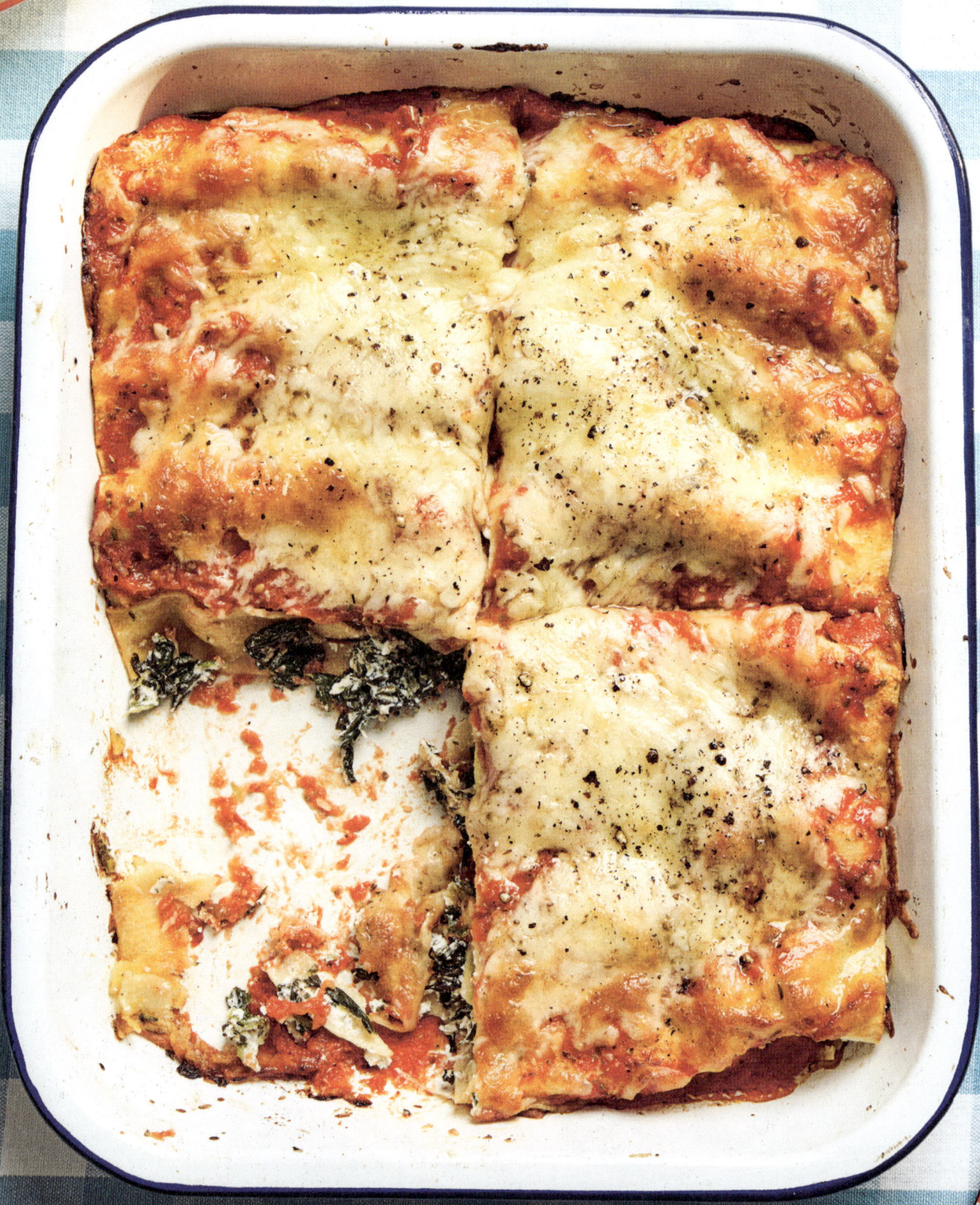

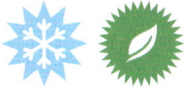

CHEAT'S SPINACH & RICOTTA CANNELLONI

SERVES 4
PREP TIME 10 minutes
COOK TIME 25 minutes

200g (7oz) frozen spinach

400g (14oz) can of chopped tomatoes

3 garlic cloves

1½ teaspoons dried oregano

1 teaspoon onion granules

250g (9oz) ricotta

juice of ½ lemon

200g (7oz) fresh lasagne sheets (about 8), halved, if large

150g (5½oz) grated mozzarella, or mozzarella and Cheddar mix

15g (½oz) Parmesan-style vegetarian cheese

salt and pepper

NOTE

If you want a cheese sauce to go over the tomato sauce, you can heat 125ml (4fl oz) semi-skimmed milk and add 150g (5½oz) light (reduced-fat) cream cheese. Stir them together to melt the cream cheese into the milk, allow it to thicken up for a couple of minutes, then pour over the assembled cannelloni and tomato sauce before topping with the mozzarella and Parmesan.

Using fresh lasagne sheets, you can wrap up creamy ricotta and spinach to replicate cannelloni tubes for a meal that's easy and quick to make at home. Of course, if you prefer, you can use dried cannelloni tubes, but personally I find it way too fiddly to stuff them when I want an easy meal, whereas with this simple method you can have them ready to go in the oven within 10 minutes. Serve this up with green salad or vegetables.

Even though this is a pasta dish, it is fine to freeze it, as the change in texture once defrosted doesn't matter so much here.

1   Preheat the oven to 220°C/200°C fan (425°F), Gas Mark 7. Add the frozen spinach to a pan of boiling water and simmer for 5 minutes, then drain and allow to cool while you prepare the sauce.

2   Put the chopped tomatoes, garlic, 1 teaspoon of the oregano, the onion granules and salt and pepper into a mini chopper, or use a stick blender, then blend into a smooth sauce.

3   In a bowl, mix the drained and cooled spinach, ricotta and lemon juice and season with salt and pepper.

4   Choose an ovenproof baking dish (I use a 25 x 20cm/10 x 8 inch dish), put in a spoonful of the sauce and spread it over the base.

5   Take a lasagne sheet, spoon 2–3 tablespoons of the ricotta mixture in a line down a long edge, then use the spoon to spread it evenly along. Roll the sheet up. Place the roll seam side down in the baking dish, then repeat with all the lasagne sheets and ricotta filling, laying them neatly in a row as you fill them.

6   Now spread the remainder of the tomato sauce over the tubes of pasta and scatter evenly with the mozzarella, then the Parmesan-style cheese and the remaining ½ teaspoon of oregano. Grind over some black pepper.

7   Bake on the middle shelf of the oven for 20 minutes, until the cheese is golden and bubbling. Let it rest for 20 minutes before serving.

PER SERVING

CALORIES	FAT	SAT FAT	CARBS	SUGARS	FIBRE	PROTEIN	SALT
406	17G	9.5G	34G	6.8G	4.4G	25G	1.1G

FAMILY FAVOURITES

4

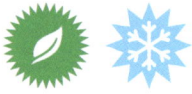

PEANUT BUTTER BREAKFAST BARS

MAKES 8
PREP TIME 5 minutes
COOK TIME 20 minutes

240g (8¾oz) oats
50g (1¾oz) dried cranberries
2 tablespoons peanut butter, smooth or crunchy
2 tablespoons honey
1 egg, lightly beaten
1 teaspoon vanilla extract

Breakfast is my youngest daughter's favourite meal and she really enjoys trying new ideas. These simple bars are fun to make together and provide a nourishing and filling start to the day. They're especially convenient as they can be grabbed on the go for a speedy option.

1 Preheat the oven to 200°C/180°C fan (400°F), Gas Mark 6.

2 Put all the ingredients into a mixing bowl and stir well to combine.

3 Line a small baking tin (I use a loaf tin) with nonstick baking paper, tip in the oat mixture and press it down into an even layer – make sure it's really packed down.

4 Bake for 20 minutes.

5 Allow to cool before slicing into 8 bars.

NOTE

You can mix up the ingredients in this to suit your own tastes, or to use up ingredients. Try adding:

finely grated orange zest

chocolate chips

seeds, such as sunflower, pumpkin, sesame, poppy, linseeds or chia seeds

1 tablespoon cocoa powder

dried fruits, such as raisins, chopped apricots or dates

½ teaspoon ground cinnamon instead of the vanilla extract

PER SERVING

CALORIES	FAT	SAT FAT	CARBS	SUGARS	FIBRE	PROTEIN	SALT
174	3.4G	0.7G	27G	4.6G	2.4G	7.3G	0.51G

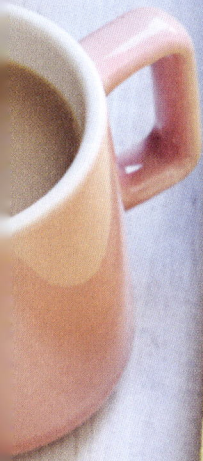

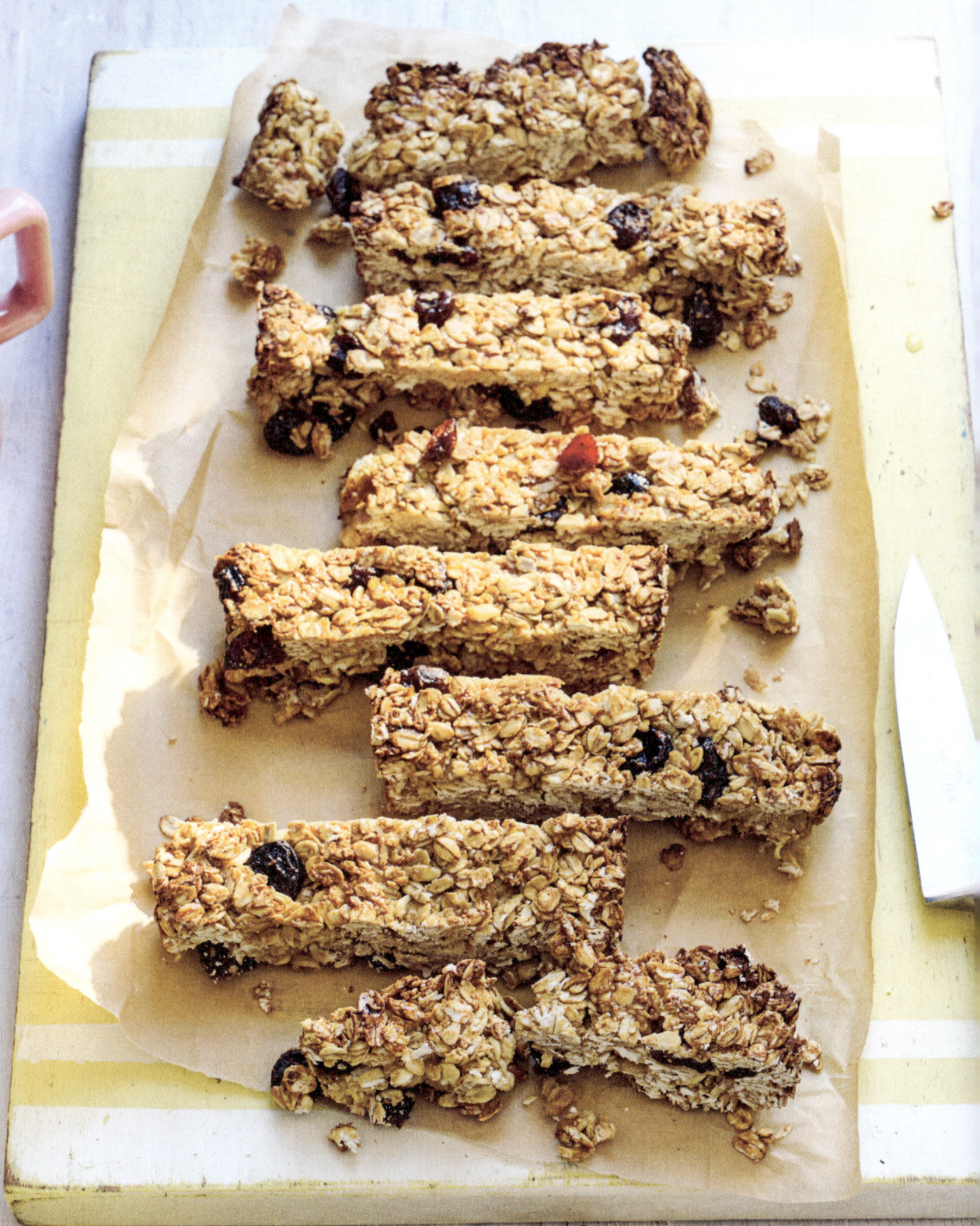

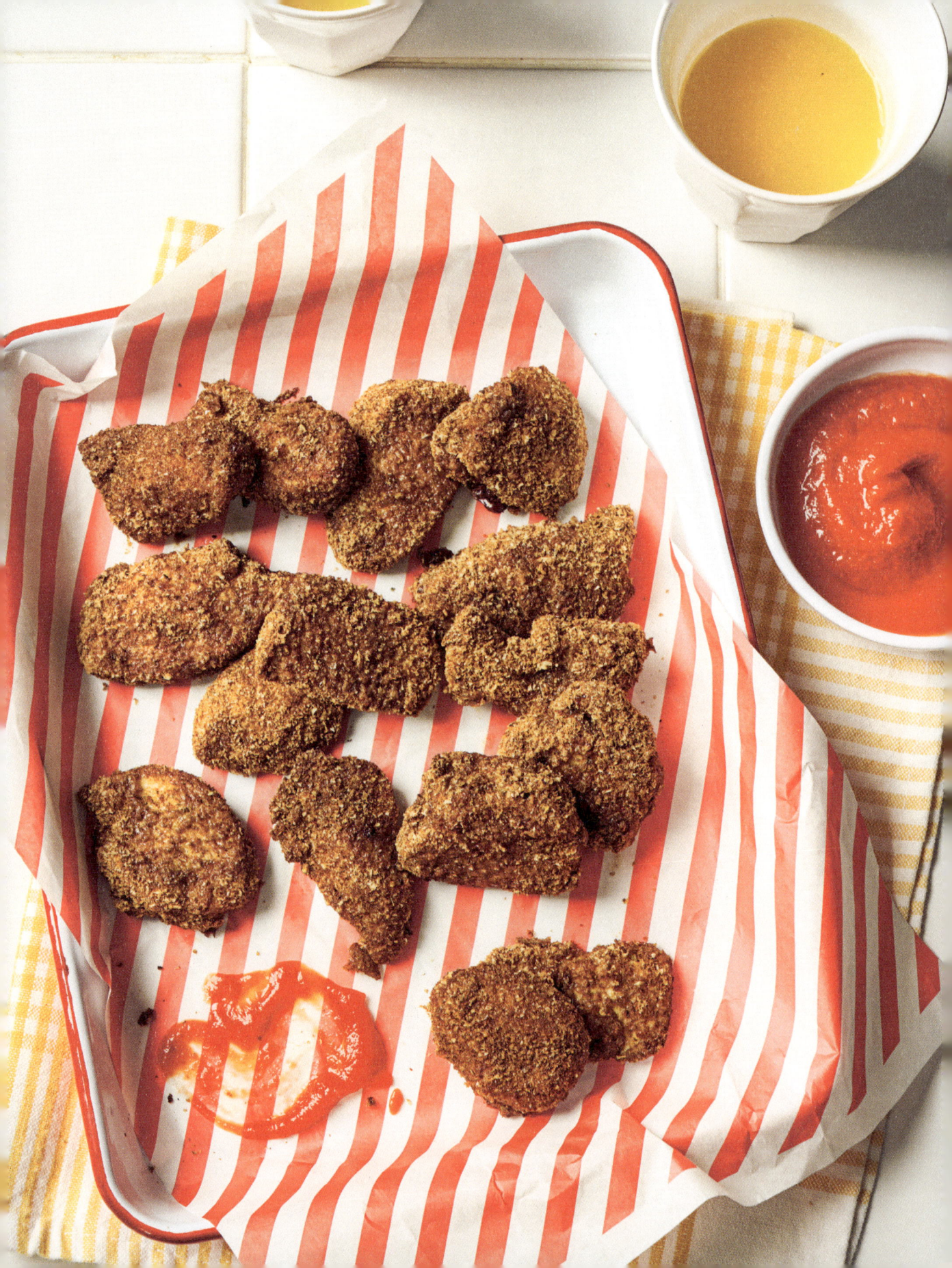

SOUTHERN 'FRIED' CHICKEN NUGGETS

SERVES 4
PREP TIME 10 minutes
COOK TIME 25 minutes

4 breakfast cereal whole wheat
  biscuits (80g/2¾oz)
1 tablespoon sweet (unsmoked)
  paprika
1 teaspoon dried oregano
1 teaspoon garlic granules
1 teaspoon onion granules
1 teaspoon dried sage
1 teaspoon dried basil
½ teaspoon coarse salt
1 chicken stock cube, crumbled
2 eggs
4 skinless chicken breasts,
  chopped into chunks
spray oil

Chicken nuggets are the guaranteed winner with my daughters and their friends, and if I have a little time, I much prefer to make my own. I think cereal makes a brilliant crispy coating for nuggets; here I've suggested whole wheat biscuits, but I also use crispy rice cereal and cornflakes, as I usually have them in the house. My girls are much better with a hint of spice now they are older, but you can easily leave the chilli out of these, if you need to. We serve these with homemade thin-cut oven chips and peas or sweetcorn.

1   Preheat the oven to 210°C/190°C fan (410°F), Gas Mark 6½.

2   Put the whole wheat biscuits, plus all the spices and herbs, salt and chicken stock cube into a food processor and whizz into fine crumbs. Tip into a shallow bowl.

3   Line a large baking tray or roasting tin with nonstick baking paper.

4   Lightly beat the eggs in a separate shallow bowl.

5   Dip each chicken chunk into the eggs, then into the crumbs to fully coat. Place on the prepared tray or tin.

6   Once you have coated all the chicken pieces, spray with oil, then bake for 25 minutes, until the coating on the chicken is crunchy.

NOTE

Make up a bigger batch of the cereal-and-spice mix for a quicker meal next time, minus the chicken stock cube, and store the mix in an airtight jar or container – crumble in the chicken stock cube just before you make the nuggets.

PER SERVING

CALORIES	FAT	SAT FAT	CARBS	SUGARS	FIBRE	PROTEIN	SALT
277	5.8G	1.4G	8.3G	1G	2.2G	47G	1.6G

SWEET CHILLI CHICKEN & MUSHROOM ORZO

SERVES 4
PREP TIME 5 minutes
COOK TIME 25 minutes

spray oil
1 large onion, peeled and finely
    sliced into half moons
2 skinless chicken breasts
    (about 150g/5½oz each)
350g (12oz) orzo
300g (10½oz) chestnut
    mushrooms, quartered
300ml (½ pint) hot chicken stock
4 tablespoons sweet chilli sauce
4 tablespoons light (reduced-fat)
    cream cheese
salt and pepper

TO SERVE (OPTIONAL)
Parmesan cheese
handful of basil leaves, torn

Sweet chilli sauce has been a favourite of mine since childhood and it is a brilliant ingredient to keep in your store cupboard. This easy orzo dish packs amazing flavour with only a handful of ingredients, and it's easy to customize with whatever pasta shape you have.

1   Spray a sauté pan lightly with oil, place over a medium heat and add the onion. Cook for 5 minutes, stirring occasionally.

2   Add the chicken breasts to the pan, increase the heat and fry on each side for 2 minutes, shuffling the onion around as you do so to prevent it from burning.

3   In a separate pan of boiling water, put the orzo on to simmer according to the packet instructions (usually 9–11 minutes, set a timer). Drain the orzo and set aside for a moment; I set the sieve over some of the leftover cooking water just to keep it warm, while I finish making the sauce.

4   Meanwhile, add the mushrooms and hot stock to the sauté pan, stir well and allow to simmer for 10 minutes.

5   Remove the cooked chicken breasts from the sauté pan and use a sharp knife to thinly slice them up, then return them to the pan. If there is still any pink showing in the middle of the chicken at this point, just simmer it in the stock for a couple more minutes until there is no more remaining.

6   Add the sweet chilli sauce and the cream cheese to the sauté pan and stir through until combined. Season with salt and pepper.

7   Tip the cooked orzo into the sauce, stir thoroughly until it's all coated, then serve in warmed bowls. Scatter with grated Parmesan and torn basil leaves, if you like.

NOTE

Other vegetables that work really well in this, as well as – or instead of – the mushrooms. Try asparagus spears cut into 2cm (¾ inch) lengths, green beans or sugar snaps stirred in at the same time as the cream cheese; or frozen or fresh spinach added when you return the sliced chicken and stirred through until defrosted or wilted; or courgettes sliced into half moons and added at the same time as the hot stock.

PER SERVING

CALORIES	FAT	SAT FAT	CARBS	SUGARS	FIBRE	PROTEIN	SALT
521	5.5G	1.9G	77G	17G	6.3G	38G	0.89G

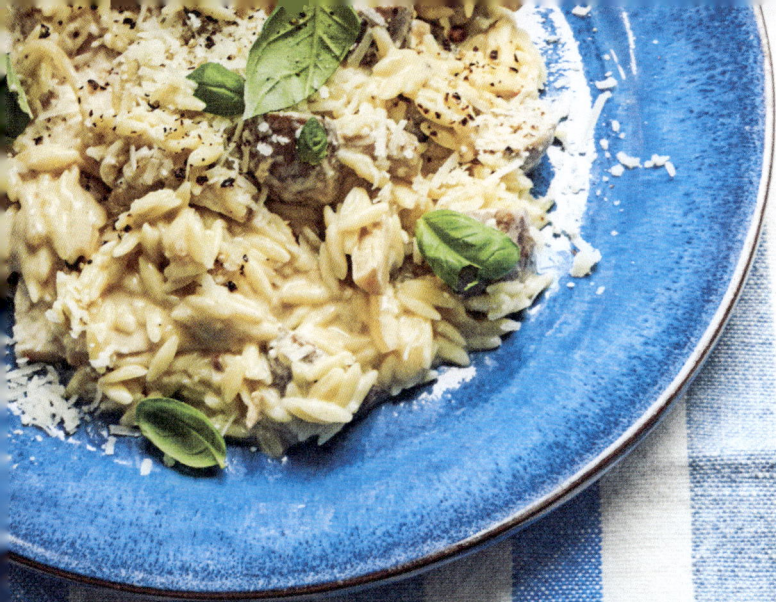

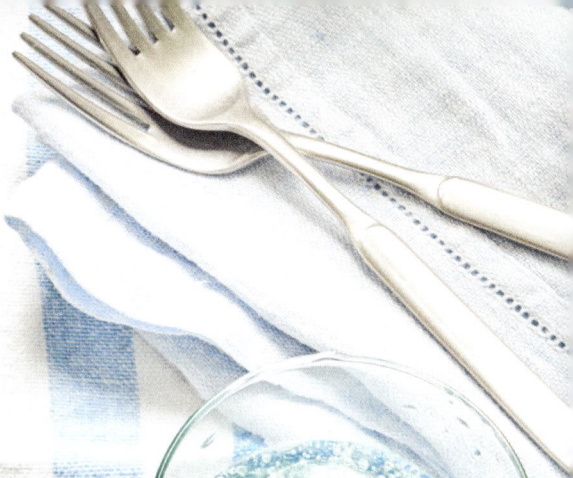

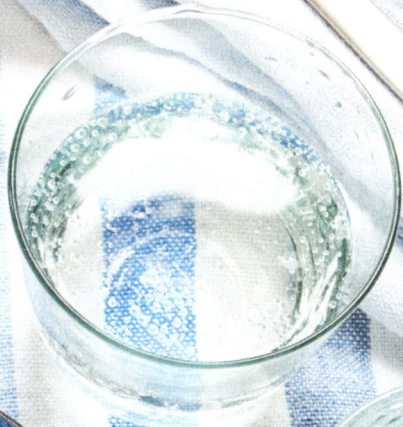

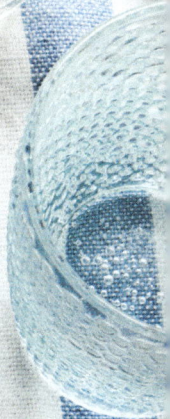

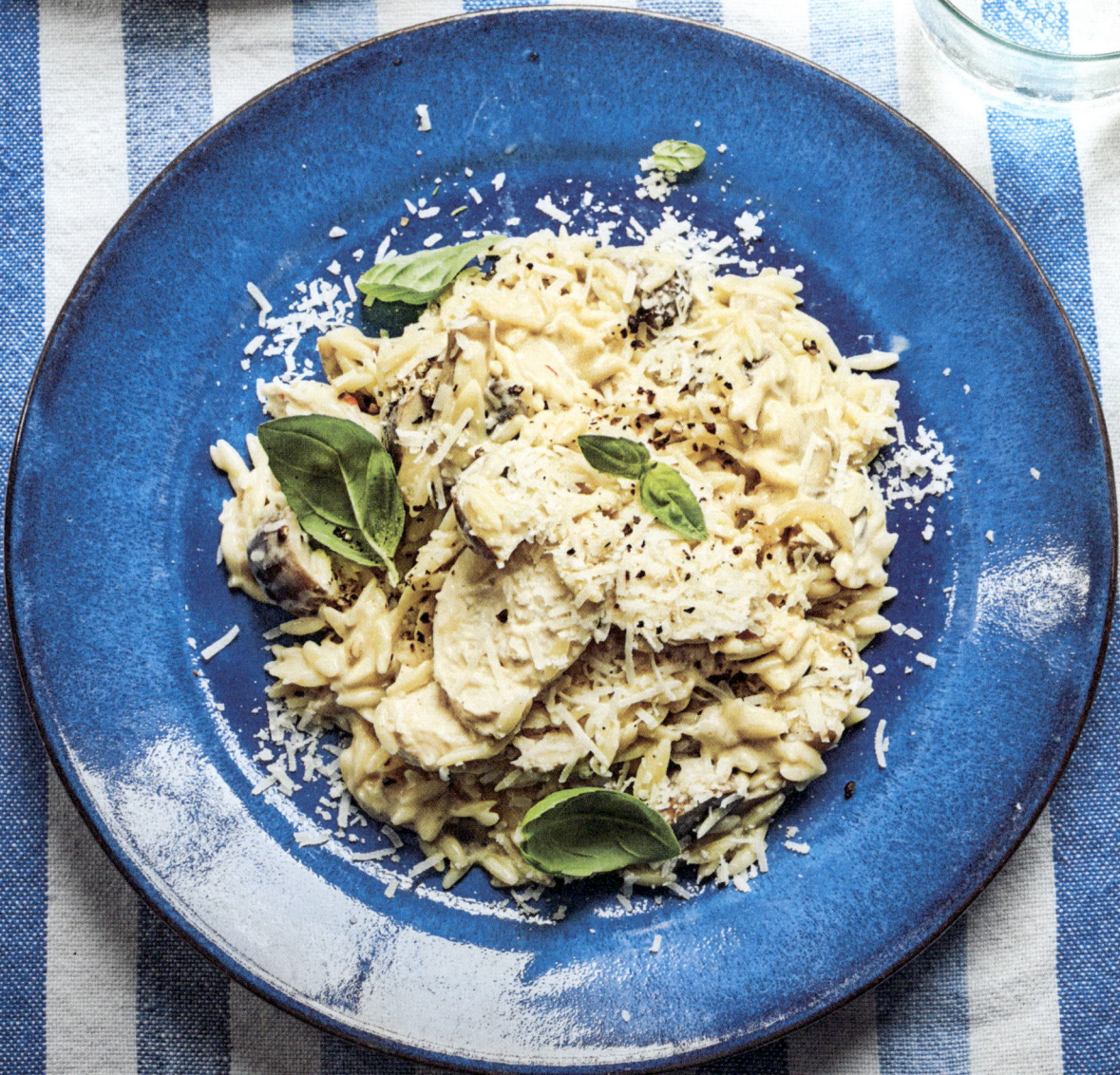

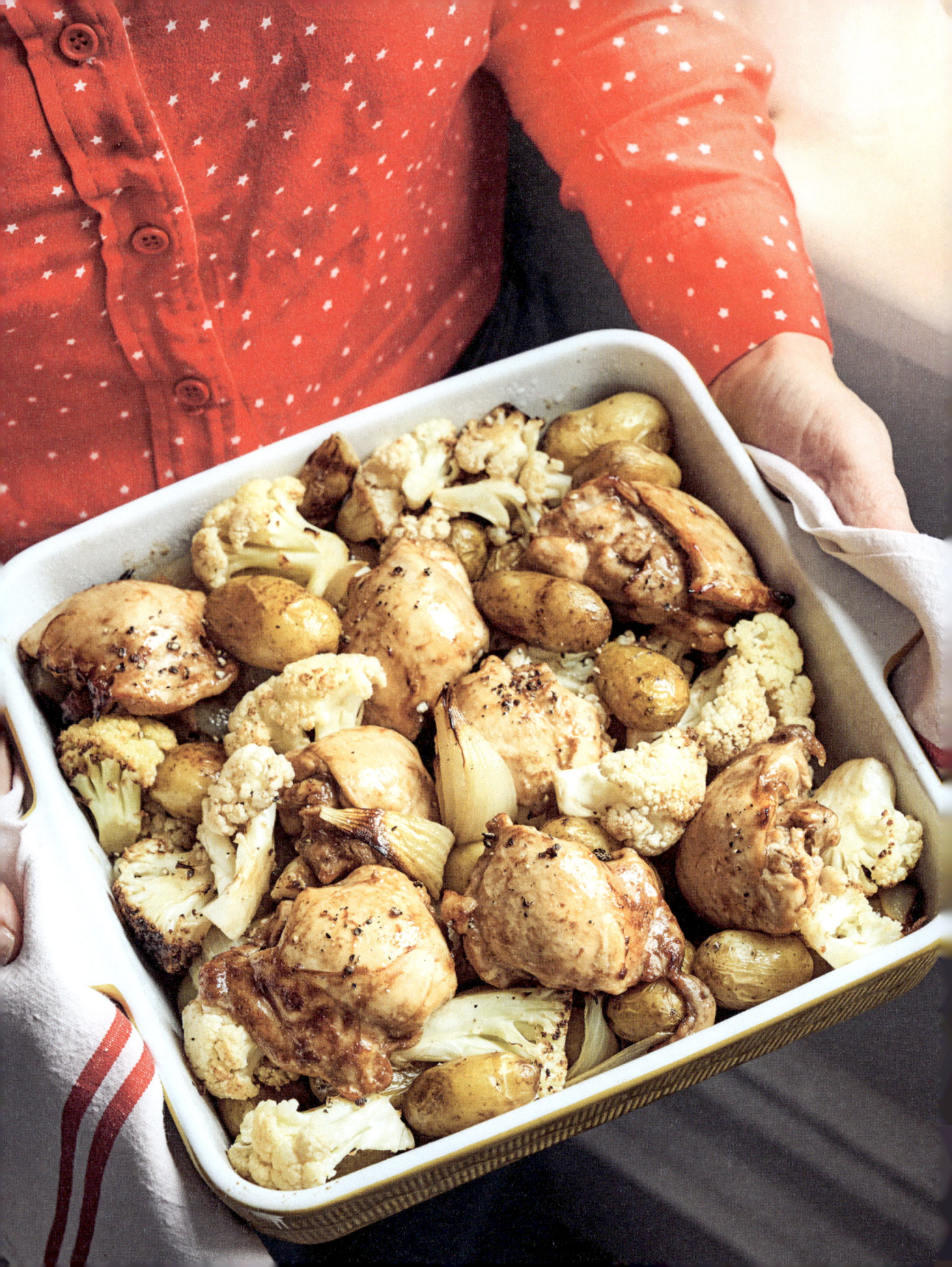

HP SAUCE CHICKEN TRAYBAKE

SERVES 4
PREP TIME 10 minutes
COOK TIME 40 minutes

8 skinless chicken thigh fillets, excess fat removed

4 tablespoons HP sauce, or other brown sauce

750g (1lb 10oz) baby potatoes, larger ones halved so they are all evenly sized

2 onions, cut into wedges

1 tablespoon olive oil

1 cauliflower, cut into bite-sized florets

salt and pepper

HP sauce, or brown sauce, is a British institution… though, at the time of writing, it is manufactured in the Netherlands! You can use an unbranded brown sauce for this, if you prefer. The base flavours of tomato, vinegar and tamarind make for a brilliant marinade and a super time-saver. If I asked either of my kids if they liked brown sauce the answer would be a resounding 'no!' but little do they know that this traybake, which they both happily wolf down, contains it! I serve this up with a side of green vegetables (broccoli, green beans, asparagus or peas).

1   Preheat the oven to 220°C/200°C fan (425°F), Gas Mark 7.

2   In a bowl, mix the chicken thigh fillets with the HP sauce.

3   Put the potatoes, onions and chicken into a large roasting tray (see note), drizzle over the olive oil and give everything a mix to coat in the oil.

4   Put into the oven and roast for 20 minutes.

5   Take the tray out of the oven, add the cauliflower, season with salt and pepper, stir everything together and return to the oven for another 20 minutes, giving everything a stir after 10 minutes, then serve.

NOTE

To ensure even cooking, everything needs to be roasted in a single layer. I use an extra-large stainless-steel roasting tin from IKEA (40 x 32cm/ 16 x 13 inches), but if you don't have one large enough, just divide the ingredients between 2 smaller roasting tins.

PER SERVING

CALORIES	FAT	SAT FAT	CARBS	SUGARS	FIBRE	PROTEIN	SALT
476	9.6G	2.3G	46G	15G	7.8G	49G	1.2G

OVERNIGHT-MARINATED ROAST BEEF DINNER

SERVES 4, with half the beef left over for sandwiches or meals during the week
PREP TIME 20 minutes, plus overnight marinating
COOK TIME 1 hour, plus resting

1kg (2lb 4oz) beef joint, such as silverside or topside

1 large or 3 small red onions, cut into wedges

1 large leek, trimmed, cleaned and sliced (see page 197)

4 carrots, peeled and cut into batons

400g (14oz) sweet potatoes, peeled and cut into chunks

spray oil

800g (1lb 12oz) potatoes, peeled and cut into 3–4 chunks, depending on size

1 beef bouillon stock cube, crumbled (I use OXO)

400ml (14fl oz) hot beef stock

2 teaspoons cornflour

1 head of broccoli, cut into florets

200g (7oz) frozen peas

horseradish sauce, to serve

A roast dinner is a great family meal, and this version just takes a little bit of forethought. Marinating the meat overnight will help to make it tender, juicy and flavoursome.

1   Put all the marinade ingredients into a large resealable freezer bag, add the joint of beef, seal the bag and shake it up to thoroughly cover the meat. Pop it in the refrigerator to marinate overnight.

2   Remove the beef from the refrigerator 1 hour before you want to start cooking.

3   Preheat the oven to 200°C/180°C fan (400°F), Gas Mark 6. Arrange the onions in the middle of a large roasting tin and place the joint of beef on top, reserving the leftover marinade in the bag. Place the leek, carrots and sweet potatoes around the beef.

4   Spray the vegetables with oil and place the roasting tin into the oven to roast (for timings, see note opposite) along with another empty roasting tray for the potatoes.

5   Put the potatoes in a large pan of boiling water and simmer for 8 minutes, then drain and allow them to steam off in the colander for a couple of minutes. Tip the potatoes back into the pan (without any water), sprinkle over the crumbled stock cube and give them a good shake, to roughen the edges. Spray with oil, tossing them around to make sure they have a light covering, then remove the empty roasting tin from the oven and tip in the potatoes. Pop these into the oven for 45–50 minutes to roast alongside the beef.

6   Pour the leftover marinade from the bag into a saucepan and bring to the boil. As soon as it's bubbling vigorously, add the hot stock. Separately, mix the cornflour with a couple of spoons of cold water in a cup or small bowl so you have a smooth liquid, then add it to the gravy. Leave the gravy simmering gently while the beef and potatoes cook (see note), stirring every now and again.

7   Once the beef is ready (you can use a meat thermometer here to check the internal temperature, see note), remove the tray from the oven, cover with foil and leave to rest for at least 10 minutes.

PER SERVING

CALORIES	FAT	SAT FAT	CARBS	SUGARS	FIBRE	PROTEIN	SALT
575	7.9G	2.2G	75G	24G	18G	42G	1.8G

FOR THE MARINADE

juice of 1 lemon

2 garlic cloves, crushed, or
  2 teaspoons garlic purée
  from a jar

2 tablespoons Worcestershire
  sauce

2 tablespoons wholegrain mustard

1 tablespoon dried rosemary, or
  finely chopped rosemary leaves

1 tablespoon balsamic vinegar

1 tablespoon olive oil

2 teaspoons onion granules

1 teaspoon coarse salt

1 teaspoon pepper

8 If the roast potatoes are nicely golden brown, switch the oven off and leave them in there to keep warm while you rest the beef.

9 Once the beef has rested, use a sharp knife to slice it as thinly as you can; try to cut it against the grain for a more tender slice. Add any juices to the gravy.

10 Bring a pan of water to the boil and add the broccoli and peas. Simmer for 4–5 minutes, then drain. Pour the gravy into a jug.

11 I like to serve the beef, potatoes and roast vegetables, along with the horseradish sauce, on a big warmed platter so everyone can help themselves. With a joint of meat this size, if you are feeding four, you should have about half left over. Keep it wrapped in foil in the refrigerator for up to 5 days: it's great for making sandwiches for a tasty lunch, or for adding to a curry during the week.

NOTE

Calculating the cooking time for a beef joint Allow 20 minutes per 450g (1lb) meat plus an extra 20 minutes, for medium-rare. The internal temperature should reach 56–60°C (133–140°F) on a meat thermometer.

Resting the beef Letting the beef rest after cooking is an important step in making sure it is tender and juicy.

Topside vs. silverside Both cuts can be used for roasting, but topside is more tender and better suited to being cooked rare or medium-rare. Silverside has more connective tissue and can be chewy if undercooked, so it's best cooked for longer and served medium or well-done for a more tender result.

For thicker gravy Take a couple of the cooked onion wedges and pieces of carrot, add them to the gravy and use a stick blender to blitz it until smooth, before continuing with the recipe.

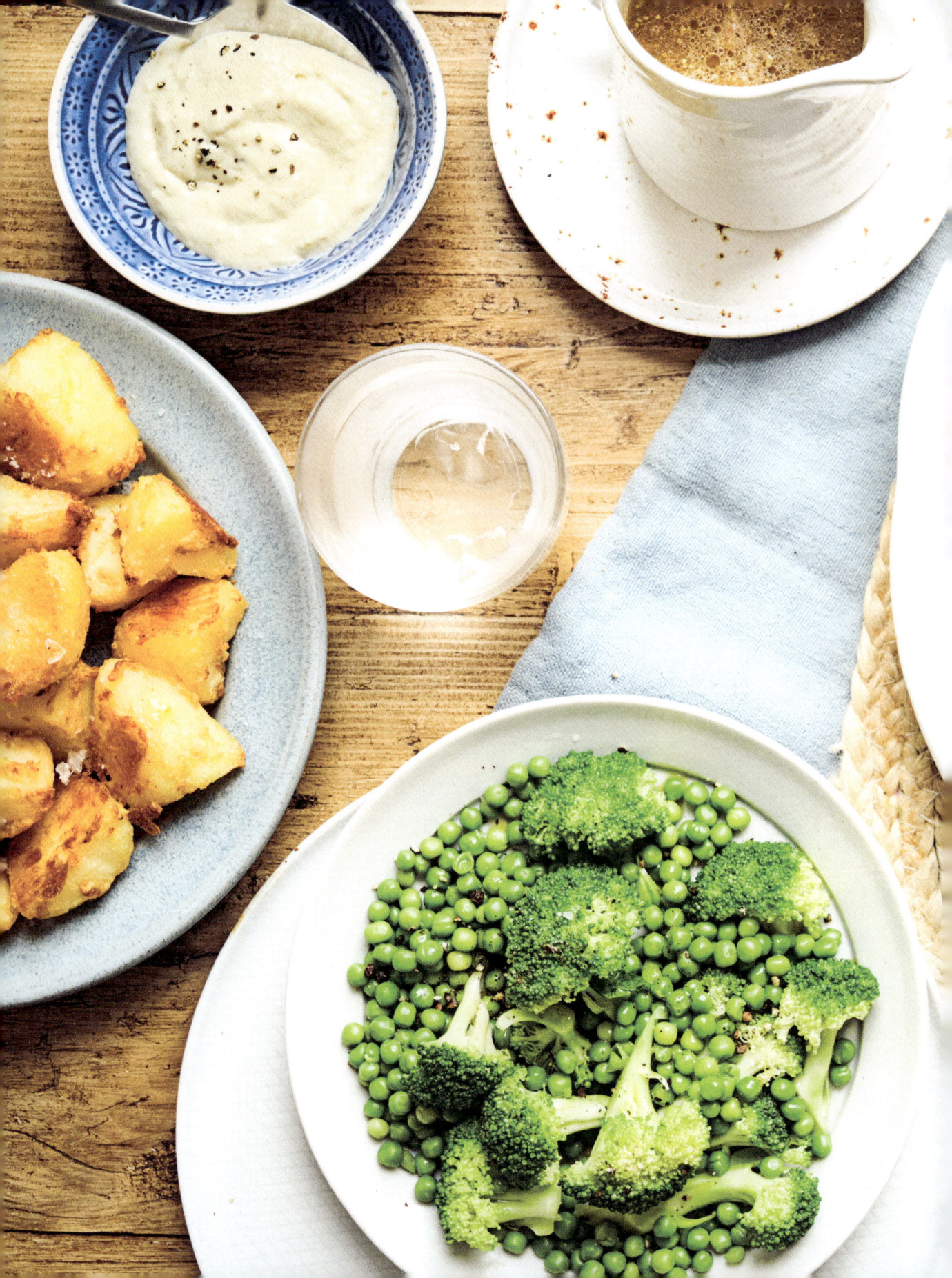

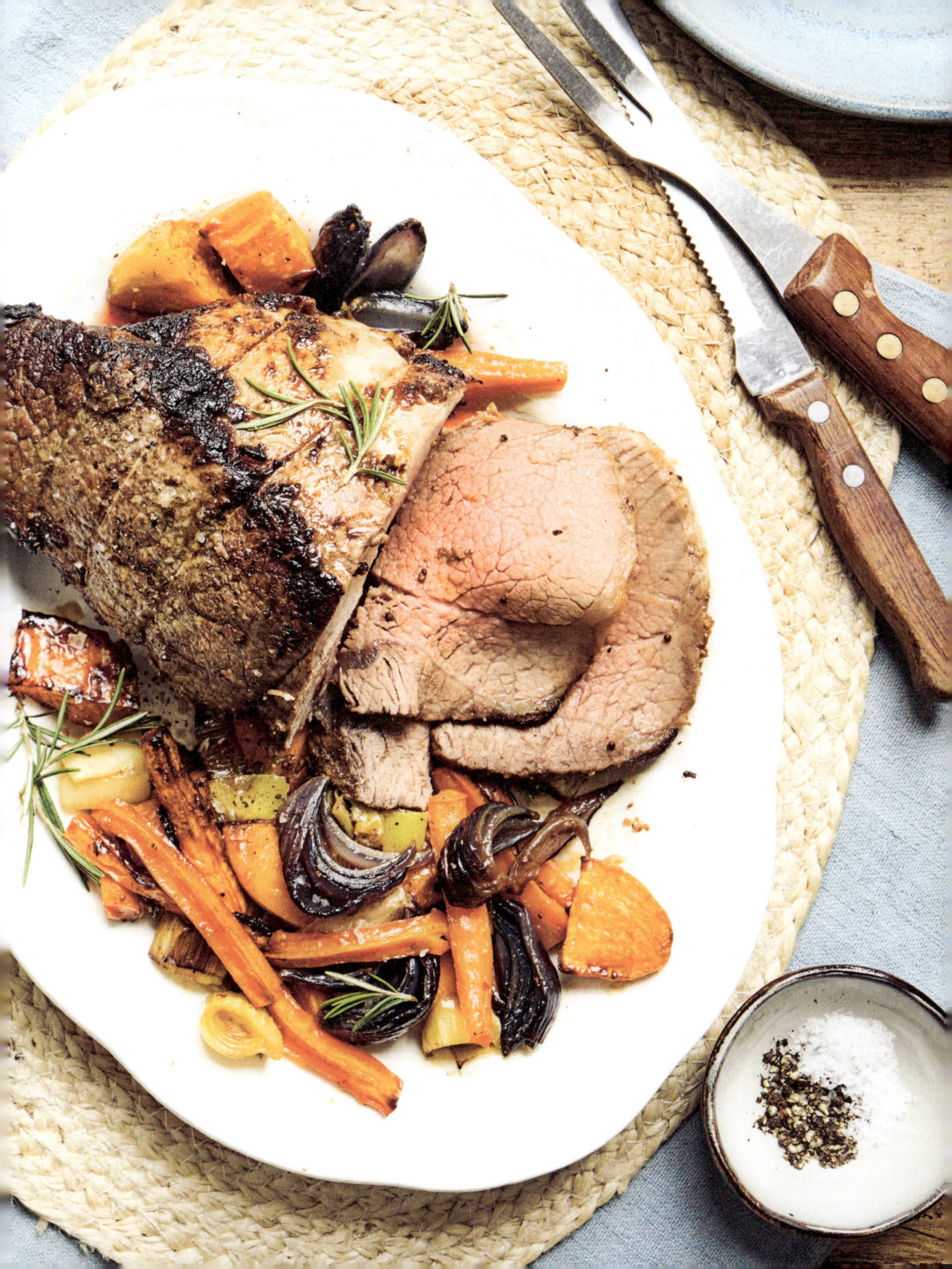

SAUCY TOMATO, BASIL & CHICKEN PENNE

SERVES 4
PREP TIME 5 minutes
COOK TIME 15 minutes

spray oil
2 skinless chicken breasts
400g (14oz) can of chopped
    tomatoes
3 garlic cloves
large handful of basil leaves
1 teaspoon coarse salt
1 teaspoon dried oregano
300g (10½oz) penne pasta,
    white or wholemeal

TO SERVE
Parmesan cheese
freshly ground black pepper

One of my quick knock-it-together dinners for the girls when I'm low on ingredients. They always eat up with no complaints, so I tend to choose this when I need a quick and stress-free dinner time!

1 Spray a sauté pan with oil and start frying the chicken breasts.

2 Put the chopped tomatoes, garlic and basil into a mini chopper and blend into a smooth sauce.

3 Once the chicken has been lightly cooked on either side, pour in the tomato sauce, add the salt and oregano and simmer for 15 minutes, until the chicken breasts are cooked through.

4 Cook the pasta in boiling water for 10–12 minutes, or until al dente.

5 Remove the chicken breasts from the sauce, thinly slice them with a sharp knife, then return them to the sauce.

6 Drain the pasta (reserve a little bit of the pasta water) and stir it into the chicken and tomato sauce. If you want to loosen it up a bit, add some of the pasta cooking water.

7 Serve in warmed pasta bowls, with Parmesan for grating and a few turns of black pepper.

NOTE

I really love a green chilli blended into this tomato sauce; if everyone eating likes a bit of spice, it makes a lovely addition. Sometimes I fry halved cherry tomatoes along with the chicken breasts, to add texture to the sauce.

PER SERVING

CALORIES	FAT	SAT FAT	CARBS	SUGARS	FIBRE	PROTEIN	SALT
442	7G	3.4G	56G	5.5G	3.6G	36G	1.9G

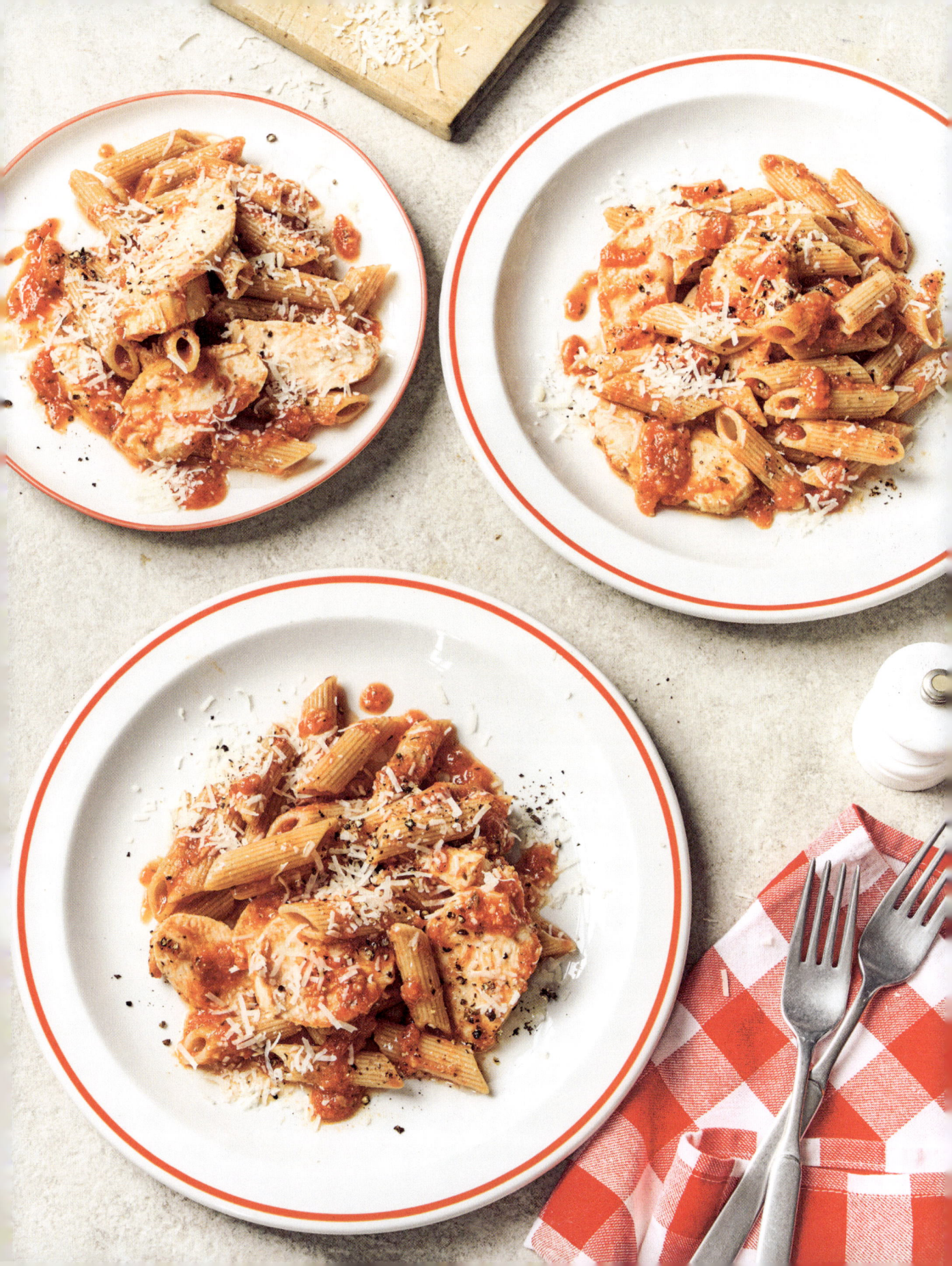

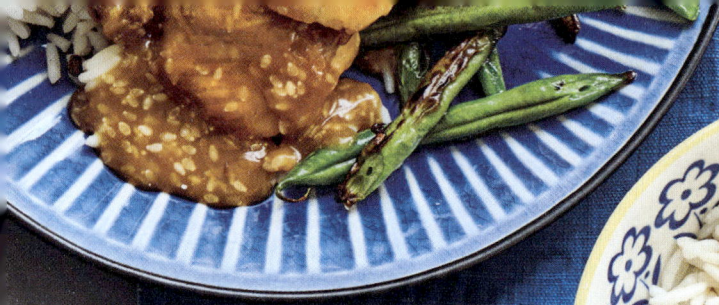

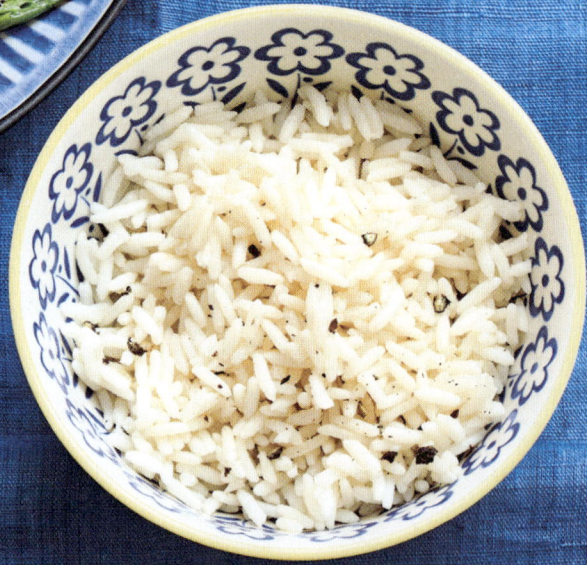

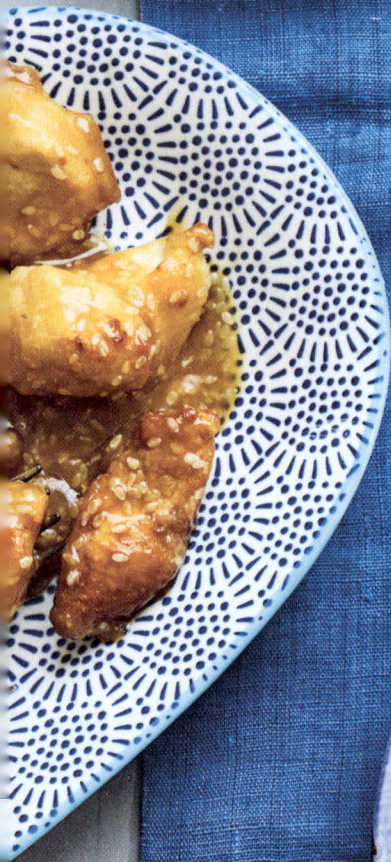

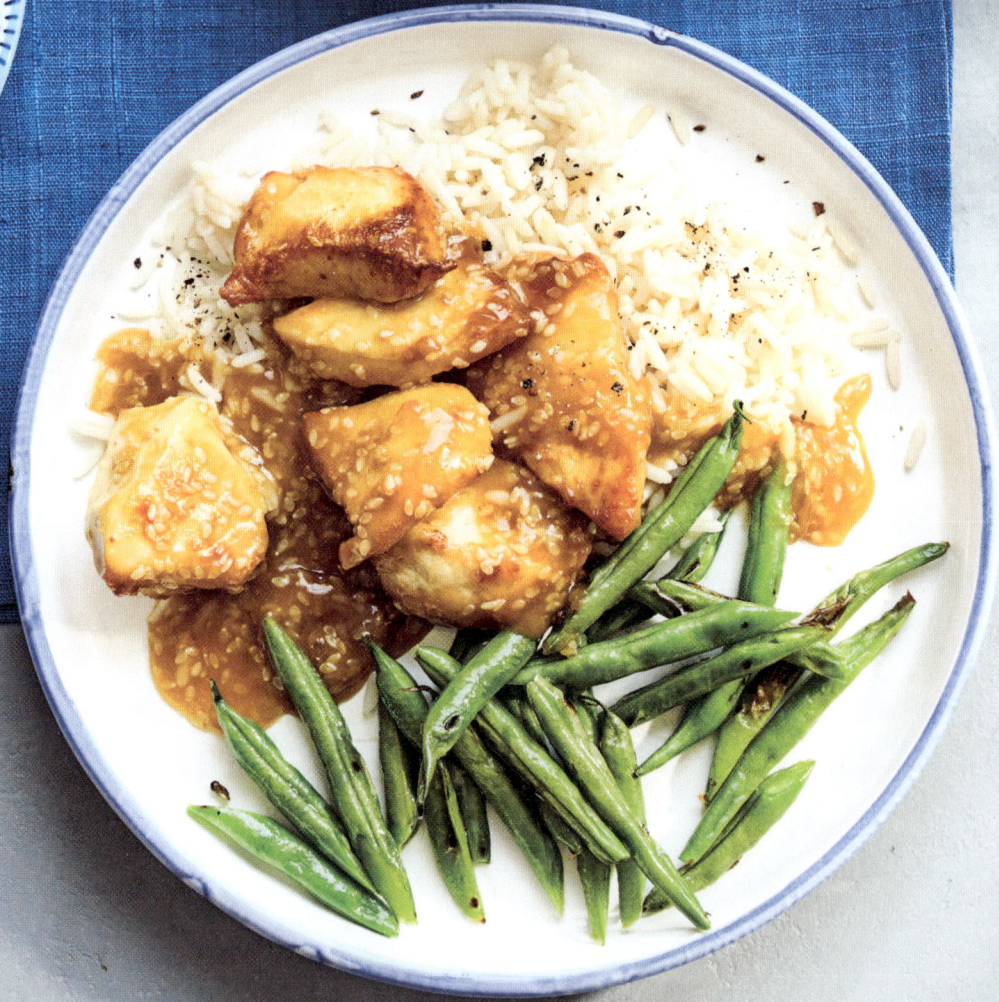

CRISPY LEMON SESAME CHICKEN WITH RICE & FRIED GREEN BEANS

SERVES 4
PREP TIME 10 minutes
COOK TIME 20 minutes

4 skinless chicken breasts, cut into chunks

2 tablespoons cornflour

spray oil

250g (9oz) long grain rice, or basmati rice

200g (7oz) fine green beans, topped and tailed

FOR THE SAUCE

finely grated zest and juice of 2 lemons

2 teaspoons cornflour

2 tablespoons honey

2 tablespoons light soy sauce

2 teaspoons sesame seeds

1 teaspoon sesame oil

NOTE

For a vegetarian version, try using tofu instead of chicken, chopped into chunks. Mix it with the cornflour, place on a baking tray lined with nonstick baking paper, spray with oil, and bake for 25–30 minutes until it is crispy on the outside and soft in the middle.

A simple flavour combination of lemon, honey and sesame brings this dish together and this has been a big hit with my kids. With a takeaway vibe to it, crisping the chicken in cornflour before mixing into the zingy sauce makes this a total all-round winner. I serve it simply with rice and whatever green vegetables we have in, or are in season, I've suggested fine green beans here, but this also works well with broccoli, asparagus, mangetout, courgette, peas, sweetcorn, carrots or whatever you fancy really!

1 Preheat the oven to 220°C/200°C fan (425°F), Gas Mark 7.

2 In a bowl, combine the chicken breast chunks with the cornflour and mix well.

3 Line a large baking tray with nonstick baking paper, spray it lightly with oil, then lay out the chicken pieces, ensuring they are not touching each other. Spray the chicken with oil.

4 Bake for 20 minutes, by which time the chicken will have cooked through, gained a golden colour and crisped up on the outside.

5 Meanwhile, make the sauce. To start with, put the lemon juice and cornflour into a small saucepan and mix until the cornflour dissolves and there are no lumps remaining. Add the rest of the sauce ingredients and cook over a medium heat for about 5 minutes, stirring constantly, until you have a thick and glossy sauce. Remove this from the heat until the chicken is ready.

6 Cook the rice according to the packet instructions. When there are 5 minutes before the chicken is ready, spray a frying pan with oil, add the green beans and stir-fry over a high heat for 5 minutes to get some slight charring on them.

7 When the chicken is cooked, put it into a clean bowl and pour over the hot lemon sauce. (If the sauce has cooled down, just bubble it for a couple of minutes to reheat.) Mix the chicken and sauce together. Serve the chicken over the rice, with the fried green beans on the side.

PER SERVING

CALORIES	FAT	SAT FAT	CARBS	SUGARS	FIBRE	PROTEIN	SALT
540	5G	1.1G	73G	11G	3.2G	49G	1.3G

PEKING-INSPIRED ROAST CHICKEN

SERVES 6
PREP TIME 5 minutes,
plus marinating
COOK TIME 1 hour 30 minutes,
plus resting

Here I have combined some of the flavours usually used for Peking duck, to add a delicious twist to roast chicken. This can be served in a variety of ways to suit the occasion. For Sunday lunch, I serve it with roast potatoes (it's especially good with Sesame Roast Potatoes, see page 194), roast carrots and seasonal green vegetables – see the note opposite for more ideas.

1 whole chicken (about 1.5kg/
  3lb 5oz)
½ orange, halved

FOR THE MARINADE
2 garlic cloves, crushed
5cm (2 inch) piece of root ginger,
  peeled and finely grated
2 tablespoons rice wine
2 tablespoons dark soy sauce
1 teaspoon Chinese 5 spice
1 tablespoon tomato purée

FOR THE SAUCE
2 tablespoons honey
1 tablespoon dark soy sauce
1 tablespoon rice wine
1 teaspoon sesame oil
juice of ½ orange

1   Make up the marinade by mixing together all the ingredients.

2   Use your fingers to loosen underneath the chicken skin over the breast, from the neck end, then cover the whole chicken in the marinade, including underneath the breast skin. Leave to marinate for at least 1 hour. You can place it in the refrigerator and leave overnight, if you want.

3   Preheat the oven to 200°C/180°C fan (400°F), Gas Mark 6.

4   Make up the sauce by mixing all the ingredients together in a small bowl.

5   Place the chicken into a roasting tin and stuff the cavity with the orange quarters. Cover with foil (try to tent this over the chicken so it does not stick to the skin) and roast for 40 minutes.

6   After 40 minutes, remove the chicken from the oven, take off the foil (reserve it) and pour the sauce over the chicken. Cover with the foil once more and roast for a further 1 hour, or depending on a calculated cooking time-to-weight of 25 minutes per 500g (1lb 2oz) plus 25 minutes. Every 15 minutes, remove the chicken from the oven and baste it all over with the sauce and juices pooling in the bottom of the roasting tin, using a spoon, turkey baster, or silicone pastry brush.

7   Remove the foil for the final 15 minutes of cooking time to allow to skin to crisp up and the sauce to caramelize over the chicken.

8   Check that the chicken is cooked through (I recommend using a meat thermometer in the thickest part of the chicken thigh: it should have reached at least 75°C/167°F). Carefully lift the chicken on to a large warmed platter or carving dish, cover again with the foil and leave to rest for 15 minutes; this keeps the juices in and the meat succulent).

9   You can now carve the chicken to serve straight away, or allow it to cool enough to strip the meat away to use later.

PER SERVING

CALORIES	FAT	SAT FAT	CARBS	SUGARS	FIBRE	PROTEIN	SALT
411	21G	5.6G	12G	12G	0.6G	42G	1.4G

NOTE

More ways to serve this chicken:

With basmati rice and sesame fried fine green beans.

With chilled noodles and crunchy veg, for a tasty salad.

In a stir-fry with mixed vegetables, over rice or noodles.

With lettuce leaves to use as wraps with sliced cucumber and shredded carrots, with sweet chilli sauce.

In fried rice with soy sauce, sesame oil, spring onions and chopped sweet peppers.

As a bao bun filling with sliced cucumbers, spring onions and hoisin sauce.

Added to a ramen broth, with noodles, soft-boiled eggs and mixed vegetables.

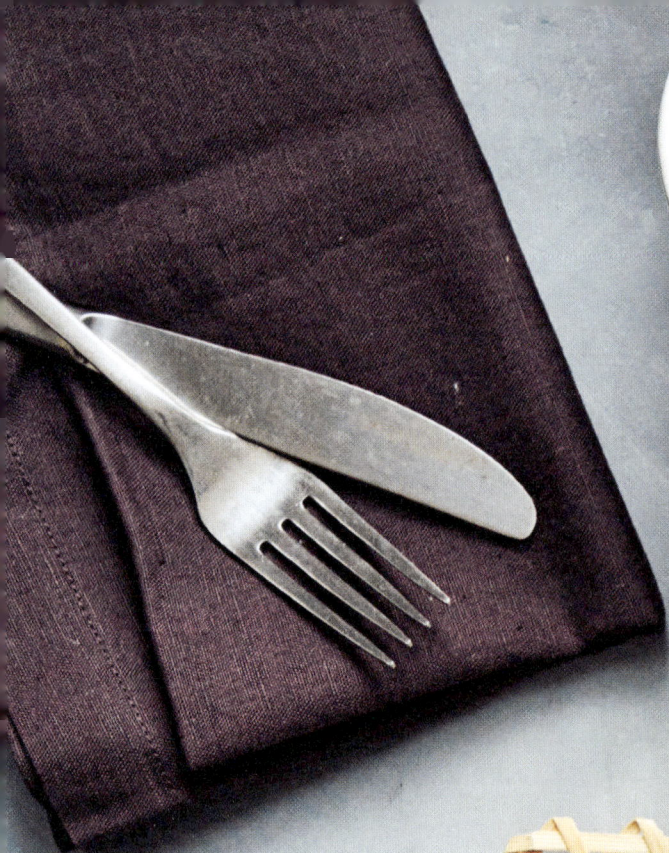

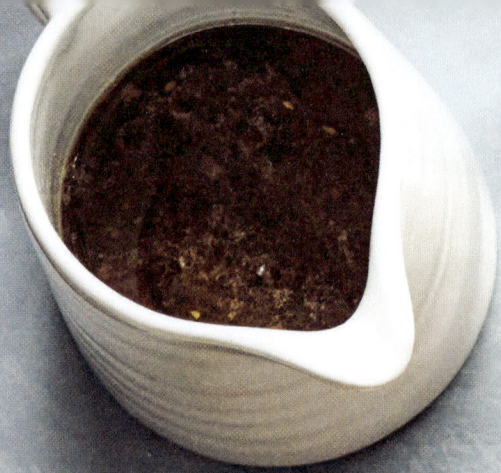

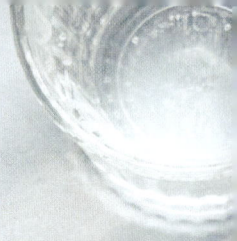

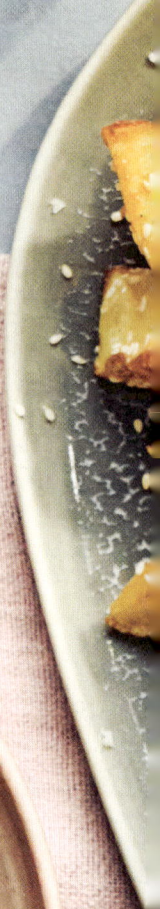

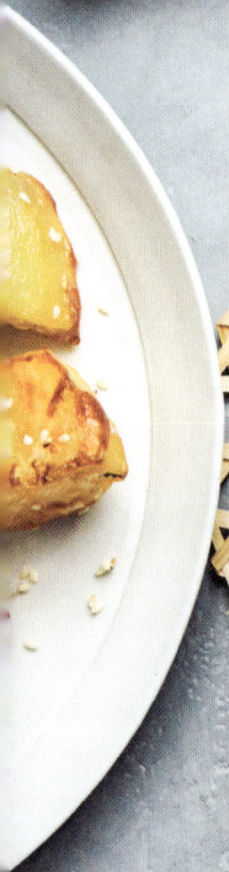

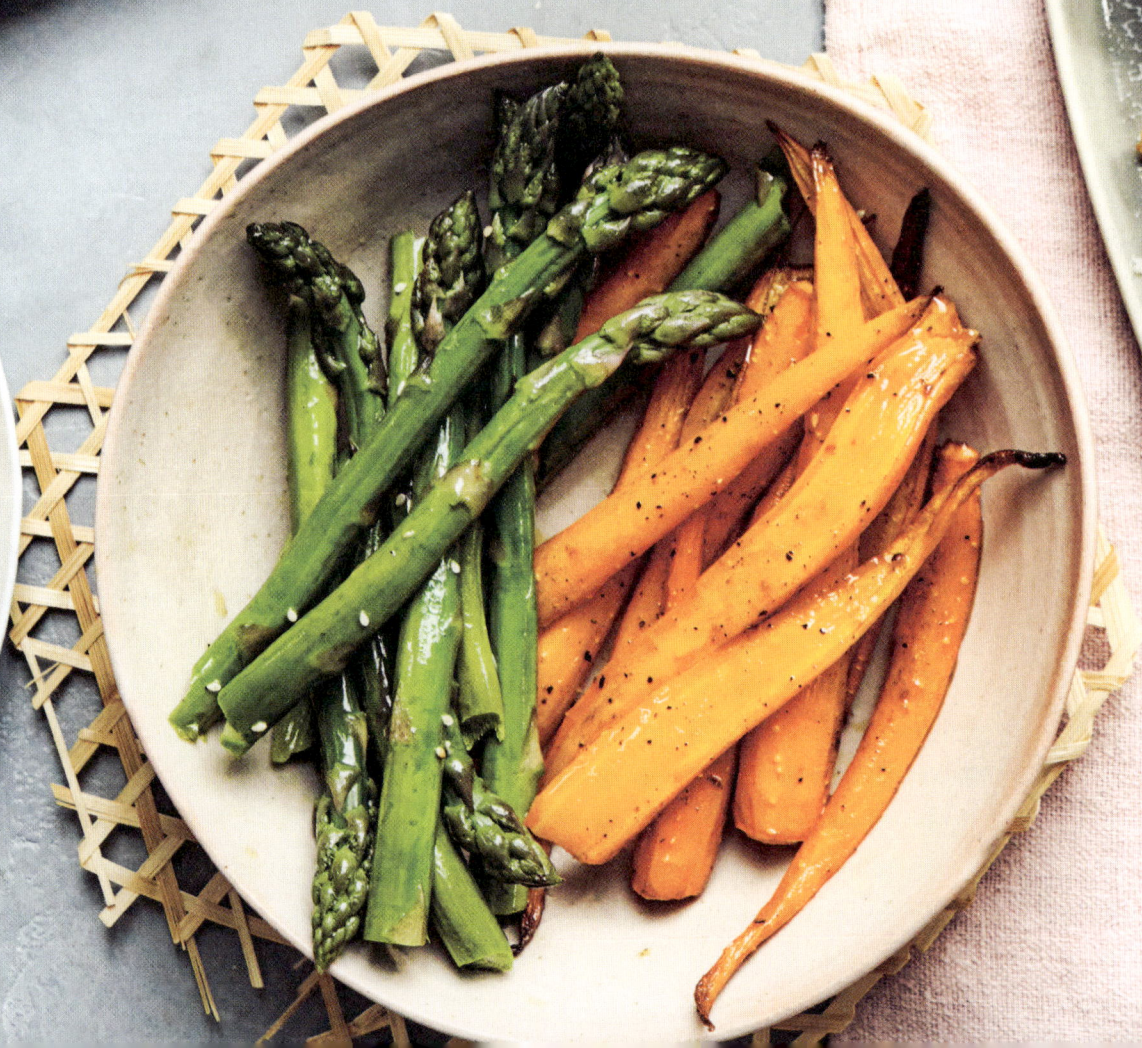

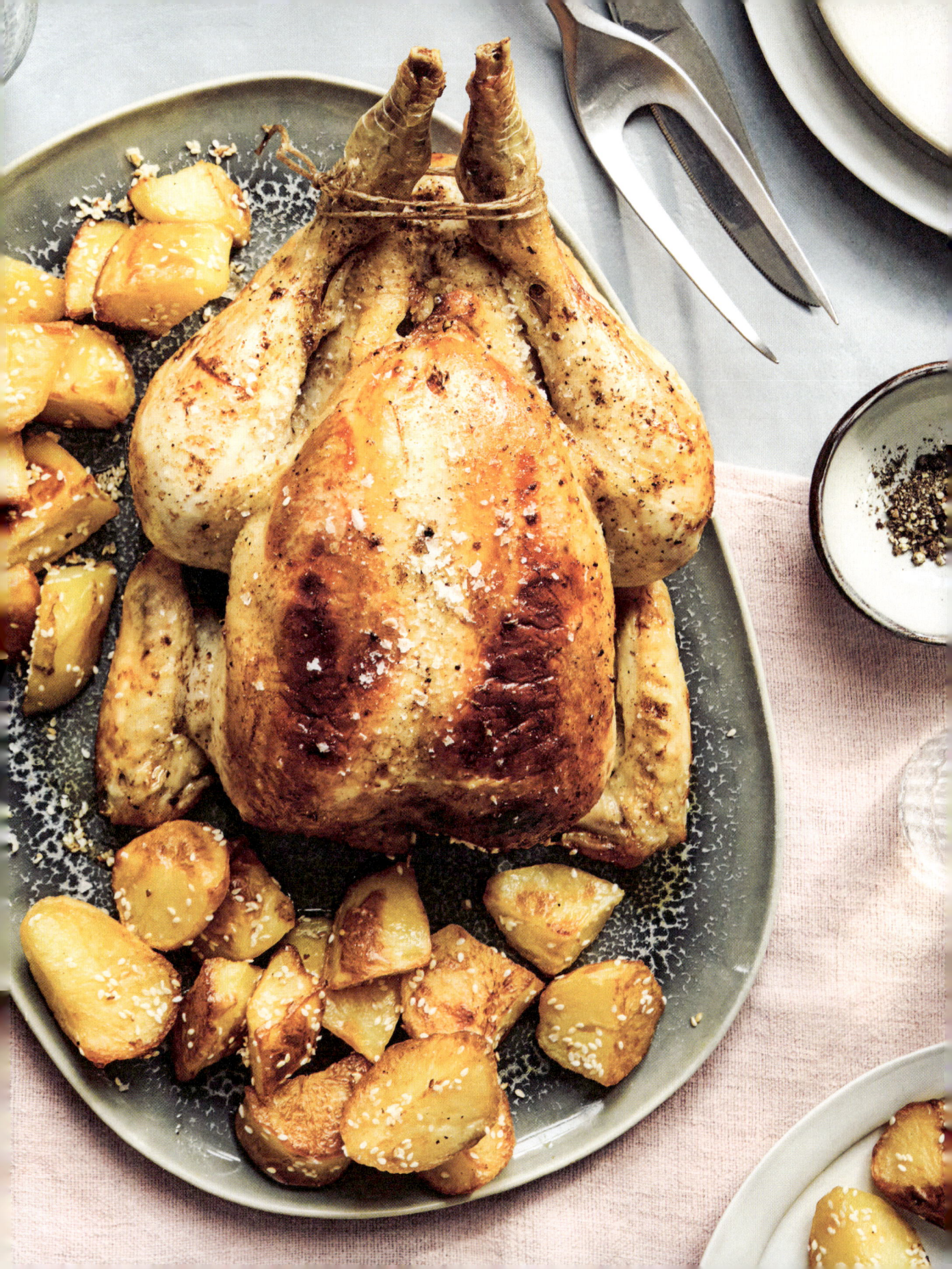

CHICKEN PAD SEE EW

SERVES 4
PREP TIME 10 minutes
COOK TIME 14 minutes

2 skinless chicken breasts (total
  weight about 300g/10½oz), cut
  into strips
1 tablespoon soy sauce
1 teaspoon sesame oil
200g (7oz) dried medium or thick
  flat rice noodles
200g (7oz) Tenderstem broccoli,
  or regular broccoli florets, cut
  into bite-sized pieces
3 eggs, lightly beaten
3 garlic cloves, crushed

FOR THE SAUCE

1 tablespoon soy sauce
1 tablespoon dark soy sauce
1 tablespoon fish sauce
1 tablespoon brown sugar
1 teaspoon sesame oil

TO SERVE (OPTIONAL)

sriracha (or other chilli) sauce
sliced spring onions

My interpretation of a classic Thai dish, which has a simple set of ingredients and is delicious and satisfying to eat, but lacking any chilli heat, which makes it a great family stir-fry. It's always important with a dish like this to have all your ingredients ready in advance, because once you are frying, everything happens quickly! I get all my sauce ingredients together in a little bowl ready to add, rather than measuring them out separately while I am cooking.

1 In a bowl, mix the chicken strips, soy sauce and sesame oil.

2 Mix the sauce ingredients in a small bowl.

3 Cook the rice noodles in a large pan of boiling water for 3 minutes until they are just tender. Immediately drain them in a colander and rinse them thoroughly under the cold tap both to ensure they are fully cooled down and to prevent them from sticking together. Set aside.

4 Put the chicken into a sauté pan or wok over a medium-high heat and stir-fry for 4 minutes. Add the broccoli pieces and stir-fry them for 1 minute.

5 Scoot the chicken and broccoli to one side of the pan, pour the eggs into the empty side and fry for about 2 minutes, breaking them up as they cook so they resemble scrambled eggs.

6 Stir together the egg, chicken and broccoli, stir through the crushed garlic and add the sauce. Stir everything together thoroughly for about a minute.

7 Toss in the cooked noodles, gently breaking them apart to coat them in the sauce, and stir-fry over a medium-high heat for 2–3 minutes while you get them mixed in with the other ingredients and heated back up. I like to serve this with chilli sauce and sliced spring onions.

NOTE

Thick, flat rice noodles are integral to this and aren't always easy to find in the British supermarkets, but you'll have your pick in an Asian supermarket, and will also generally find them in larger mainstream supermarkets.

PER SERVING

CALORIES	FAT	SAT FAT	CARBS	SUGARS	FIBRE	PROTEIN	SALT
399	7.6G	1.8G	44G	5.2G	6.1G	36G	2.1G

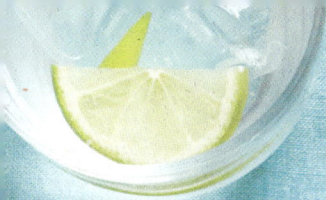

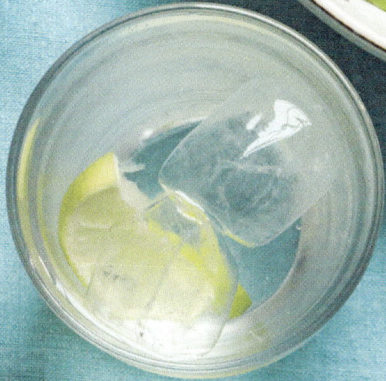

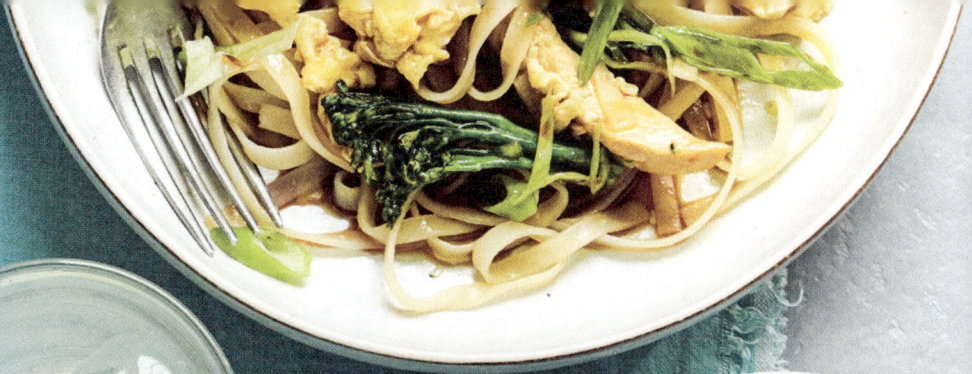

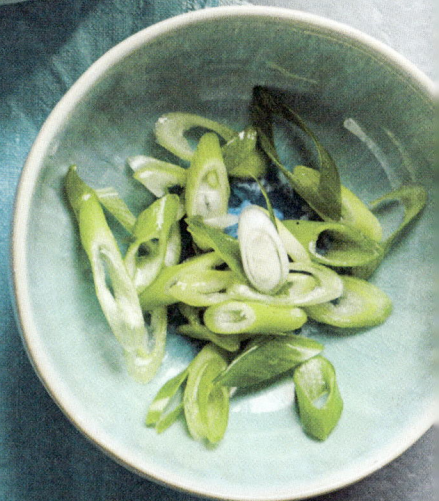

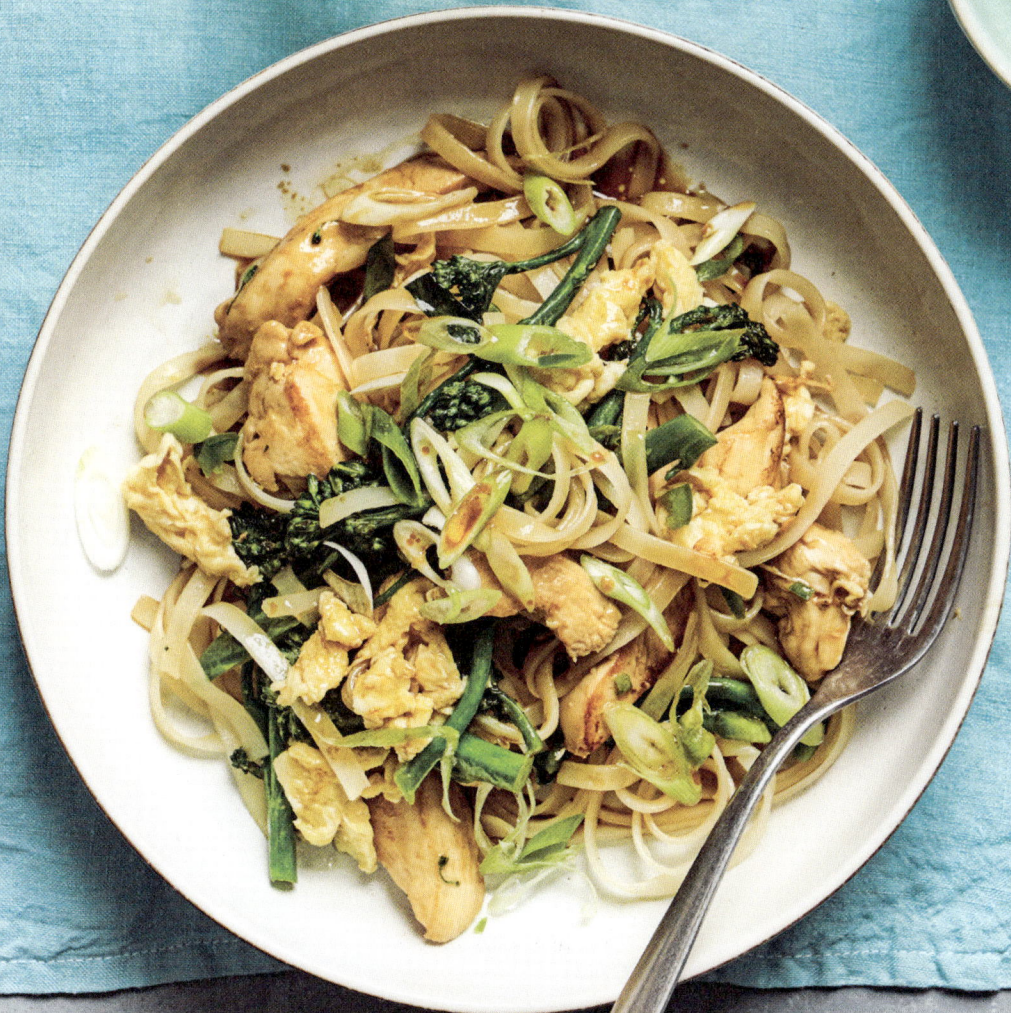

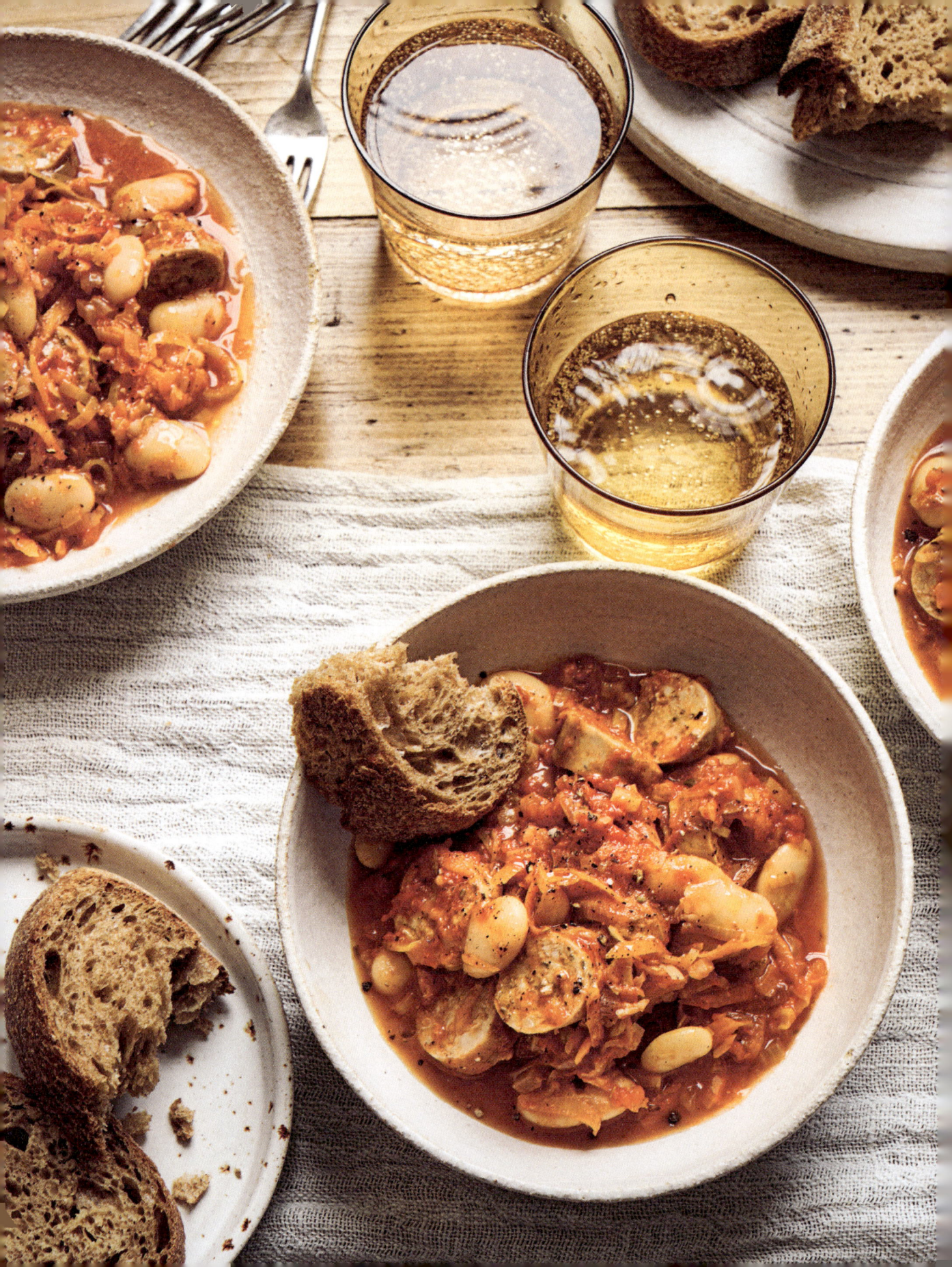

SAUSAGE, ROSEMARY & BUTTER BEAN RAGU

SERVES 4
PREP TIME 10 minutes
COOK TIME 42 minutes

spray oil

8 light (reduced-fat) sausages

1 red onion, finely chopped

1 leek, trimmed, cleaned and finely chopped (see page 197)

2 garlic cloves, crushed

2 tablespoons dried rosemary, or finely chopped rosemary leaves

400g (14oz) can of chopped tomatoes

250ml (9fl oz) hot chicken stock

1 tablespoon balsamic vinegar

1 teaspoon dried basil

1 teaspoon garlic granules

2 carrots, grated

2 x 400g cans of butter beans, drained and rinsed

salt and pepper

A flavour-filled one-pot with a simple herby taste, this works well for the whole family. The recipe specifies reduced-fat sausages, but you can choose whatever sausages work for your family, whether that's smaller chipolatas or a more hearty Cumberland sausage. This pairs well with slice of fresh crusty bread.

1   Spray a sauté pan or flameproof casserole dish with oil and fry the sausages for 5 minutes over a high heat, to get some good browning on the outsides.

2   Add the onion and leek to the pan and fry over a medium heat for 10 minutes, stirring every now and again.

3   Add the crushed garlic and rosemary and stir-fry for another 2 minutes.

4   Add the chopped tomatoes, hot stock, balsamic vinegar, dried basil, garlic granules and grated carrots to the pan. Simmer gently for 10 minutes.

5   Add the butter beans, season with salt and pepper and simmer gently for a further 15 minutes.

6   Remove the sausages from the pan and slice each into around 8 pieces, then return to the pan. Stir well and serve.

NOTE

If you want to make a vegetarian version, swap the sausages for veggie sausages, cooked according to the packet instructions. Start the recipe from step 2 and add the cooked veggie sausages into the ragu in step 6. You will also need to swap the chicken stock for vegetable stock.

PER SERVING

CALORIES	FAT	SAT FAT	CARBS	SUGARS	FIBRE	PROTEIN	SALT
374	7.9G	2.7G	37G	18G	15G	28G	2G

CHICKEN & CAULIFLOWER PASANDA

SERVES 4
PREP TIME 15 minutes
COOK TIME 27 minutes

spray oil

1 onion, finely chopped

3 skinless chicken breasts (total weight about 450g/1lb), cut into chunks

3 garlic cloves, crushed

2.5cm (1 inch) piece of root ginger, peeled and finely grated

1 teaspoon tomato purée

1 tablespoon garam masala

1 teaspoon ground turmeric

½ teaspoon mild chilli powder

¼ teaspoon ground cinnamon

½ teaspoon salt

25g (1oz) creamed coconut, dissolved in 150ml (¼ pint) boiling water

250g (9oz) fat-free Greek yogurt

2 tablespoons ground almonds

1 small cauliflower, cut into bite-sized florets

TO SERVE (OPTIONAL)

2 tablespoons flaked almonds

300g (10½oz) basmati rice

handful of coriander

If I'm cooking a curry for the whole family, I'll usually opt for a mild, creamy chicken variety... and try to sneak some extra vegetables into the sauce. Pasanda is one of my favourite mild curries, the sauce lightly flavoured by ground almonds for a slightly sweet, nutty flavour, as well as extra creaminess. Serve with fluffy basmati rice and mini naans on the side, if you wish, though note this will increase the calories.

1   Spray a sauté pan or shallow flameproof casserole dish, which has a lid, with oil and fry the onion for 5 minutes.

2   Add the chicken pieces and stir-fry for a further 3 minutes to seal (which means when you can see no traces of pink on the outside).

3   Add the garlic, ginger, tomato purée, spices and salt to the pan and stir-fry everything over a medium heat for 2 minutes.

4   Pour in the creamed coconut, dissolved in its measured boiling water, then stir in the yogurt and ground almonds. Simmer for 10 minutes.

5   Meanwhile, put the flaked almonds in a dry frying pan and fry them for a few minutes until golden-brown and fragrant, then set aside.

6   Cook the rice according to the packet instructions.

7   Add the cauliflower florets to the curry, stir them through, pop on the lid and simmer for 5–7 minutes, until the cauliflower is tender but not overcooked. Serve over the rice, scattered with the toasted almonds and coriander.

NOTE

Creamed coconut comes as a solid bar and is formed from finely ground coconut flesh. It's fantastic for curries, because you can just take however much you like from the bar to get the flavour and texture you want. Sometimes I find it more useful than canned coconut milk, if I just want a little coconut flavour and creaminess without adding the whole can.

PER SERVING

CALORIES	FAT	SAT FAT	CARBS	SUGARS	FIBRE	PROTEIN	SALT
394	14G	4.2G	19G	10G	5.8G	46G	1G

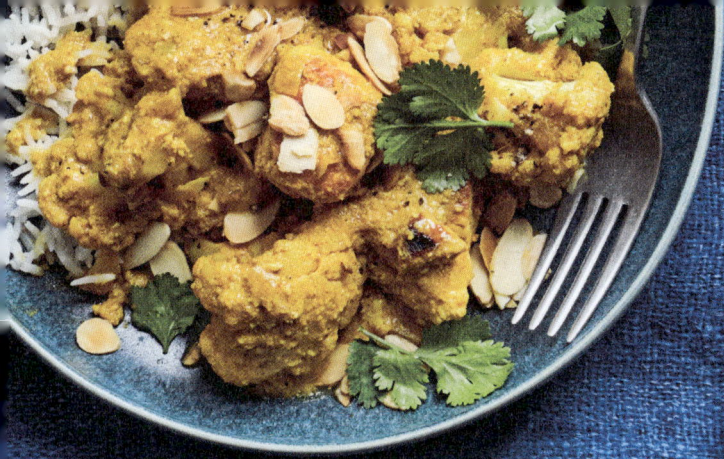

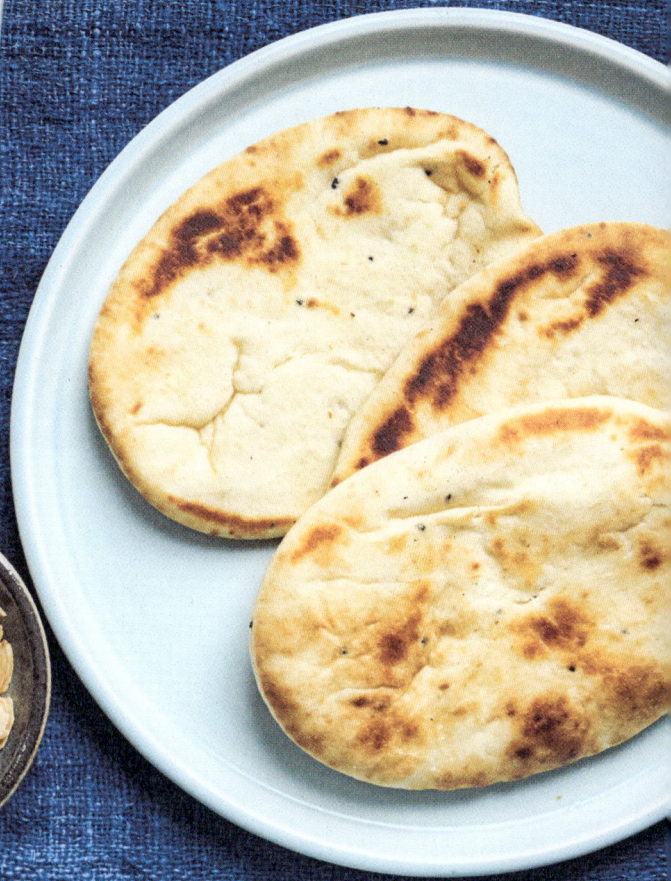

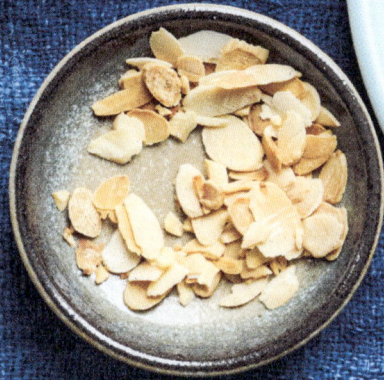

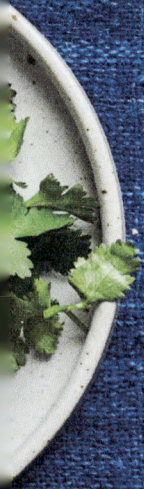

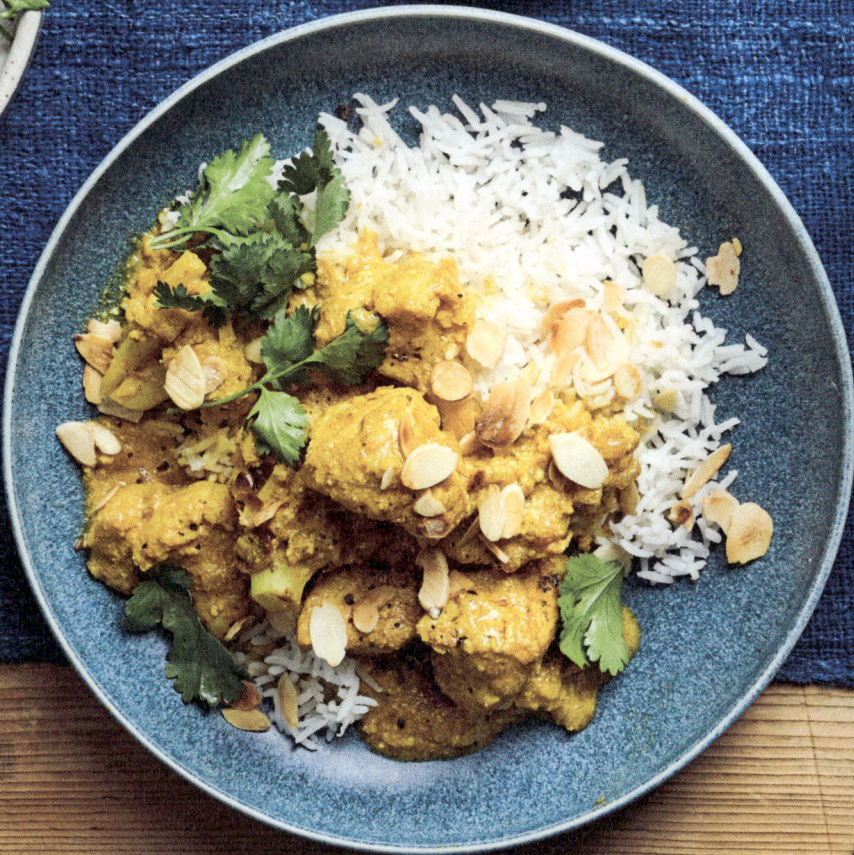

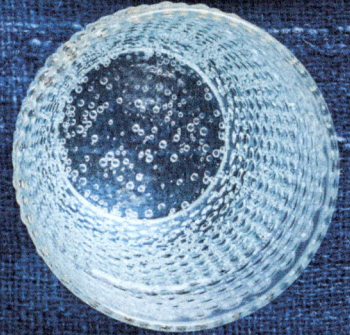

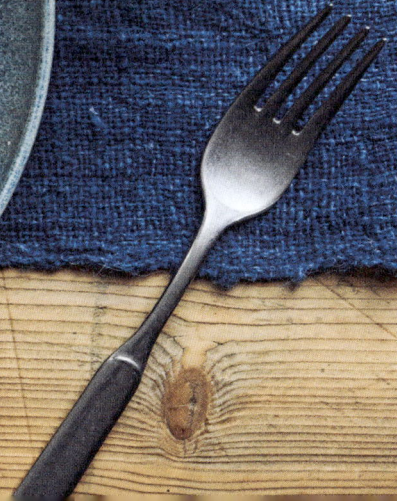

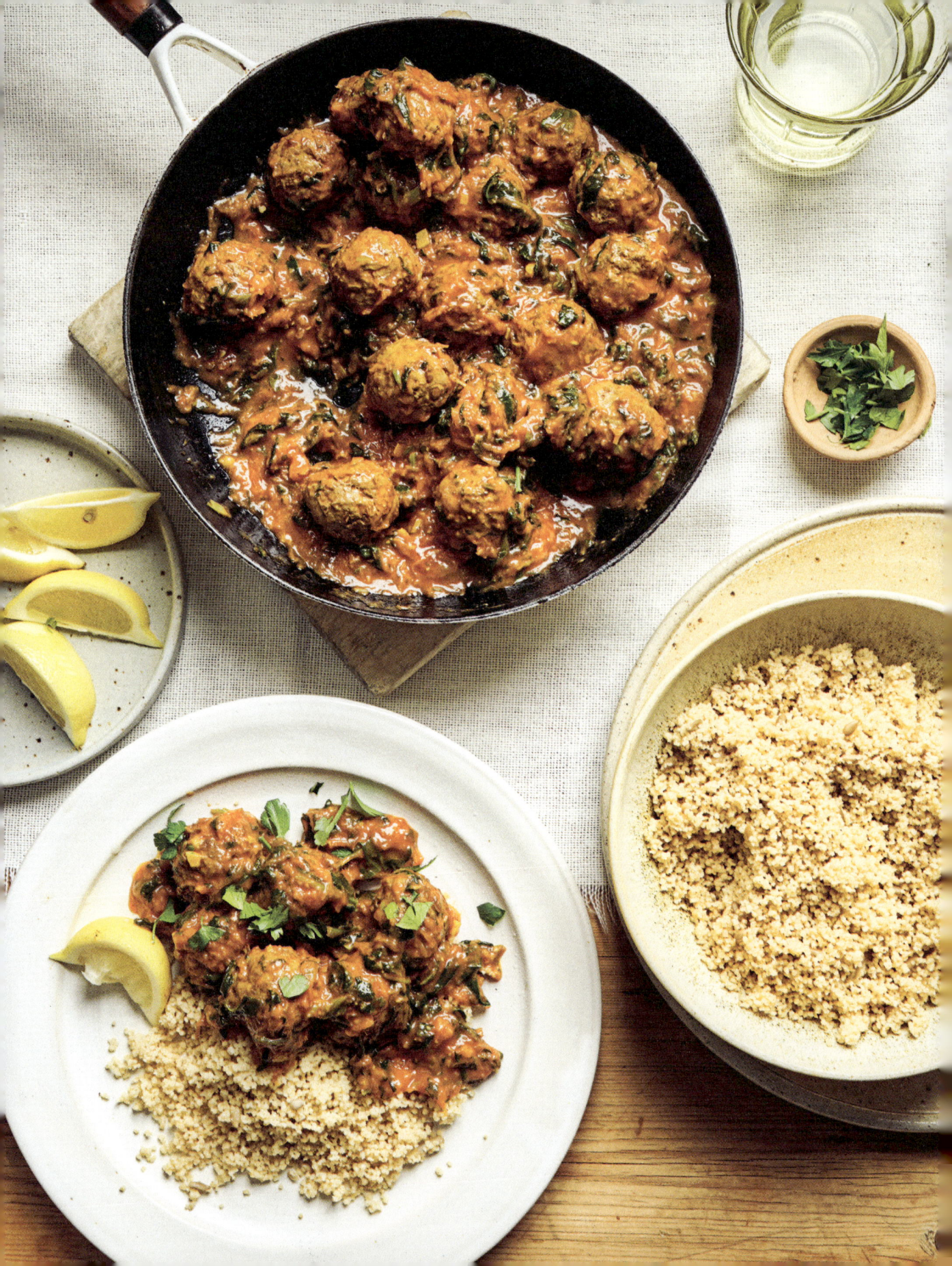

CHERMOULA MEATBALLS WITH COUSCOUS

SERVES 4
PREP TIME 20 minutes
COOK TIME 15 minutes

A great way to get kids to try some new flavours, in the familiar form of a meatball. Adding lentils gives these both filling-power and more nutritional content, plus it makes the meat stretch further. Serve this up with your family's favourite green vegetables.

FOR THE MEATBALLS

500g (1lb 2oz) lean minced beef (less than 5 per cent fat)
400g (14oz) can of green lentils, drained and rinsed
1 garlic clove, crushed
1 tablespoon Chermoula Spice Blend (see page 205)
½ teaspoon coarse salt

FOR THE SAUCE

spray oil
1 garlic clove, crushed
1 tablespoon Chermoula Spice Blend (see page 205)
2 carrots, grated
500g (1lb 2oz) tomato passata
1 tablespoon honey
1 beef stock cube
100g (3½oz) frozen spinach
salt and pepper

FOR THE COUSCOUS

250g (9oz) wholewheat couscous
3 tablespoons sunflower seeds

TO SERVE

handful of chopped parsley leaves
1 lemon, cut into wedges

1 Preheat the oven to 220°C/200°C fan (425°F), Gas Mark 7.

2 To make the meatballs, mix all the ingredients in a bowl, using your hands to bring everything together and mash in the lentils a little bit.

3 Line a large baking tray with nonstick baking paper and shape the meatballs: I make around 24 from this mixture, each about 3cm (1¼ inch) in diameter, and place them on the prepared tray.

4 Bake the meatballs for 15 minutes.

5 Meanwhile, make the sauce. Spray a frying pan with oil and fry the garlic, chermoula and grated carrots together for 2 minutes. Add the passata and honey, then crumble in the beef stock cube. Simmer for 10 minutes.

6 Add the spinach to the sauce to defrost and, when it has, add the meatballs, too. Season with salt and pepper

7 Prepare the couscous according to the packet instructions, and, once it is ready, stir through the sunflower seeds. Divide the couscous between 4 warmed bowls, top with the meatballs and sauce, scatter with parsley and serve with lemon wedges on the side.

NOTE

Chermoula is a North African spice blend of herbs, spices and seasonings. You can find it in many UK supermarkets, but if not, it's very easy to make your own (see page 205). It has a great combination of flavours and can be used as a marinade, rub or in a sauce.

PER SERVING

CALORIES	FAT	SAT FAT	CARBS	SUGARS	FIBRE	PROTEIN	SALT
593	12G	3.6G	67G	17G	15G	44G	1.6G

CAJUN-STYLE CHICKEN BURGER WITH SWEETCORN SALSA & CHIPS

SERVES 4
PREP TIME 25 minutes
COOK TIME 40 minutes

900g (2lb) Maris Piper potatoes, peeled and cut into 1cm (½ inch) thick chips

spray oil

1 tablespoon Cajun seasoning

2 skinless chicken breasts, halved crossways through the middle to create 2 equal halves

1 egg

50g (1¾oz) breadcrumbs

1 onion, finely chopped

300g (10½oz) can of sweetcorn, drained

4 brioche burger buns (or see recipe introduction)

4 slices of burger cheese (optional)

salt and pepper

NOTE

For a tasty burger sauce, mix 4 tablespoons fat-free Greek yogurt with 2 tablespoons tomato ketchup, 1 tablespoon Dijon mustard, 1 teaspoon honey, 1 teaspoon apple cider vinegar and ½ teaspoon each of garlic and onion granules. Season with salt and pepper and add a dash of hot sauce, if you fancy. Chill for 30 minutes before serving.

A chicken burger always goes down well in my family and this crispy, lightly spiced coating is one of our favourite versions. We enjoy this burger in brioche buns, but you can choose a wholemeal roll for a healthier option.

1   Preheat the oven to 220°C/200°C fan (425°F), Gas Mark 7. Put the chips into a large saucepan of water, then bring to the boil and simmer for 3 minutes. Drain and leave in a colander for a few minutes to dry out.

2   Line a large baking tray with nonstick baking paper and spray with oil. Spread the chips out on one tray in an even layer and spray generously with oil.

3   Sprinkle the Cajun seasoning over the chicken, and season with salt and pepper.

4   Lightly beat the egg in a bowl and put the breadcrumbs in another bowl (I use shallow pasta bowls, because they give you space to dip the chicken). Season the breadcrumbs with salt and pepper.

5   Dip the seasoned chicken breasts first into the egg, then into the breadcrumbs, making sure to cover all sides. Lay on the prepared tray. Spray them well with oil.

6   Bake the chips and chicken for 25 minutes. Halfway through cooking, turn the chips to allow them to brown on both sides, and remove the chicken from the oven. Bake the chips for another 5–10 minutes until golden and crisp on the outside and fluffy on the inside.

7   Meanwhile, prepare the sweetcorn salsa. Spray a frying pan with oil and fry the onion gently for about 10 minutes, then add the sweetcorn. Fry for another 5 minutes.

8   Cut the burger buns in half, and lightly toast them by putting them in the oven for a couple of minutes. Make up the burgers with the cheese slices (if using), chicken and burger sauce, if you fancy (see note), then serve alongside the chips and sweetcorn salsa.

PER SERVING (WITHOUT CHEESE OR BURGER SAUCE)

CALORIES	FAT	SAT FAT	CARBS	SUGARS	FIBRE	PROTEIN	SALT
533	7.2G	1.7G	78.7G	9.5G	9.1G	33.7G	0.93G

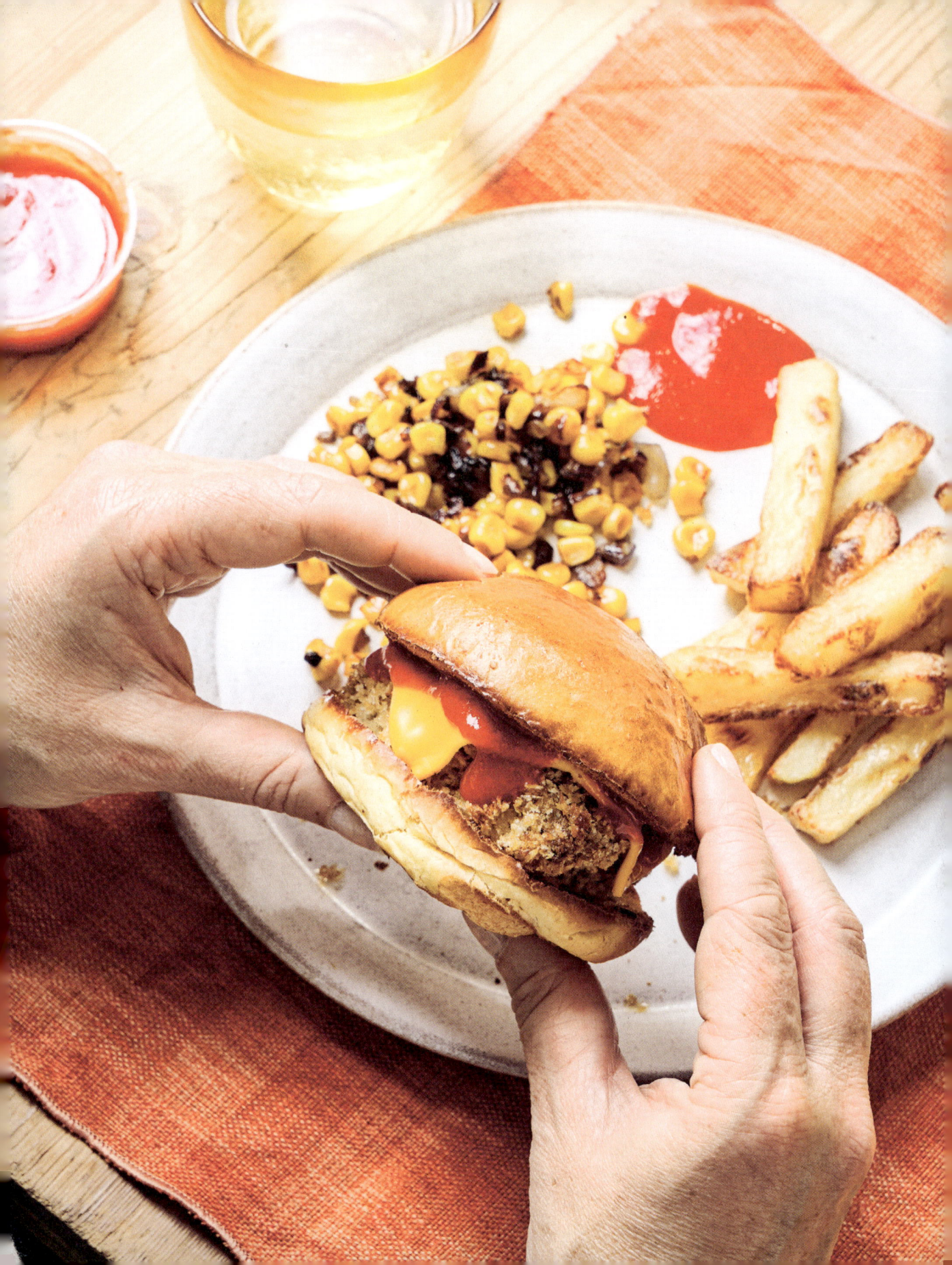

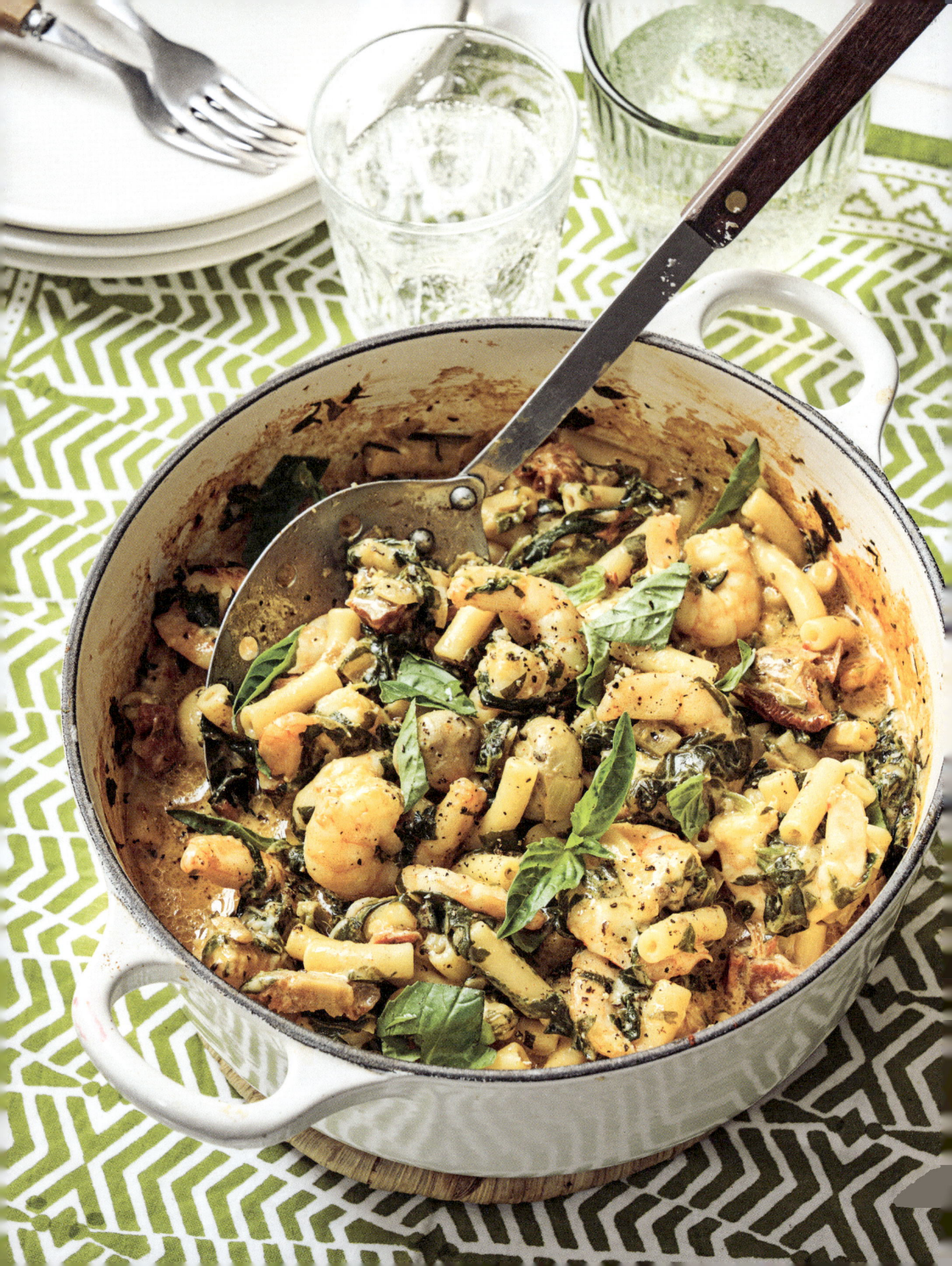

MARRY ME MACARONI

SERVES 4
PREP TIME 10 minutes
COOK TIME 30 minutes

spray oil

1 onion, finely chopped

3 garlic cloves, crushed

100g (3½oz) sundried tomatoes, drained of oil and patted with kitchen paper, then finely chopped

200g (7oz) baby button mushrooms

1 tablespoon tomato purée

2 teaspoons sweet (unsmoked) paprika

1 teaspoon dried oregano

600ml (20fl oz) hot chicken stock

250g (9oz) macaroni

100g (3½oz) frozen spinach, or 2 large handfuls of fresh baby spinach

360g (12½oz) raw king prawns

150g (5½oz) light (reduced-fat) cream cheese

30g (1oz) Parmesan cheese, finely grated

small handful of basil leaves, shredded

salt and pepper

1 lemon, cut into 4 wedges, to serve

You may have seen the 'marry-me chicken' recipe which went viral on social media. It was chicken cooked in a very creamy sauce with paprika, sundried tomatoes and basil. This is my own lighter version, with prawns and macaroni – a delicious combination.

1 Spray a deep pan which has a lid – ideally a flameproof casserole dish – with oil and fry the onion for 5 minutes (you will need a pan deep enough to hold all the pasta). Add the garlic, sundried tomatoes and mushrooms. Stir-fry for 2 minutes.

2 Add the tomato purée, paprika and oregano and stir-fry for 1 more minute. Pour in the hot stock, tip in the macaroni and simmer for 15 minutes, covered, stirring every few minutes.

3 Now add the spinach, put the lid back on and simmer for another 5 minutes. Check the macaroni is cooked (if it isn't, simmer for a minute or two longer, adding a splash of hot water if it is drying out).

4 Meanwhile, spray a frying pan with oil and fry the prawns over a high heat for 2–3 minutes until fully pink. Set aside.

5 Once the macaroni is fully cooked, add the cream cheese, Parmesan and prawns and season with salt and pepper. Stir thoroughly to combine. Scatter with the basil and serve with a lemon wedge on the side.

NOTE

Make this vegetarian by omitting the prawns and swapping the Parmesan for a Parmesan-style vegetarian cheese. You could also add:

In step 1 Chopped sweet peppers, sliced or chopped courgettes or cherry tomatoes, halved or quartered.

In step 3 Asparagus spears cut into bite-sized pieces, or broccoli or cauliflower florets.

In step 4 Carrots, grated or finely chopped, or fresh or frozen peas.

PER SERVING

CALORIES	FAT	SAT FAT	CARBS	SUGARS	FIBRE	PROTEIN	SALT
593	12G	3.6G	67G	17G	15G	44G	1.6G

WARM & SNUG

5

CHRISTMAS GRANOLA

MAKES 8
PREP TIME 5 minutes
COOK TIME 15 minutes

160g (5¾oz) porridge oats
40g (1½oz) flaked almonds
2 tablespoons pumpkin seeds
2 tablespoons sunflower seeds
finely grated zest of 1 large orange
½ teaspoon ground cinnamon
¼ teaspoon coarse salt
1 egg, lightly beaten
2 tablespoons honey
30g (1oz) dried cranberries

I eat granola for breakfast nearly every day, as a topping for Greek yogurt and fruit rather than the main component of my bowl. I find the extra crunch, flavour and touch of sweetness from the granola really makes the yogurt and fruit enjoyable and filling. This recipe has the deliberately festive flavours of orange, cinnamon and cranberry, but can equally be enjoyed at any time of year!

1   Preheat the oven to 200°C/180°C fan (400°F), Gas Mark 6.

2   In a bowl, mix the oats, almonds, pumpkin seeds, sunflower seeds, orange zest, cinnamon and salt.

3   Add the egg and the honey and stir thoroughly to make sure that everything is well combined.

4   Spread over a baking tray to create a thin layer, then bake for 15 minutes, using a wooden spoon to stir it halfway through cooking to break it up and try to stop it from clumping too much, as well as to help everything become evenly toasted.

5   Take out of the oven, give it another good stir, breaking up any large chunks, then add the cranberries. Leave it on the tray to completely cool.

6   Once fully cooled, transfer to an airtight container. This will keep for up to 3 weeks.

NOTE

There are a load of ways you can customize this to your own tastes:

Nuts and seeds Add chopped walnuts, pecans, pistachios, cashews, hazelnuts, peanuts, chia seeds, flaxseeds and linseeds.

Dried fruit In addition to – or instead of – cranberries, you can add raisins, chopped apricots, dates or dried cherries.

Spices Add a pinch of ground nutmeg, ground ginger or ground cardamom.

Sweeteners You can substitute honey for maple syrup, agave nectar or brown rice syrup, adjusting the quantity to taste.

Other flavours Add 1 tablespoon peanut or almond butter, 1 teaspoon vanilla extract, or a handful of dark chocolate chips or chunks. If you mix in the chocolate while the granola is still slightly warm, it will melt slightly and create satisfying chocolate clusters.

PER SERVING

CALORIES	FAT	SAT FAT	CARBS	SUGARS	FIBRE	PROTEIN	SALT
181	8.3G	1G	19G	5.8G	3.4G	5.8G	0.19G

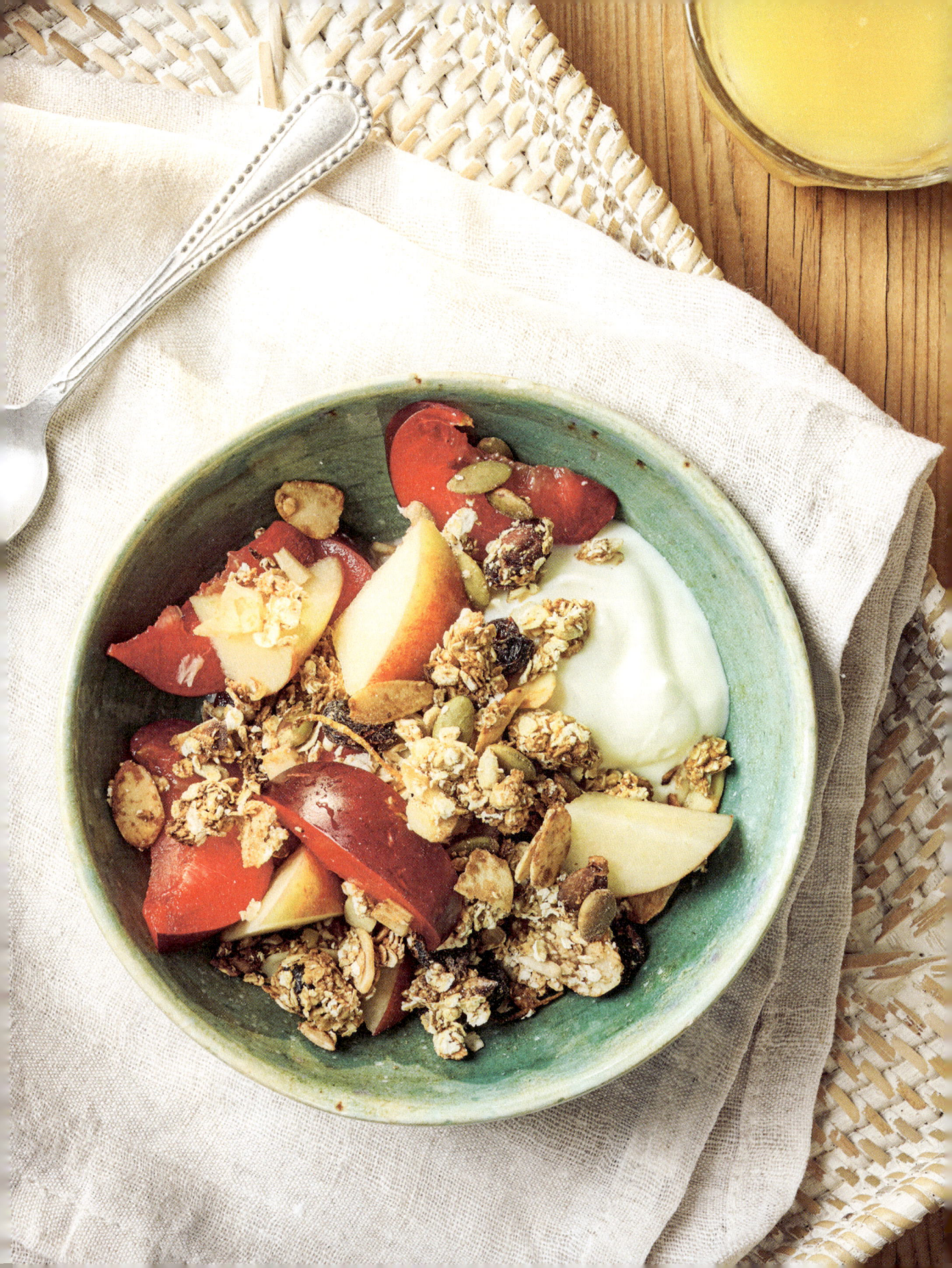

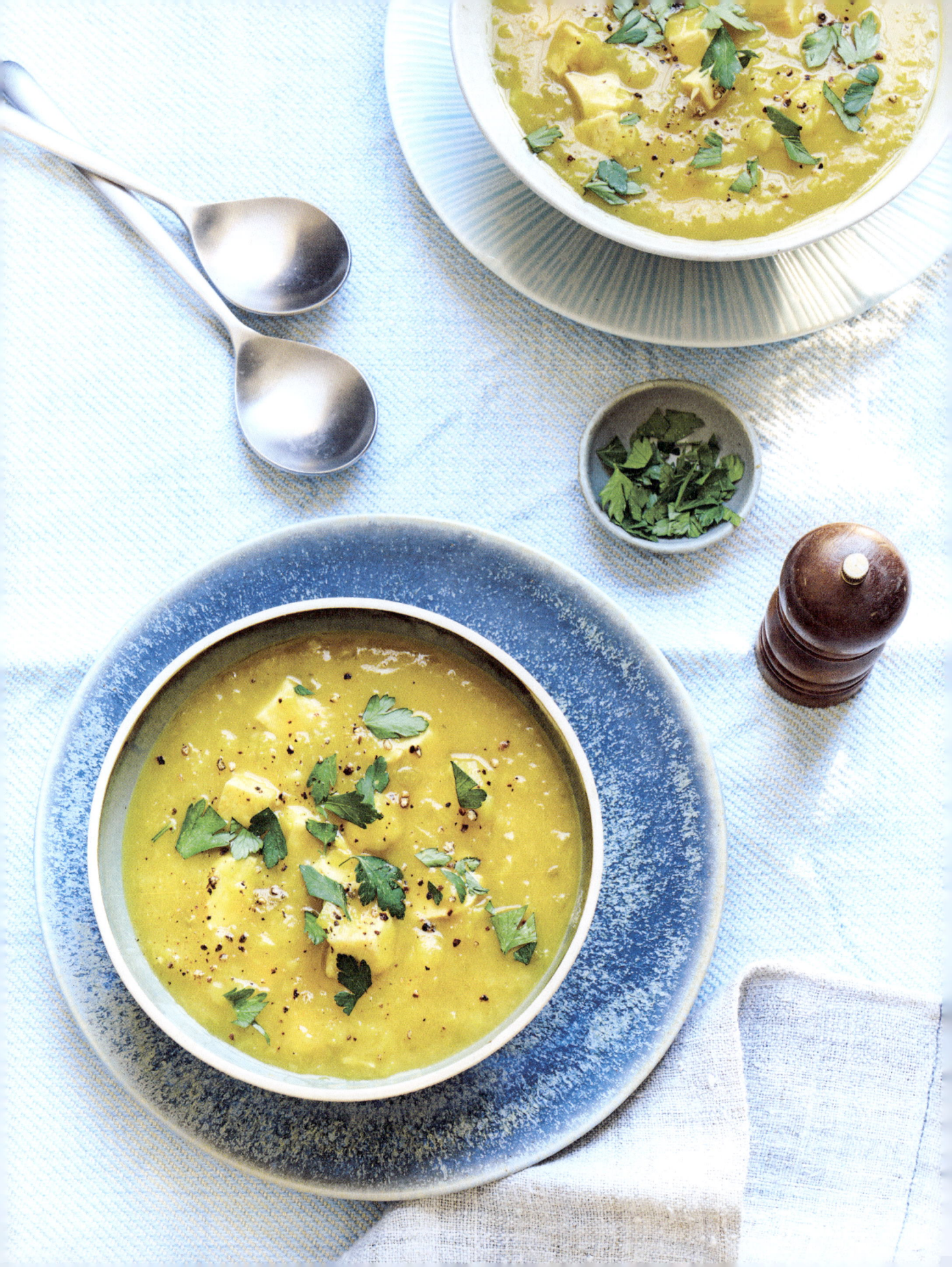

WINTERTIME BLUES-BUSTING CURRIED CHICKEN & LEEK SOUP

SERVES 2
PREP TIME 10 minutes
COOK TIME 26 minutes

2 teaspoons (10g/¼ oz) butter

1 skinless chicken breast

1 onion, finely chopped

2 leeks, trimmed, cleaned and sliced (see page 197)

2 celery sticks, finely chopped

1 teaspoon curry powder

¼ teaspoon ground turmeric

1 litre (1¾ pints) hot chicken stock

2 potatoes (total weight around 300g/10½oz), peeled and chopped into dice-sized cubes

small handful of parsley leaves

salt and pepper

I probably spend more time than I should trying to pinpoint the ultimate comfort soup! I really believe that soup is the best medicine when you are feeling under the weather with the usual winter sore throats, sniffles, coughs and colds. This soup is designed to be a bowl full of comfort for those times, or just when you're in need of warming nourishment on a chilly day. Gentle, warming spices and a nourishing, filling chicken broth certainly hit the spot for me.

1   Melt the butter in a large saucepan over a medium heat. Add the chicken breast, onion, leeks and celery and fry for 10 minutes, stirring and turning the chicken breast occasionally.

2   Add the curry powder and turmeric and stir-fry for 1 minute.

3   Pour in the hot stock, add the potatoes and simmer for 15 minutes, until the potatoes are tender.

4   Remove the chicken breast from the pan, then use a stick blender to blend the soup until it is your desired consistency (smooth, or slightly chunky). Add the parsley.

5   Chop up the chicken breast, then return it to the soup and season with salt and pepper. Serve in warmed bowls.

NOTE

Add sliced carrots or finely chopped sweet potato or butternut squash at the same time as the potatoes, to increase the vegetable content of this soup, or throw in a couple of handfuls of baby spinach before blending, for an extra vitamin boost.

PER SERVING

CALORIES	FAT	SAT FAT	CARBS	SUGARS	FIBRE	PROTEIN	SALT
412	6.8G	3.5G	38G	15G	15G	12G	1.8G

CHILLI GNOCCHI CAULIFLOWER CHEESE

SERVES 4
PREP TIME 10 minutes
COOK TIME 34 minutes

spray oil

1 red chilli, deseeded and finely chopped

1 garlic clove, crushed

2 tablespoons gochujang

500ml (18fl oz) semi-skimmed milk

250ml (9fl oz) hot vegetable stock

500g (1lb 2oz) gnocchi

100g (3½oz) light (reduced-fat) cream cheese

1 cauliflower (about 400g/14oz), cut into bite-sized florets

120g (4¼oz) mature Cheddar cheese

salt and pepper

handful of chopped parsley leaves, to serve

Indulgent-tasting comfort food at its best. A deep warmth from the gochujang harmonizes with a silky, cheesy sauce, tender cauliflower and chewy, satisfying gnocchi to make a perfect winter warmer! Serve this up with extra green vegetables on the side.

1 Preheat the oven to 220°C/200°C fan (425°F), Gas Mark 7.

2 Spray a deep, flameproof casserole dish with oil and fry the chilli and garlic for 1 minute, then stir through the gochujang and fry gently for about 30 seconds.

3 Pour in the milk and hot stock and stir everything together, then bring to a simmer.

4 Tip in the gnocchi, simmer for 2 minutes, then add the cream cheese and simmer gently for 5 more minutes, stirring. Add the cauliflower florets and half the Cheddar. Season with salt and pepper and simmer gently for 5 minutes. By this point, the sauce should have thickened up.

5 Remove the pan from the heat, sprinkle over the remaining cheese, then bake in the oven for 20 minutes. You can transfer the mixture to an ovenproof dish at this point if you need to (if your original pan wasn't ovenproof), just add the remaining cheese when the contents of the pan are in the dish.

6 After 20 minutes, the cheese should be melted and bubbling on top and the sauce will be rich and creamy. Serve immediately, scattered with parsley and sprinkled with black pepper.

NOTE

Gochujang is a Korean fermented red pepper paste known for its unique sweet, spicy and umami flavour. Different brands vary in spiciness and depth of flavour. Authentic tubs from Korean supermarkets, some larger mainstream supermarkets and online often taste better than smaller, western market-targeted jars. Its popularity has surged in the UK, making it more accessible. If you can't find it locally, it's readily available online.

PER SERVING

CALORIES	FAT	SAT FAT	CARBS	SUGARS	FIBRE	PROTEIN	SALT
521	17G	10G	64G	13G	7.1G	23G	1.7G

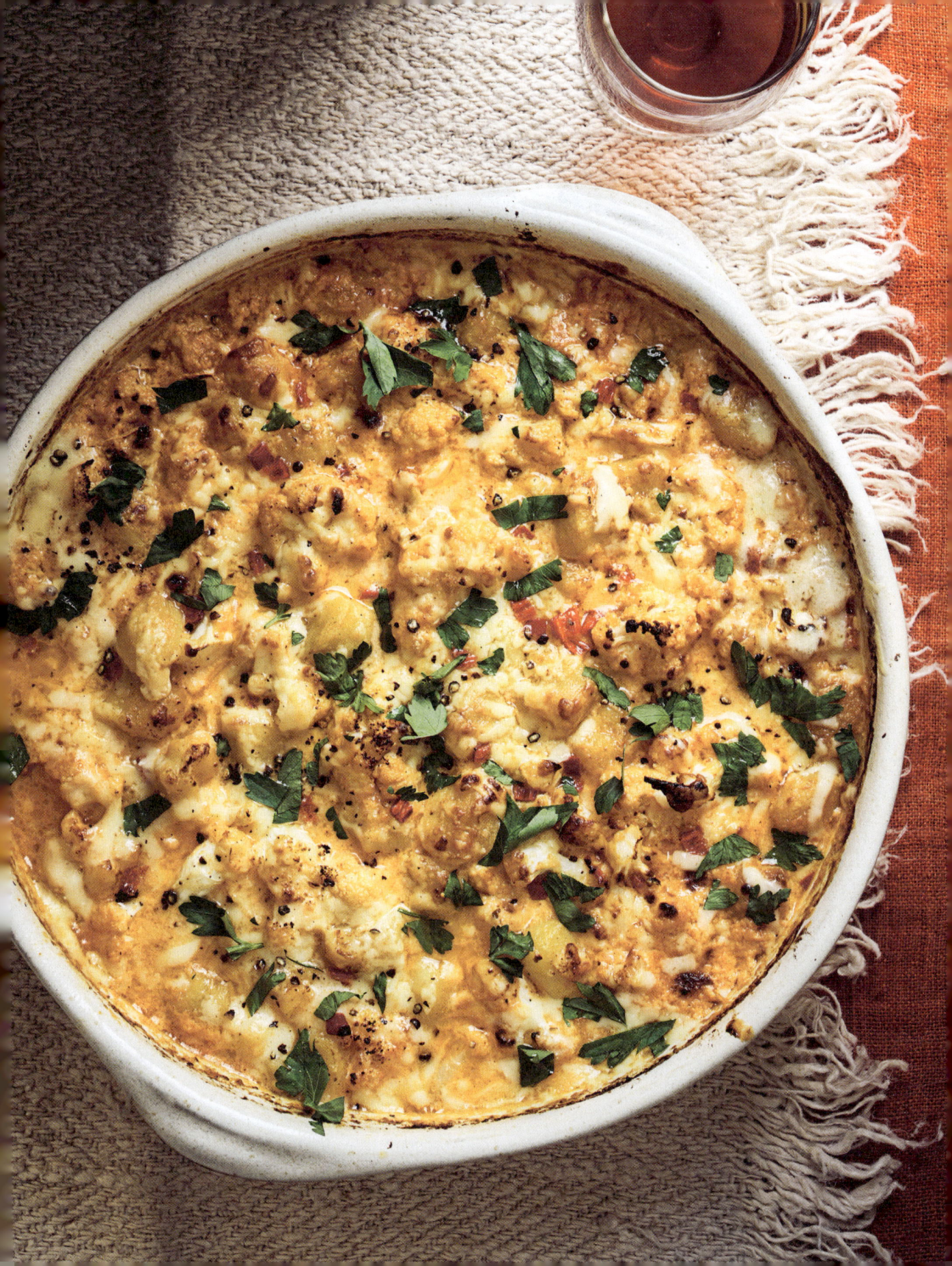

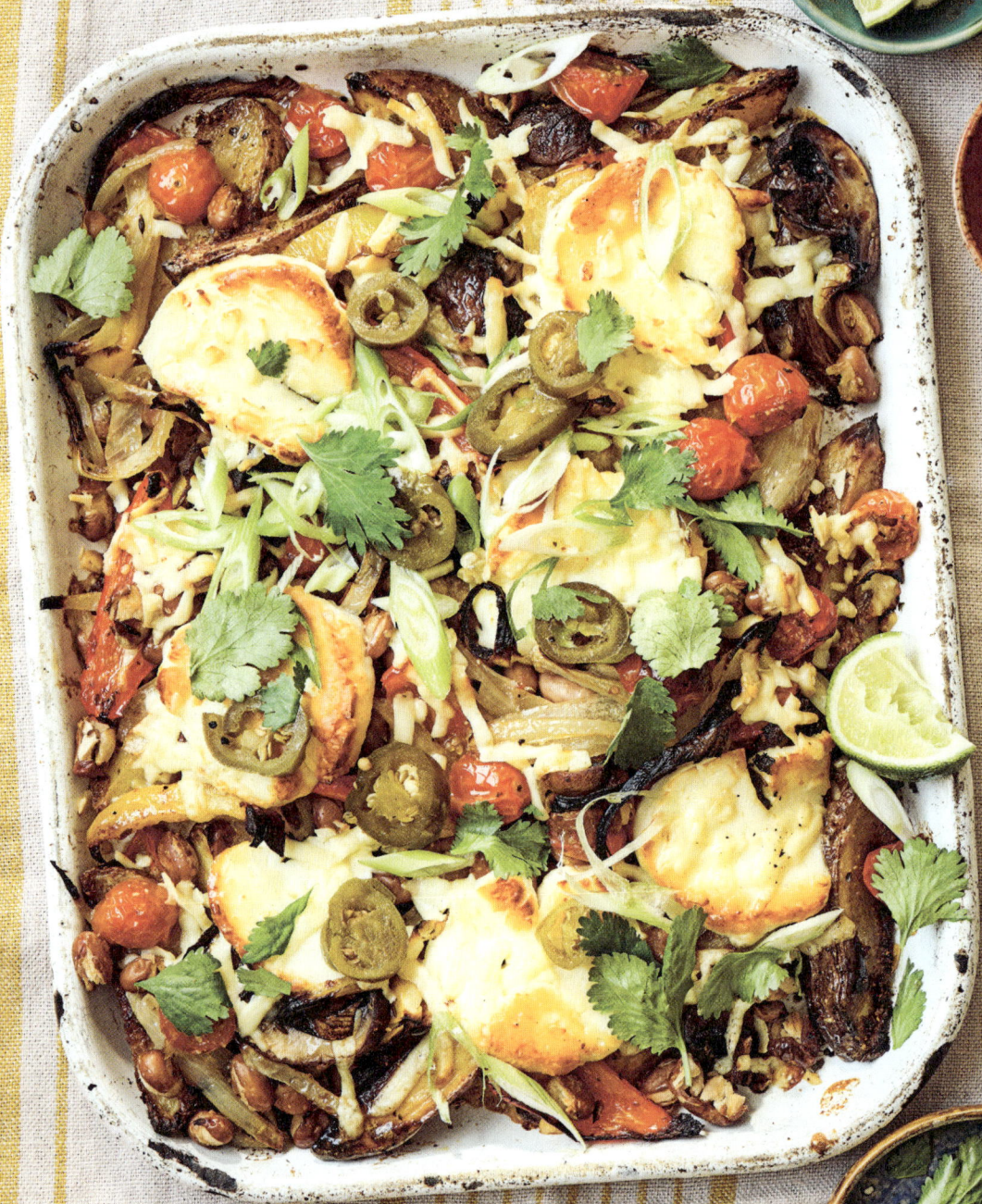

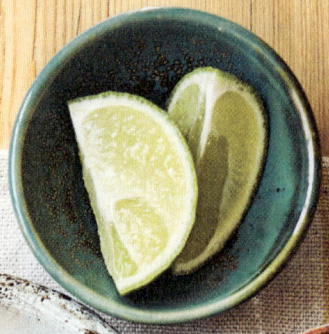

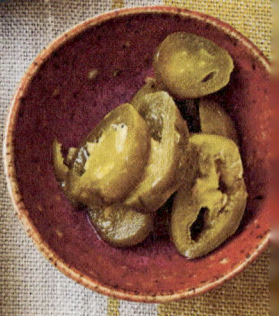

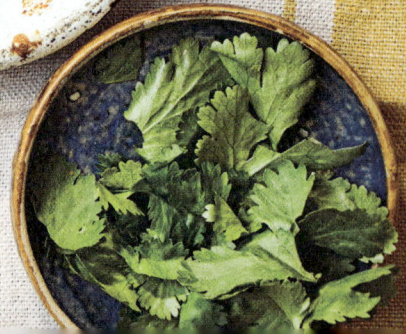

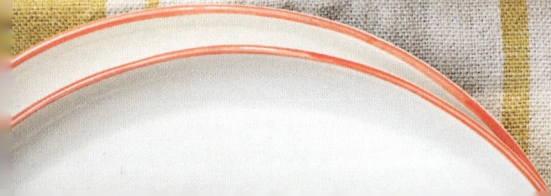

MEXICAN-STYLE LOADED WEDGES WITH HALLOUMI

SERVES 4
PREP TIME 15 minutes
COOK TIME 35 minutes

1kg (2lb 4oz) potatoes (I use Maris Piper for this), washed but skin left on, cut into wedges

spray oil

2 onions, finely sliced

3 sweet peppers (red, yellow and orange), deseeded and cut into strips

300g (10½oz) closed cup mushrooms, sliced

200g (7oz) cherry tomatoes, halved

400g (14oz) can of pinto beans, drained and rinsed

175g (6oz) halloumi cheese, chopped into cubes

60g (2¼oz) Cheddar cheese, grated

3 tablespoons pickled jalapeños

2 spring onions, finely sliced

small handful of coriander

salt and pepper

1 lime, cut into quarters, to serve

FOR THE SPICE MIX

2 tablespoons smoked paprika

1 tablespoon onion granules

1 tablespoon garlic granules

1 tablespoon dried oregano

2 teaspoons ground cumin

2 teaspoons chilli flakes

1 teaspoon coarse salt

A vibrant and satisfying dish, perfect for sharing, of tasty wedges loaded up with spiced roasted vegetables, tangy halloumi, beans and melted cheese. As well as tasting delicious, this looks great.

1   Preheat the oven to 220°C/200°C fan (425°F), Gas Mark 7.

2   Put the potato wedges on a large baking tray, spray with oil, then season with salt and pepper.

3   Tip the sliced onions into another deep baking tray and add the peppers, mushrooms and cherry tomatoes.

4   Combine the spice mix ingredients in a small bowl, then sprinkle it all over the chopped-up vegetables. Mix thoroughly, then spray with oil.

5   Place the wedges on the top shelf of the oven and the tray of spiced vegetables on the middle shelf. Bake for 20 minutes.

6   Remove both trays from the oven. Shuffle the potato wedges around the tray to allow them to brown more evenly. Add the drained pinto beans to the vegetables, mix, then scatter the halloumi cubes on top. Return both trays to the oven for 10 minutes. Preheat the grill to high.

7   Choose a large warmed ovenproof platter, or individual bowls. Put the potato wedges on the base (check they are cooked through first), spoon over the vegetables and halloumi, scatter over the grated Cheddar, then grill for a few minutes to melt and brown it a little, if you wish. Scatter over the jalapeños, spring onions and coriander, pop on the lime wedges and serve.

NOTE

There are plenty of other toppings and sauces you could add to these wedges. Try chopped avocado, or Guacamole (see page 200), drained and rinsed black beans, sweetcorn, pickled red onions, soured cream or fat-free Greek yogurt, salsa, chipotle mayo and/or hot sauce.

PER SERVING

CALORIES	FAT	SAT FAT	CARBS	SUGARS	FIBRE	PROTEIN	SALT
576	19G	11G	63G	18G	17G	29G	3.5G

IRISH SEAFOOD CHOWDER

SERVES 4
PREP TIME 10 minutes
COOK TIME 30 minutes

This hearty and nourishing chowder will definitely warm your cockles! A little indulgence, in the form of double cream, makes it really special. Delicious on its own, or served with lovely chunky slices of bread.

1 tablespoon (15g/½oz) butter

1 leek, trimmed, cleaned and finely chopped (see page 197)

1 large onion, finely chopped

1 teaspoon coarse salt

4 smoked bacon medallions, finely chopped

1 teaspoon dried thyme

400g (14oz) white potatoes, peeled and cut into 1cm (½ inch) cubes

1 litre (1¾ pints) hot fish stock

¼ teaspoon freshly ground black pepper

100ml (3½fl oz) double cream

150g (5½oz) skinless smoked haddock fillet, chopped

150g (5½oz) skinless white fish fillet, such as cod, chopped

165g (5¾oz) raw king prawns

chives, to serve

1   Melt the butter in a large pot, or flameproof casserole dish which has a lid, and add the leek, onion and salt. Put the lid on the pan and sweat for 10 minutes over a medium-low heat, stirring occasionally.

2   Add the bacon and thyme and stir-fry for 3 minutes over a medium heat. Stir in the chopped potatoes, then the hot stock and pepper.

3   Bring to the boil, then reduce the heat to a simmer, cover with a lid and simmer for 12 minutes.

4   Pour in the cream, add the fish and prawns, stir well and simmer gently for 5 minutes.

5   Divide between 4 warmed bowls and scatter with chopped chives.

NOTE

You can personalize this recipe with your favourite seafood, or any you have in the freezer. Sometimes, if pre-packaged fish is more than I need for a recipe, I chop leftovers and pop them in a freezer bag for fish pie, or my next batch of chowder. Here, I have outlined the suggested cooking times of different varieties, so you can add them to the chowder accordingly:

Salmon Cook bite-sized chunks for 5 minutes, or add sliced smoked salmon to the finished bowls.

Mussels Cook for 5–6 minutes; ensure you remove the beards and clean them thoroughly before adding them to the pot.

Clams Cook thoroughly cleaned and rinsed clams for 7–10 minutes.

Crab meat Cook fresh or canned crab for 5 minutes.

Scallops Cook bite-sized chunks for 3–5 minutes.

Squid Cook rings or slices for 2–3 minutes.

PER SERVING

CALORIES	FAT	SAT FAT	CARBS	SUGARS	FIBRE	PROTEIN	SALT
437	20G	11G	24G	7.1G	4.6G	37G	4.25G

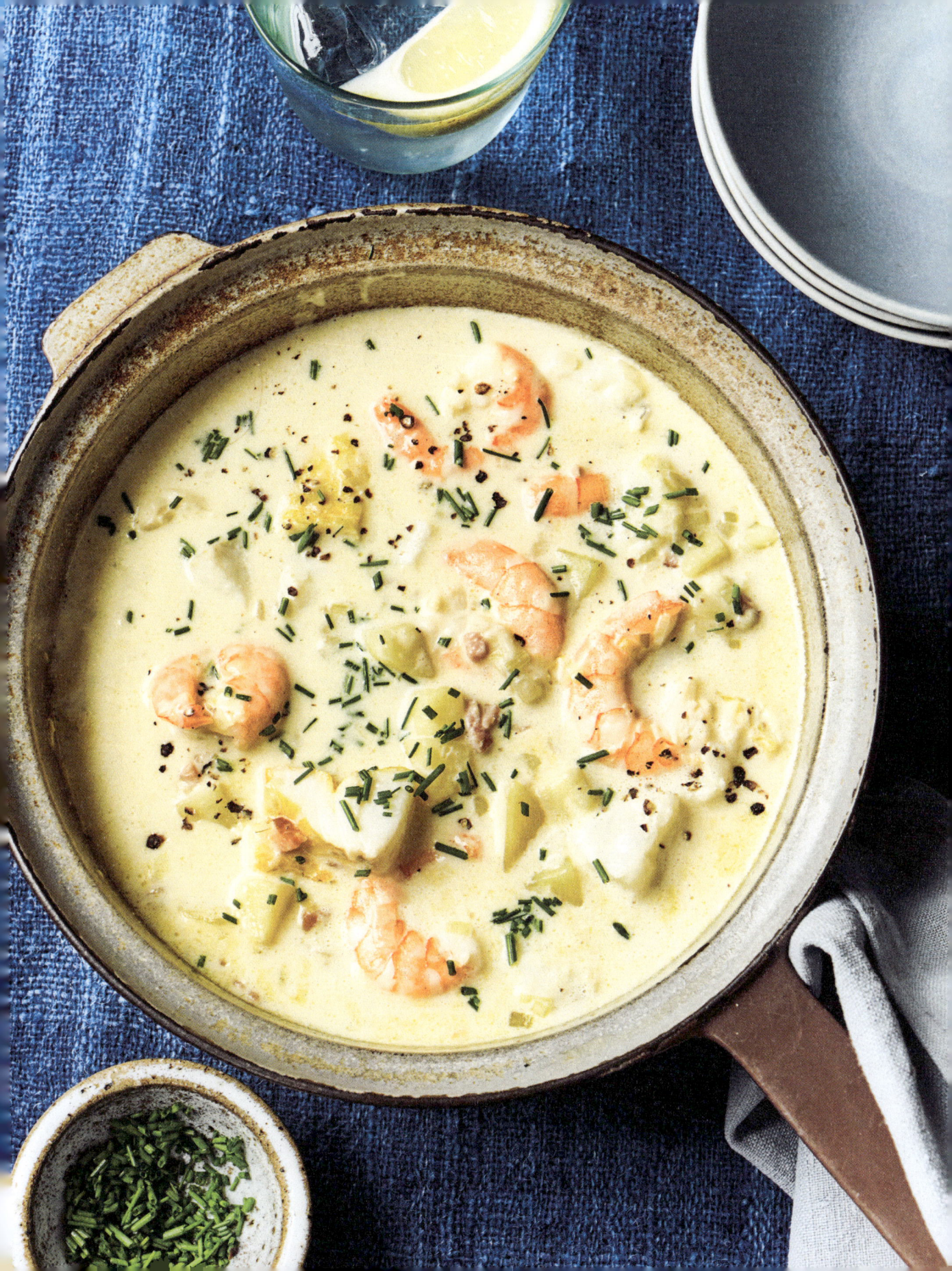

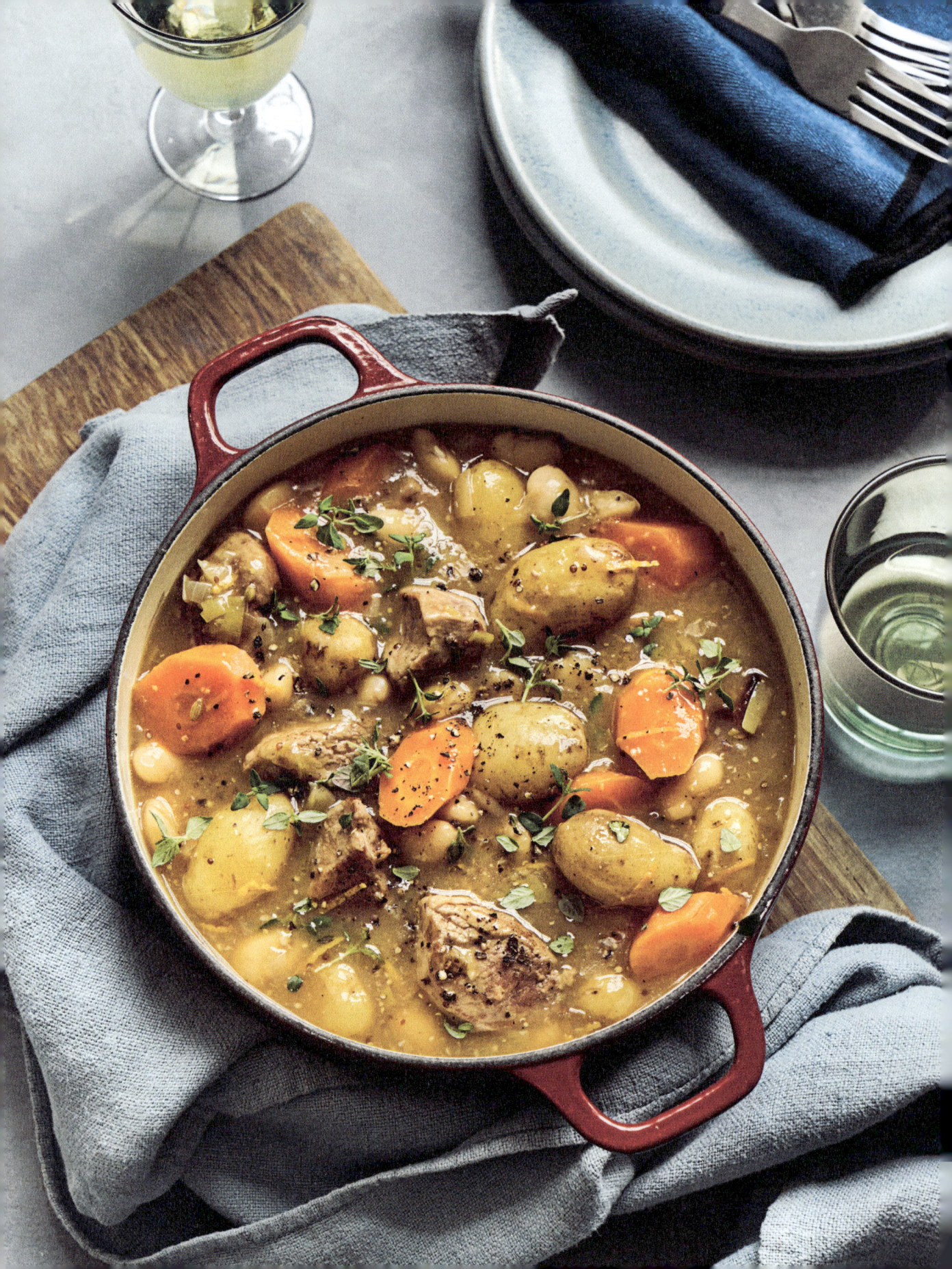

RICH PORK & ORANGE STEW

SERVES 6
PREP TIME 20 minutes
COOK TIME 55 minutes

A comforting one-pot dish that is the perfect way to warm up on a chilly winter evening. With its tender pork, zesty orange and touch of fennel, this stew boasts deep flavours with a subtle hint of festivity. Serve it with leafy greens, such as kale or chard, for a satisfying meal that's both comforting and nourishing.

spray oil

1 pork tenderloin/fillet (total weight 400–500g/1lb), chopped into small pieces

1 onion, finely chopped

1 leek, trimmed, cleaned and chopped (see page 197)

2 garlic cloves, crushed

¼ teaspoon fennel seeds

600ml (20fl oz) hot beef stock

750g (1lb 10oz) baby potatoes, halved if necessary to make them bite-sized

300g (10½oz) carrots, sliced on the diagonal

2 tablespoons cornflour

2 tablespoons water

finely grated zest and juice of 1 orange

2 tablespoons honey

1 tablespoon dark soy sauce

1 tablespoon wholegrain mustard

1 tablespoon balsamic vinegar

1 teaspoon dried thyme, or fresh thyme leaves

2 x 400g (14oz) cans of butter beans, drained and rinsed

salt and pepper

1 Spray a deep flameproof casserole dish with oil and fry the pork, onion and leek for 8 minutes. Add the garlic and fennel seeds and stir-fry for another minute.

2 Pour in the hot stock, then add the baby potatoes and carrots and bring to a simmer.

3 Mix the cornflour in a small bowl with the measured water until smooth, then add to the pan. Add the orange zest and juice, honey, soy sauce, mustard, balsamic vinegar and thyme, bring to a simmer, then leave to simmer for 30 minutes.

4 Add the butter beans and simmer for a further 15 minutes. Season with salt and pepper, then serve.

NOTE

You can boost the filling-power of this stew with plenty of other winter vegetables, if you like. Squash, swede, beetroot, parsnips, spinach and cabbage all make great additions. I find pork tenderloin to be good value and a convenient size, but you can use other cuts if you prefer, such as loin steaks, if you trim away excess fat and chop them. If you don't eat pork, try this with the same weight of skinless chicken thigh fillets instead.

PER SERVING

CALORIES	FAT	SAT FAT	CARBS	SUGARS	FIBRE	PROTEIN	SALT
380	3.8G	1.4G	48G	16G	13G	32G	1.3G

KEEMA CURRY

A fantastic one-pan minced beef curry, with flavours mild enough to be popular with the whole family. This is an easy recipe to double up, so you have leftovers for the freezer, too. I usually serve this with basmati rice.

SERVES 6
PREP TIME 5 minutes
COOK TIME 40 minutes

spray oil

1 onion, finely chopped

500g (1lb 2oz) lean minced beef (less than 5 per cent fat)

3 tablespoons tomato purée

2 teaspoons ginger purée from a jar

2 teaspoons garlic purée from a jar

1½ teaspoons garam masala

1½ teaspoons ground cumin

1½ teaspoons ground coriander

1 teaspoon mild chilli powder

½ teaspoon ground turmeric

400g (14oz) can of chopped tomatoes

400g (14oz) can of green lentils, drained and rinsed

200ml (7fl oz) hot beef stock

2 tablespoons Worcestershire sauce

1 tablespoon mango chutney

2 carrots, peeled and grated

200g (7oz) frozen peas

1 teaspoon coarse salt

½ teaspoon pepper

TO SERVE
fat-free Greek yogurt
chopped mint leaves

1. Spray a sauté pan with oil and fry the onion for 8 minutes, until softened.

2. Add the minced beef and stir-fry for 5 minutes, breaking up clumps as you go, to brown it.

3. Stir in the tomato, ginger and garlic purées, garam masala, cumin, coriander, chilli powder and turmeric and fry for 1 minute. Add the chopped tomatoes, lentils, hot stock, Worcestershire sauce, mango chutney and carrots (I just grate them into the curry while it's simmering, rather than preparing them in advance). Stir well and simmer for 20 minutes.

4. Tip in the peas, season with the salt and pepper and simmer for another 5 minutes.

5. Serve with a dollop of yogurt and a scattering of chopped mint.

NOTE

Sometimes I add a can of light (reduced-fat) coconut milk to this, which gives lovely extra flavour. If I'm adding coconut milk, I add a crumbled beef stock cube, but not the 200ml (7fl oz) hot beef stock.

You can bulk this out with your favourite vegetables to make it go further. Fry mushrooms, peppers or cubes of sweet potato or regular potato just before the garlic and ginger, or add grated courgette, fresh or frozen spinach or sliced roasted peppers from a jar along with the peas.

PER SERVING

CALORIES	FAT	SAT FAT	CARBS	SUGARS	FIBRE	PROTEIN	SALT
267	5.9G	2G	22G	15G	7.6G	27G	2.1G

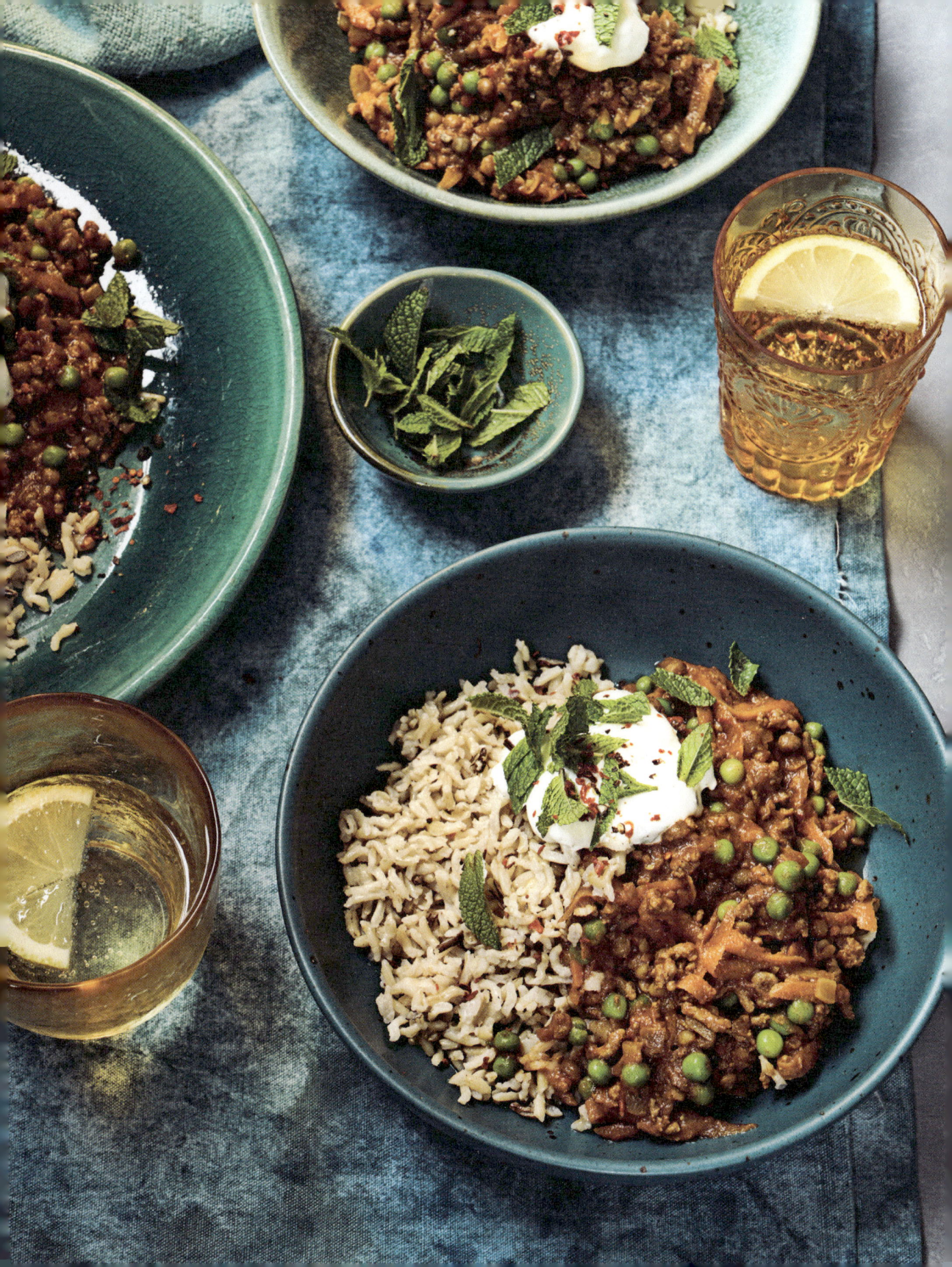

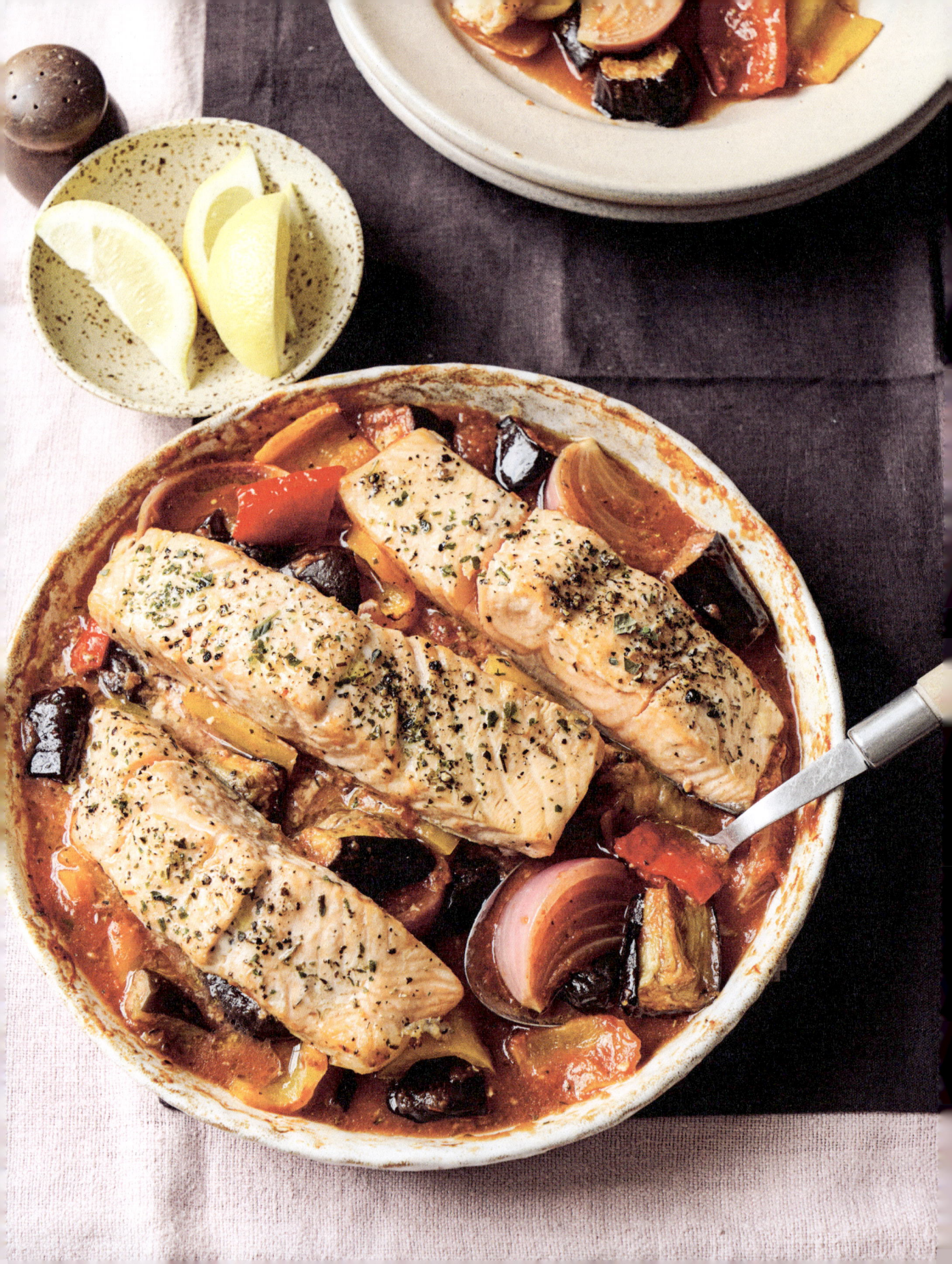

ROAST SALMON WITH RATATOUILLE

SERVES 4
PREP TIME 10 minutes
COOK TIME 25 minutes

4 salmon fillets
chopped parsley leaves, to serve

FOR THE RATATOUILLE
spray oil
2 aubergines, chopped into about 3cm (1¼ inch) chunks
3 sweet peppers (red, yellow and orange), deseeded and chopped into large chunks
1 large red onion, cut into wedges
500g (1lb 2oz) tomato passata
200ml (7fl oz) hot vegetable stock
2 garlic cloves, finely chopped or crushed
1 tablespoon balsamic vinegar
3 teaspoons dried Italian herbs
salt and pepper

The ratatouille here isn't made in a traditional way, but as it's so very hands-off — and the end result tastes great — it's my perfect recipe. Pairing it with salmon makes a satisfying meal which is nutritious, warming and comforting.

1   Preheat the oven to 220°C/200°C fan (425°F), Gas Mark 7.

2   Spray a baking tray with oil and spread the aubergine pieces out in a single layer, then spray the aubergines with oil so they are lightly covered.

3   Tip the peppers into another deep baking dish with the onion, passata, hot stock, garlic, balsamic vinegar and 2 teaspoons of the Italian herbs. Season with salt and pepper and give it a stir.

4   Place the aubergines on the top shelf of the oven and the other vegetables on the middle shelf and set a timer for 13 minutes.

5   Place the salmon fillets skin side down on another baking tray, sprinkle over the remaining teaspoon of Italian herbs and season with salt and pepper. After the vegetables have been baking for 13 minutes, give the aubergines a toss and stir the vegetables in the passata. Put everything back into the oven, including the salmon, and cook for a further 12 minutes.

6   Remove everything from the oven, check that the aubergines are cooked through (they should be soft and fudgy, not springy), then stir them into the passata mix. Divide the ratatouille between 4 warmed pasta bowls and place a salmon fillet on top of each portion. Scatter with parsley and serve.

NOTE

If you want an extra element to increase the filling-power of this dish, you can cook pasta (orzo works well here) and stir it through the ratatouille before serving, or serve it with couscous.

PER SERVING

CALORIES	FAT	SAT FAT	CARBS	SUGARS	FIBRE	PROTEIN	SALT
377	22G	4G	12G	11G	6.3G	30G	0.4G

SAUSAGE, APPLE & LEEK STEW

SERVES 4
PREP TIME 15 minutes
COOK TIME 40 minutes

spray oil
8 light (reduced-fat) sausages
   (see note)
1 onion, finely chopped
2 large leeks, trimmed, cleaned
   and chopped (see page 197)
3 garlic cloves, crushed
1 teaspoon dried thyme
1 large apple, peeled, cored and
   chopped
500g (1lb 2oz) new potatoes, cut
   into bite-sized chunks
600ml (20fl oz) hot chicken stock
1 teaspoon Dijon mustard
1 teaspoon honey
salt and pepper

A comforting combination of flavours, savoury leek and sweet apple are so good alongside sausages. This is a one-pot meal, but I'd usually cook green vegetables to serve with it: broccoli, green beans and peas all work well. Or if you want to get some extra veg into this, add sliced carrots at the same time as the potatoes.

1 Spray a sauté pan, which has a lid, with oil and fry the sausages for 10 minutes, to get the outsides nice and brown.

2 Add the onion and leeks and fry for 10 minutes, stirring regularly.

3 Now stir in in the garlic and thyme, add the apple, potatoes, hot stock, mustard and honey, season with salt and pepper and stir well. Cover the pan with a lid and simmer for 20 minutes before serving.

NOTE

I have specified light (reduced-fat) sausages, to keep the calories down in this meal, but of course you can use whatever sausages you like. If I'm cooking this for the whole family, I tend to use chipolatas because my daughters prefer them. You can always add more if 2 chipolatas per person is not enough here. Reduced-fat sausages still taste great and are available usually as a supermarket own-brand product.

PER SERVING

CALORIES	FAT	SAT FAT	CARBS	SUGARS	FIBRE	PROTEIN	SALT
422	16G	5.4G	41G	17G	8G	24G	2.9G

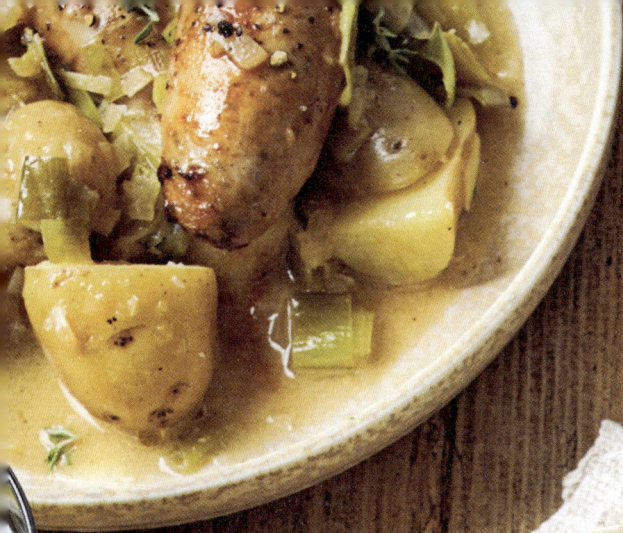

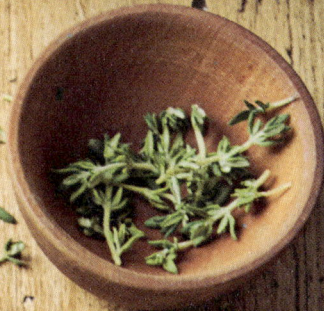

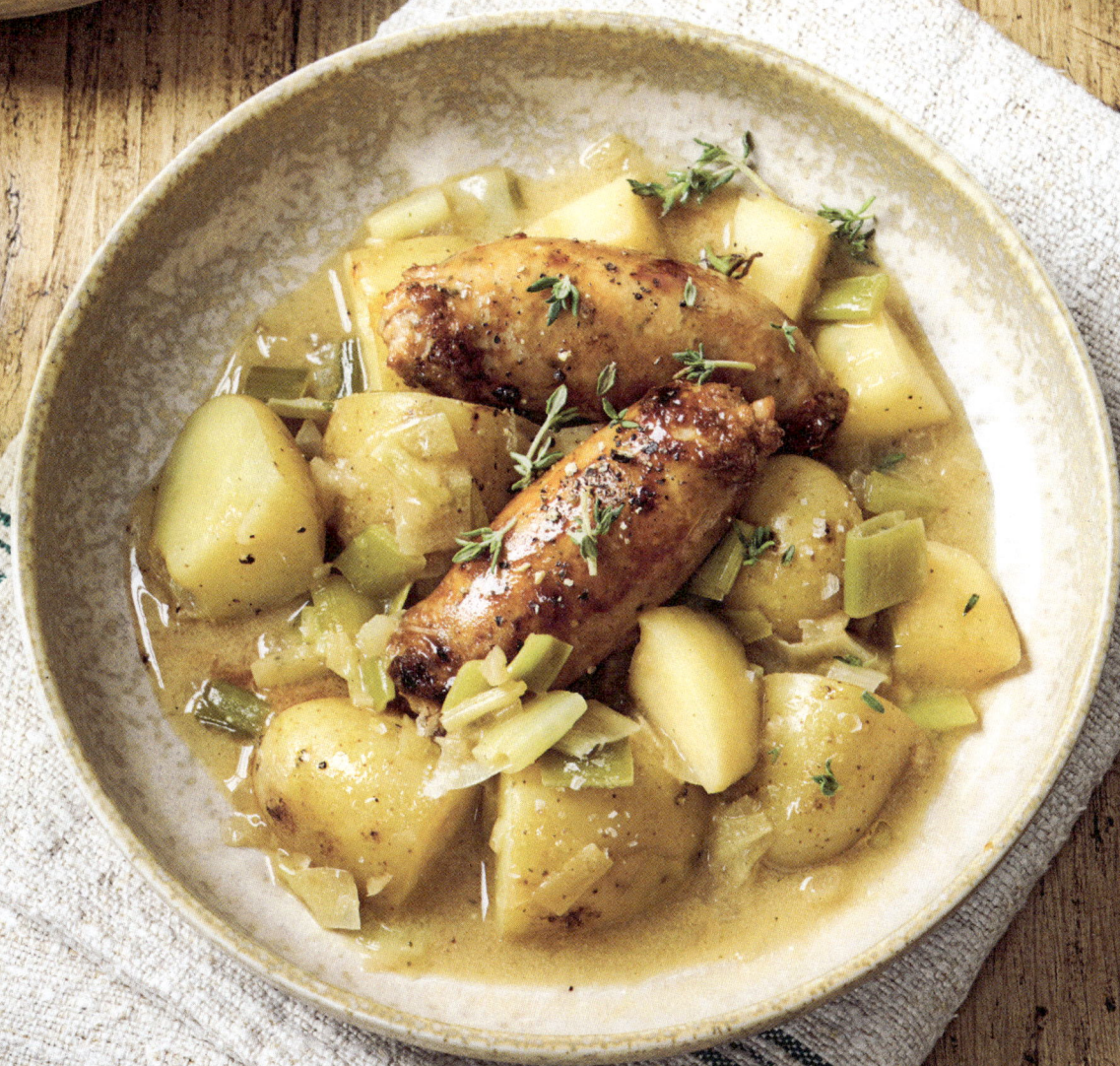

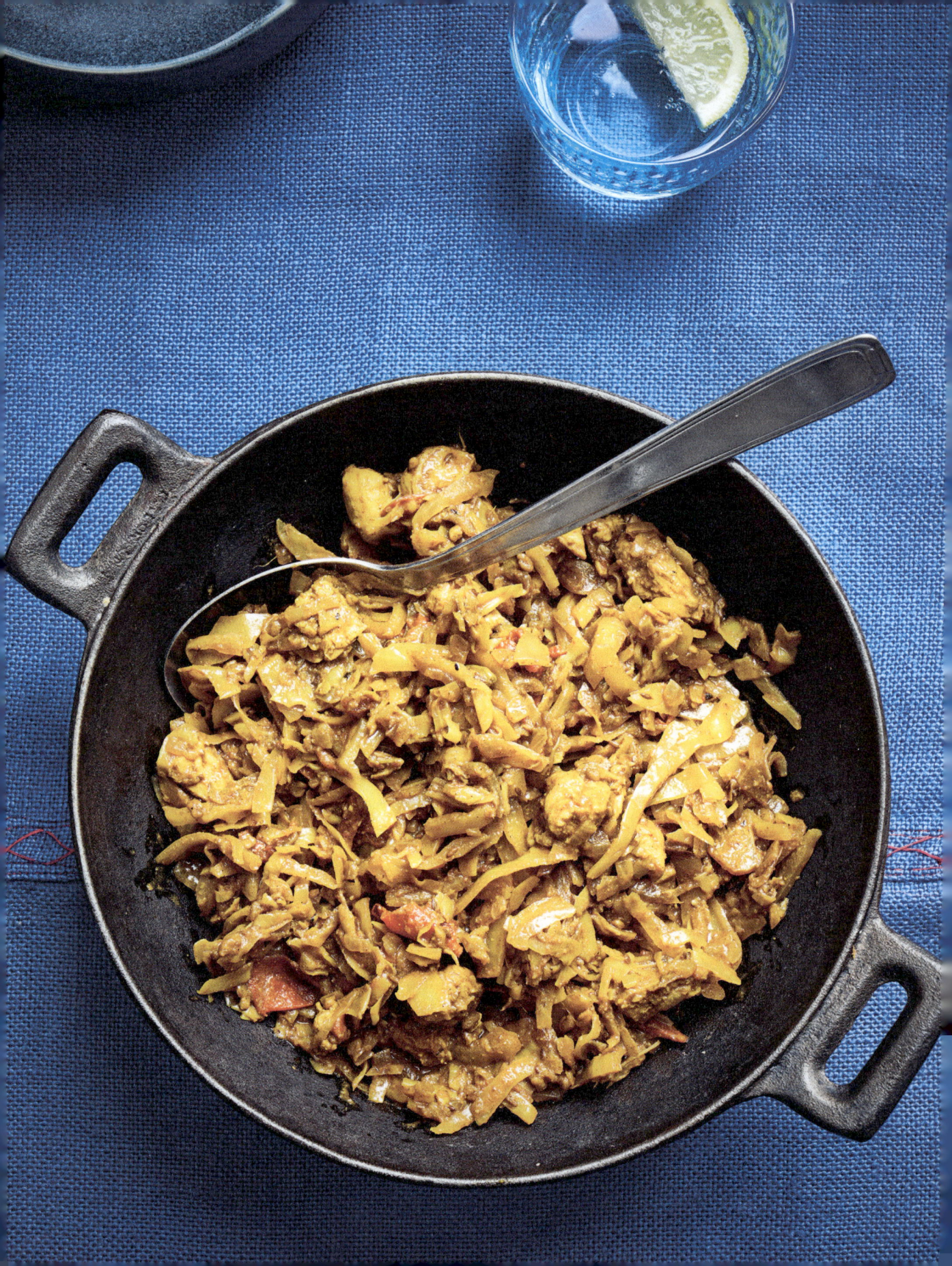

FRAGRANT CHICKEN & CABBAGE CURRY

SERVES 4
PREP TIME 20 minutes
COOK TIME 42 minutes

2 teaspoons vegetable oil
½ teaspoon fenugreek seeds
½ teaspoon cumin seeds
3 cardamom pods
1 cinnamon stick
½ teaspoon pepper
1 bay leaf
2 onions, finely chopped
½ white cabbage, shredded
   (see note)
1 teaspoon ground turmeric
3cm (1¼ inch) piece of root ginger,
   peeled and finely grated
3 garlic cloves, crushed
2 green chillies, deseeded and
   finely chopped
2 salad tomatoes, chopped
500g (1lb 2oz) skinless, boneless
   chicken thigh fillets, excess fat
   removed, chopped
2 teaspoons ground cumin
2 teaspoons ground coriander
2 teaspoons chilli powder
1 teaspoon coarse salt
50ml (1¾fl oz) water
1 teaspoon garam masala

This fragrant, dry curry combines tender chicken and cabbage, which is in season during the winter months in the UK. With warming spices and a simple cooking method, it's a quick and satisfying meal. It's also a great way to use up leftover cabbage; I often have half a cabbage left over from making coleslaw.

1 Heat the oil in a sauté pan, which has a lid, and fry the fenugreek, cumin seeds, cardamom pods, cinnamon stick, pepper and bay leaf for 2 minutes.

2 Add the onions and stir-fry for 3 minutes, then tip in the cabbage and stir-fry for 10 minutes.

3 Add the turmeric, ginger, garlic and chillies and stir-fry for 2 minutes. Now tip in the tomatoes, stir, place the lid on the pan and cook gently for 5 minutes.

4 Now add the chicken, stir well, put the lid back on and simmer for 10 minutes.

5 Add the ground cumin, coriander, chilli powder, salt and measured water, stir well and simmer for a final 10 minutes with the lid off. Stir through the garam masala before serving.

NOTE

For this recipe, the best way to chop the cabbage is to slice it thinly into shreds or strips, then roughly chop it into smaller pieces. This is how I do it:

Remove any tough or damaged outer leaves.

Cut the cabbage in half through its core, then cut out the core from each half. Lay the halves flat on a chopping board.

Use a sharp knife to slice the cabbage across into fine strips.

Chop the strips into smaller pieces.

PER SERVING

CALORIES	FAT	SAT FAT	CARBS	SUGARS	FIBRE	PROTEIN	SALT
239	6.4G	1.3G	12G	9.3G	6.6G	29G	1.6G

HARISSA SPAGHETTI BOLOGNESE

SERVES 4
PREP TIME 5 minutes
COOK TIME 40 minutes

spray oil

1 onion, finely chopped

4 garlic cloves, crushed

500g (1lb 2oz) extra-lean minced beef

2 tablespoons tomato purée

1 tablespoon harissa paste

400g (14oz) can of chopped tomatoes (either a regular can puréed until smooth with a stick blender, or use a fine tomato polpa)

1 tablespoon dried mixed herbs

1 tablespoon balsamic vinegar

1 teaspoon sugar

salt and pepper

300g (10½oz) spaghetti

TO SERVE

chopped parsley leaves, or torn basil leaves

finely grated Parmesan cheese (optional)

freshly ground black pepper

Just a little extra twist turns a simple Bolognese into a more complex meal, with added warmth and depth.

1 Spray a frying pan with oil and fry the onion for 8 minutes until softened, then add the garlic and stir-fry for another minute.

2 Add the minced beef and stir-fry, breaking up any clumps and browning the meat for about 5 minutes.

3 Stir in the tomato purée and harissa paste and stir-fry for 2 minutes. Add the tomatoes, mixed herbs, balsamic vinegar and sugar, stir well, then simmer for 25 minutes, stirring occasionally. Season with salt and pepper.

4 Cook the spaghetti according to the packet instructions, then drain and stir it into the Bolognese to coat the spaghetti with the sauce. Serve in warmed pasta bowls, topped with the herbs, Parmesan, if you like, and black pepper.

NOTE

Harissa is a spicy and aromatic North African chilli paste. It's usually made from a blend of roasted sweet red peppers, hot chillies, garlic, olive oil and spices, such as cumin, coriander and caraway. The paste adds depth of flavour and heat to dishes and most supermarkets sell it; my favourite is rose harissa.

PER SERVING

CALORIES	FAT	SAT FAT	CARBS	SUGARS	FIBRE	PROTEIN	SALT
480	7.3G	2.9G	62G	11G	5G	38G	0.4G

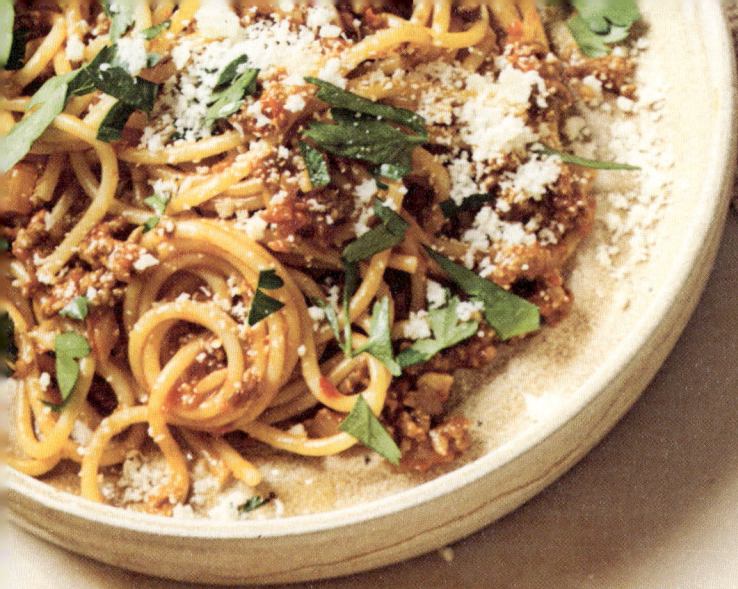

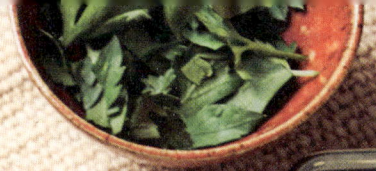

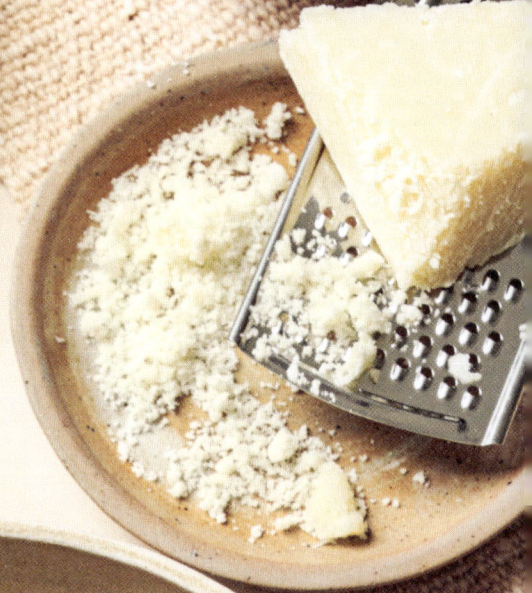

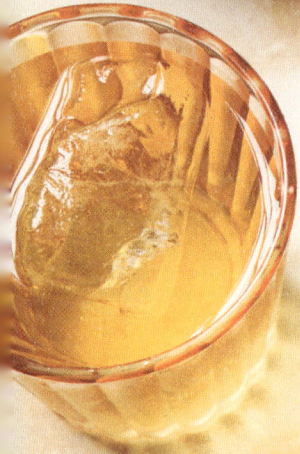

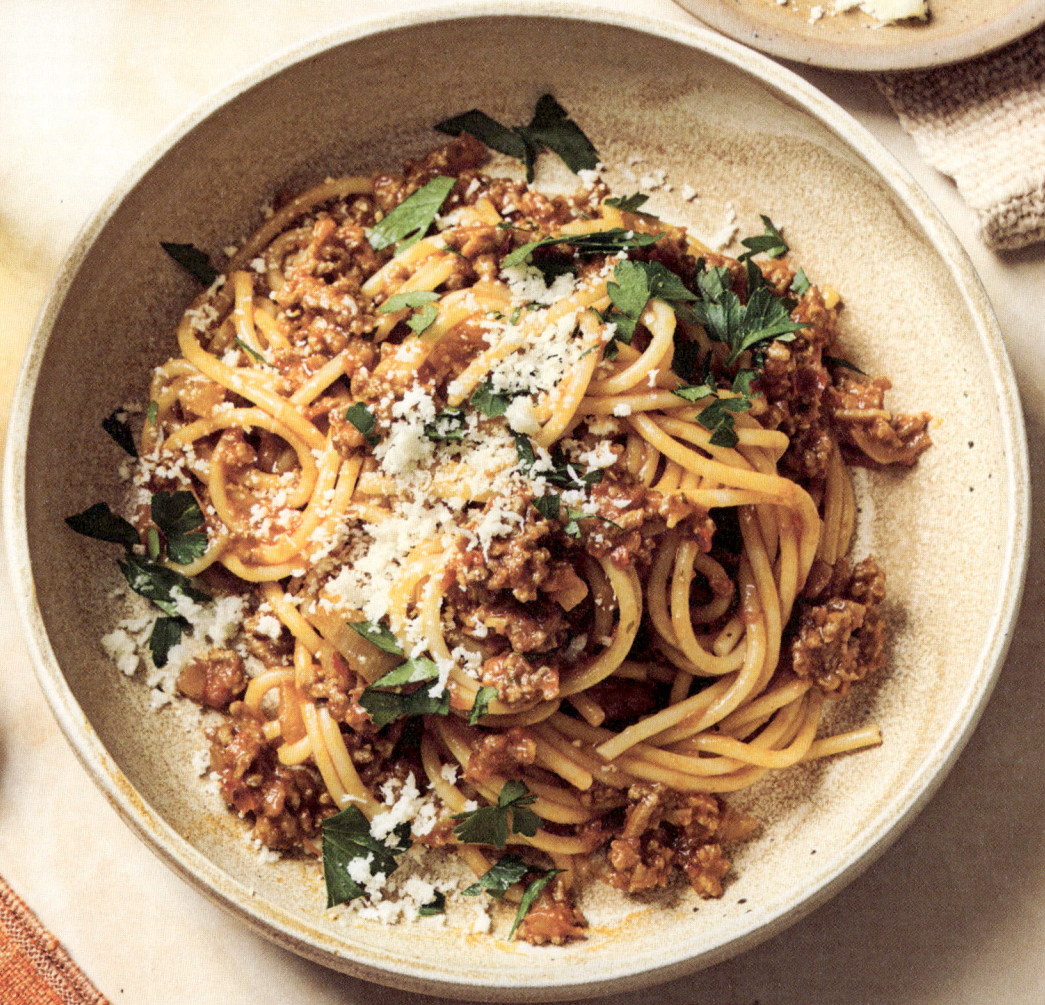

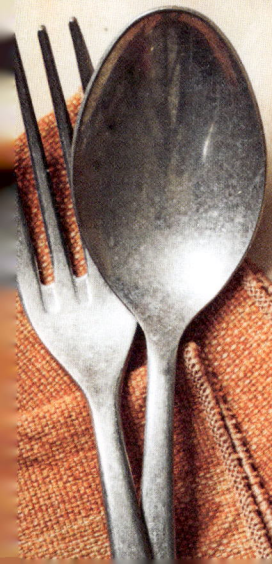

SLOW-COOKER WINNERS

6

GARLIC-PARMESAN CHICKEN & SPUDS

SERVES 4
PREP TIME 5 minutes
COOK TIME 3–4 hours (high);
7–8 hours (low)

4 skinless chicken breasts (about 150g/5½oz each), chopped

800g (1lb 12oz) red potatoes, washed but skin left on, cut into 2cm (¾ inch) chunks

2 garlic cloves, crushed

1 tablespoon dried Italian seasoning

1 teaspoon sweet (unsmoked) paprika

1 tablespoon (15g/½oz) butter, melted

100ml (3½fl oz) hot chicken stock

90g (3¼oz) Parmesan cheese, finely grated

1 head of broccoli, broken up into florets

salt and pepper

chopped parsley leaves, to serve

Simple but effective, this is a great family-friendly option when you need something easy to prepare. Tender potatoes and chicken with garlic, herbs and Parmesan are flavourful and fuss-free.

1 Put all the ingredients apart from the Parmesan, broccoli and parsley into the slow-cooker, season with salt and pepper, stir to combine, then add half the Parmesan and stir again. Set on high for 3–4 hours, or low for 7–8 hours.

2 When there are 30 minutes left before the end of the cooking time, place the broccoli florets on top of the other ingredients, replace the lid and cook for the final 30 minutes.

3 Serve with the remaining Parmesan and parsley sprinkled over.

NOTE

Red potatoes with the skins left on are a great source of dietary fibre, but you can peel them, if you prefer.

PER SERVING

CALORIES	FAT	SAT FAT	CARBS	SUGARS	FIBRE	PROTEIN	SALT
510	13G	7.2G	36G	3.6G	6.6G	58G	1.9G

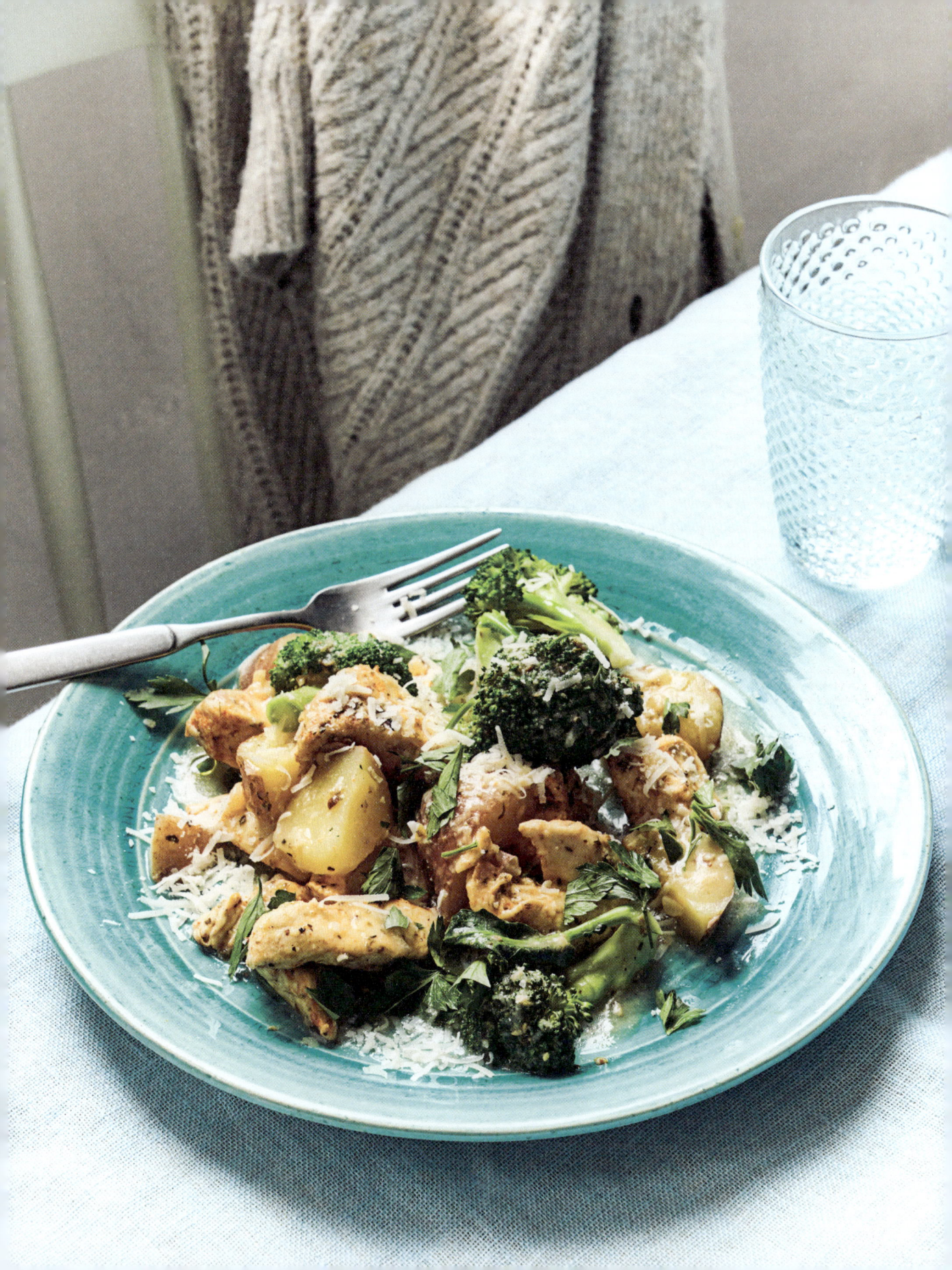

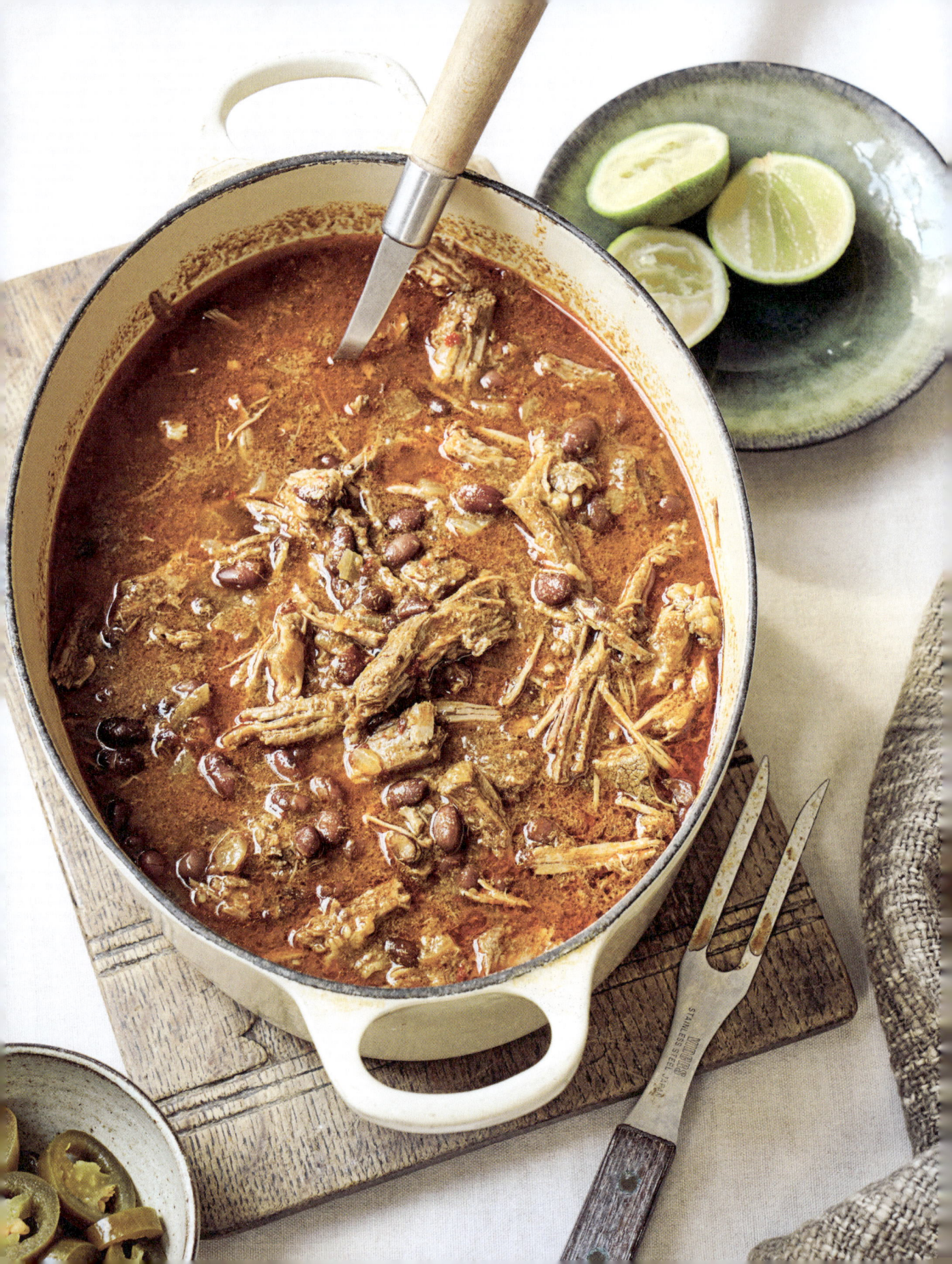

BARBACOA BEEF & BLACK BEANS

SERVES 6
PREP TIME 10 minutes
COOK TIME 6 hours (high); 8–9 hours (low)

800g (1lb 12oz) lean beef stewing steak

2 x 400g (14oz) cans of black beans, drained and rinsed

1 red onion, finely chopped

4 garlic cloves, crushed

500ml (18fl oz) hot beef stock

3 tablespoons chipotle chilli paste

2 tablespoons tomato purée

1 tablespoon apple cider vinegar

1 tablespoon ground cumin

1 tablespoon dried oregano

1 teaspoon ground coriander

1 teaspoon coarse salt

½ teaspoon pepper

¼ teaspoon ground cloves

juice of 2 limes

This Mexican-style dish has a smoky and rich chipotle chilli sauce, which perfectly complements tender, fall-apart beef, while black beans bulk it up and add texture, extra fibre and filling-power. It's a very versatile dish, perfect to serve with rice, over a jacket potato, with a simple side salad, or roasted vegetables such as peppers, onions, courgette or aubergine. I like to top it with pickled jalapeños, too.

1   Put all the ingredients into the slow-cooker pot, reserving half the lime juice. Mix well.

2   Cook on high for 6 hours, or low for 8–9 hours.

3   Once cooked, the beef should be tender and easy to pull apart. Shred any larger pieces with 2 forks.

4   Just before serving, stir through the remaining lime juice.

NOTE

To make this in an oven, preheat it to 180°C/160°C fan (350°F), Gas Mark 4. Place the ingredients into a casserole dish with a tight-fitting lid, or cover tightly with foil, and cook for 3 hours. Check it halfway through and add more beef stock if you think it is drying out.

If the dish looks like it has a lot of liquid, remove the lid for the final 30–60 minutes of cooking time (whether in the slow-cooker or oven) to allow it to reduce. For slow-cookers, placing a clean tea towel under the lid can also help absorb excess moisture and thicken the sauce.

PER SERVING

CALORIES	FAT	SAT FAT	CARBS	SUGARS	FIBRE	PROTEIN	SALT
286	6.5G	2.1G	14G	6.4G	8.4G	38G	1.6G

BBQ BEER PULLED BEEF BRISKET

SERVES 6
PREP TIME 10 minutes
COOK TIME 6–7 hours, plus
10 minutes (high); 10–12 hours,
plus 10 minutes (low)

800g (1lb 12oz) beef brisket
   (see note)
1 large onion, chopped or sliced

FOR THE RUB
1 tablespoon ground coriander
1 tablespoon cumin seeds
1 tablespoon mustard seeds
1 tablespoon smoked paprika
1 tablespoon dark brown sugar
1 teaspoon coarse salt
½ teaspoon pepper
½ teaspoon cayenne pepper

FOR THE SAUCE
330ml (11fl oz) can of beer (ale or
   lager, see recipe introduction)
100ml (3½fl oz) beef stock
4 tablespoons tomato purée
3 tablespoons red wine vinegar
1 tablespoon Worcestershire
   sauce
1 tablespoon dark soy sauce
1 tablespoon dark brown sugar
4 garlic cloves, crushed

A slow-cooker is the perfect tool to turn a beef brisket into delicious, tender pulled beef. The beer-infused sauce has a blend of savoury, sweet and smoky flavours, which hit the spot every time. I tend to use ale in this recipe, but you can use lager if you prefer: both will yield a delicious sauce. You can serve this up in a multitude of ways: I love it in a wrap with homemade coleslaw, alongside homemade chips, over rice with nacho-style toppings, such as pickled jalapeños, grated cheese, spring onion, salsa and refried beans, served in a bread roll with pickles and cheese, as a jacket potato topping, or just with a hearty salad.

1   Put all the rub ingredients into a small bowl and mix them together.

2   Cut away any string from the brisket, unroll it and cut away any large bits of fat. Massage the rub into the brisket (I do this over the slow-cooker bowl, so any bits fall directly in there), then place the brisket in the slow-cooker bowl.

3   Put all the sauce ingredients in a small saucepan and bring to the boil. Reduce the heat so it's bubbling, but not enough to boil over, and cook for about 10 minutes to reduce the amount of liquid.

4   Add the onion to the slow-cooker with the beef and pour over the sauce to cover. Cook on high for 6–7 hours, or low for 10–12 hours.

5   At the end of the cooking time, the beef should be tender and easy to pull. Shred it into the sauce using 2 forks. As you shred, the meat will absorb the sauce and juices, especially if you leave it for a few minutes after shredding. If you think there is too much sauce, you can transfer it to a saucepan over a high heat and bubble it vigorously to reduce what is remaining.

6   You can serve this straight away with your accompaniments of choice (see recipe introduction), or reheat it when you need it.

NOTE

In the UK, a beef brisket is a relatively cheap cut of meat and can usually be picked up in supermarkets as well as from the butcher. The supermarket cuts are usually 800g–1kg (1lb 12oz–2lb 4oz). It is usually a pretty lean piece of beef, but if you want to keep the fat content down, it's easy to trim away any peripheral fat with a sharp knife.

PER SERVING

CALORIES	FAT	SAT FAT	CARBS	SUGARS	FIBRE	PROTEIN	SALT
280	9.4G	3.5G	13G	11G	3G	31G	1.7G

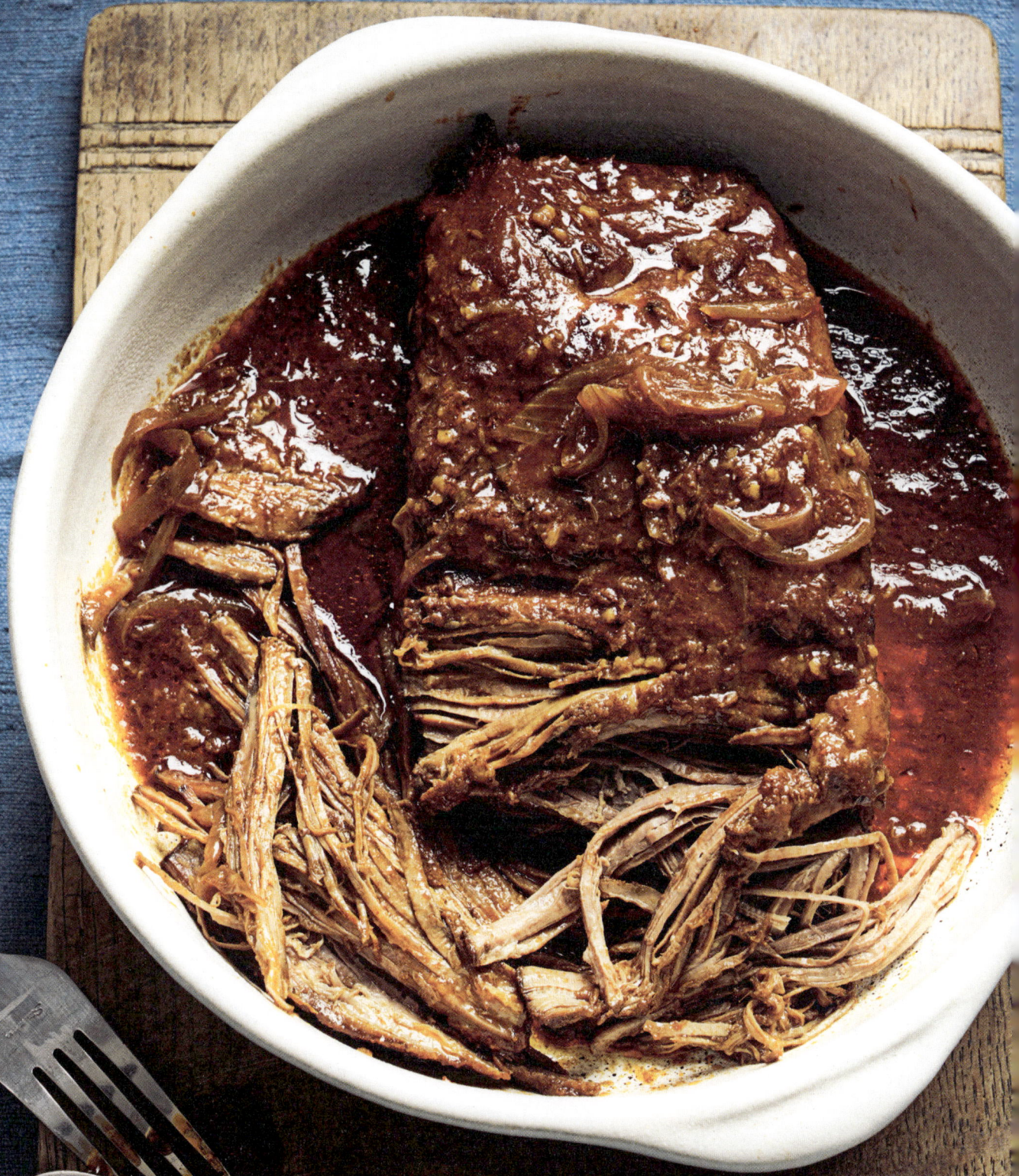

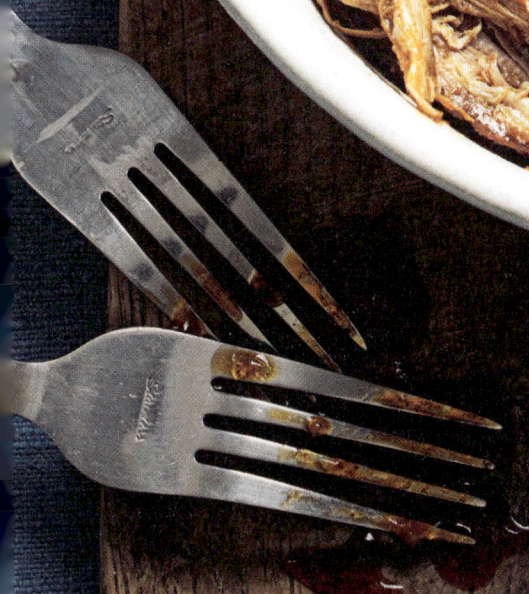

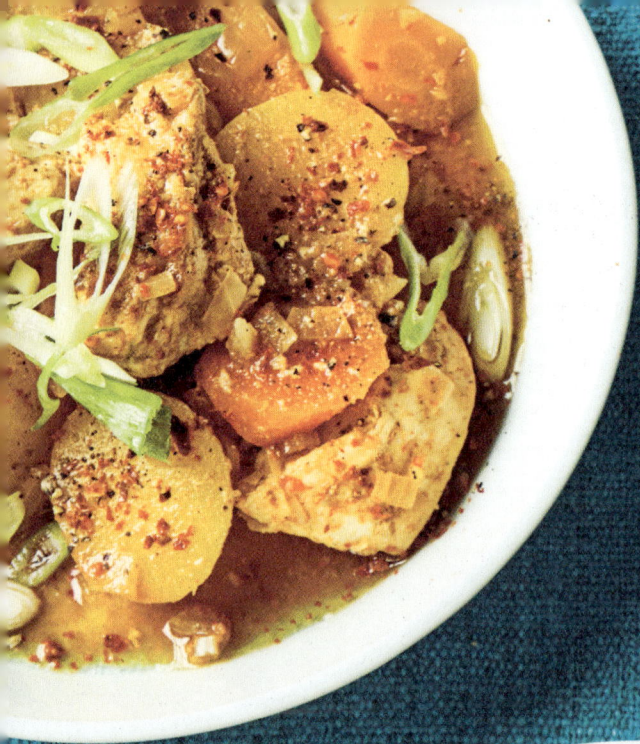

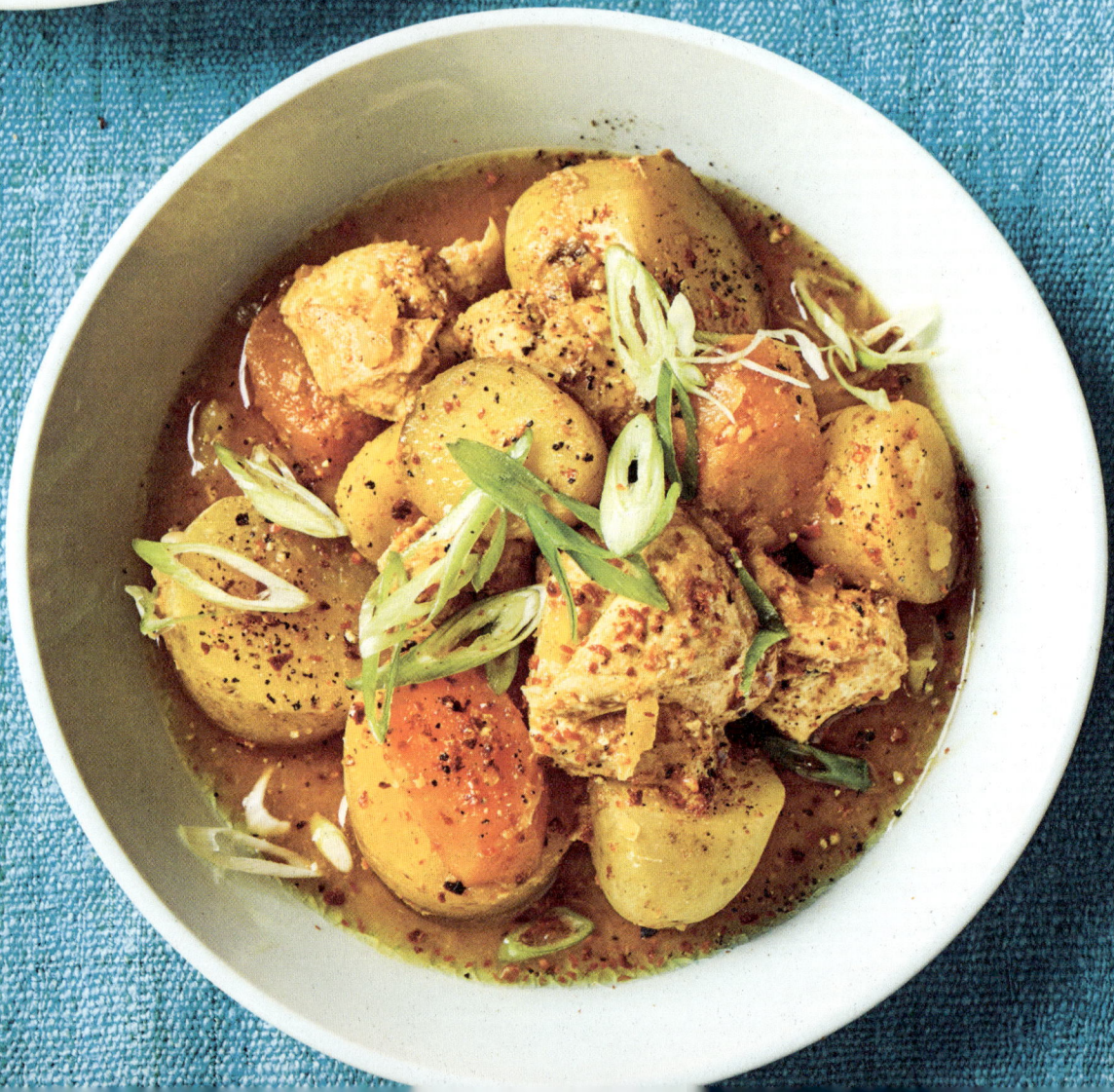

KOREAN-INSPIRED BRAISED CHICKEN & POTATOES

SERVES 4
PREP TIME 10 minutes
COOK TIME 4 hours (high);
7 hours (low)

500g (1lb 2oz) skinless chicken thigh fillets, fat removed, chopped
1 large onion, chopped
1kg (2lb 4oz) potatoes, cut into large chunks
2 carrots, sliced on the diagonal
4 spring onions, sliced, to serve

FOR THE SAUCE
2 tablespoons gochujang
4 garlic cloves, crushed
2 tablespoons soy sauce
2 tablespoons rice wine
1 tablespoon honey
1 teaspoon chilli flakes
½ teaspoon ground ginger
¼ teaspoon pepper
200ml (7fl oz) water

This recipe is inspired by dakdoritang, a spicy, savoury, hearty Korean braised chicken dish.

1   First, make up the sauce by stirring together all the sauce ingredients in a medium-large bowl.

2   Add the chicken and onion to the sauce and stir to coat.

3   Place the potato chunks and carrots in the slow-cooker bowl, cover with the chicken mix, then cook on high for 4 hours, or low for 7 hours, stirring halfway through the cooking time.

4   Garnish with the spring onions, then serve.

NOTE

This recipe would traditionally use gochugaru (Korean chilli flakes). I haven't found these in my local supermarkets, so I have substituted regular chilli flakes in this recipe, but if you can get hold of gochugaru, feel free to swap it in. You can adjust the level of spiciness by increasing or decreasing the amount of gochujang and chilli flakes to suit your taste.

PER SERVING

CALORIES	FAT	SAT FAT	CARBS	SUGARS	FIBRE	PROTEIN	SALT
425	4.4G	1.2G	59G	20G	9G	32G	1.7G

BEEF & GINGER RAMEN

SERVES 4
PREP TIME 10 minutes
COOK TIME 3–4 hours (high);
6–7 hours (low)

400g (14oz) lean braising steak

500ml (18fl oz) hot beef stock

2 garlic cloves, crushed

2½cm (1 inch) piece of root ginger,
   peeled and finely grated, or
   2 teaspoons ginger purée from
   a jar

2 tablespoons oyster sauce

1 tablespoon dark soy sauce

1 tablespoon brown sugar

2 teaspoons rice vinegar

4 spring onions, white and green
   parts separated, finely sliced

2 carrots, julienned or cut into
   thin matchsticks

1 sweet red pepper, deseeded and
   finely sliced

4 packets of instant ramen
   noodles

This tasty noodle dish – with an extremely flavoursome sauce – got the seal of approval from my whole family. I use a low-cost braising steak to make the sauce, then add vegetables and noodles at the end to retain a bit of texture in the vegetables and ensure the noodles aren't overcooked.

1   Take a moment to chop up your braising steak a little bit more: it's usually in fairly large chunks and you want it a bit smaller for this recipe (I cut each chunk into 2–3 smaller pieces).

2   Put the steak, hot stock, garlic, ginger, oyster sauce, dark soy sauce, brown sugar, rice vinegar and white parts of the spring onions into the slow-cooker bowl.

3   Cook on high for 3–4 hours, or on low for 6–7 hours.

4   When there are 30 minutes before you are ready to eat, add the carrots and red pepper and give everything a brief stir. Pop the lid back on, turn the slow-cooker to high (if it was on low) and leave to cook. Set a timer for 15 minutes.

5   After 15 minutes, add the noodles and push them down into the liquid. Set a timer for 7 minutes, after which time turn each noodle nest over to submerge the dry side into the liquid, then cook for a further 8 minutes.

6   At the end of cooking, give the noodles a stir and, if there are any noodles still clumpy or dry, use a spoon to push them into the liquid and leave them cooking for a few minutes more. Stir again and, if the noodles are all cooked, serve scattered with the green parts of the spring onions.

NOTE

I think the vegetables are much nicer here if they are added near the end of cooking, but you can add them from the beginning if you prefer. You can also cook your noodles separately in a pan of boiling water and then just mix them in once cooked, if you find that easier. Feel free to add some different vegetables: try mushrooms, sugar snap peas, fine green beans, baby sweetcorn, courgette matchsticks, pak choi or water chestnuts.

PER SERVING

CALORIES	FAT	SAT FAT	CARBS	SUGARS	FIBRE	PROTEIN	SALT
500	6.1G	2.6G	80G	9.8G	4.1G	29G	2.1G

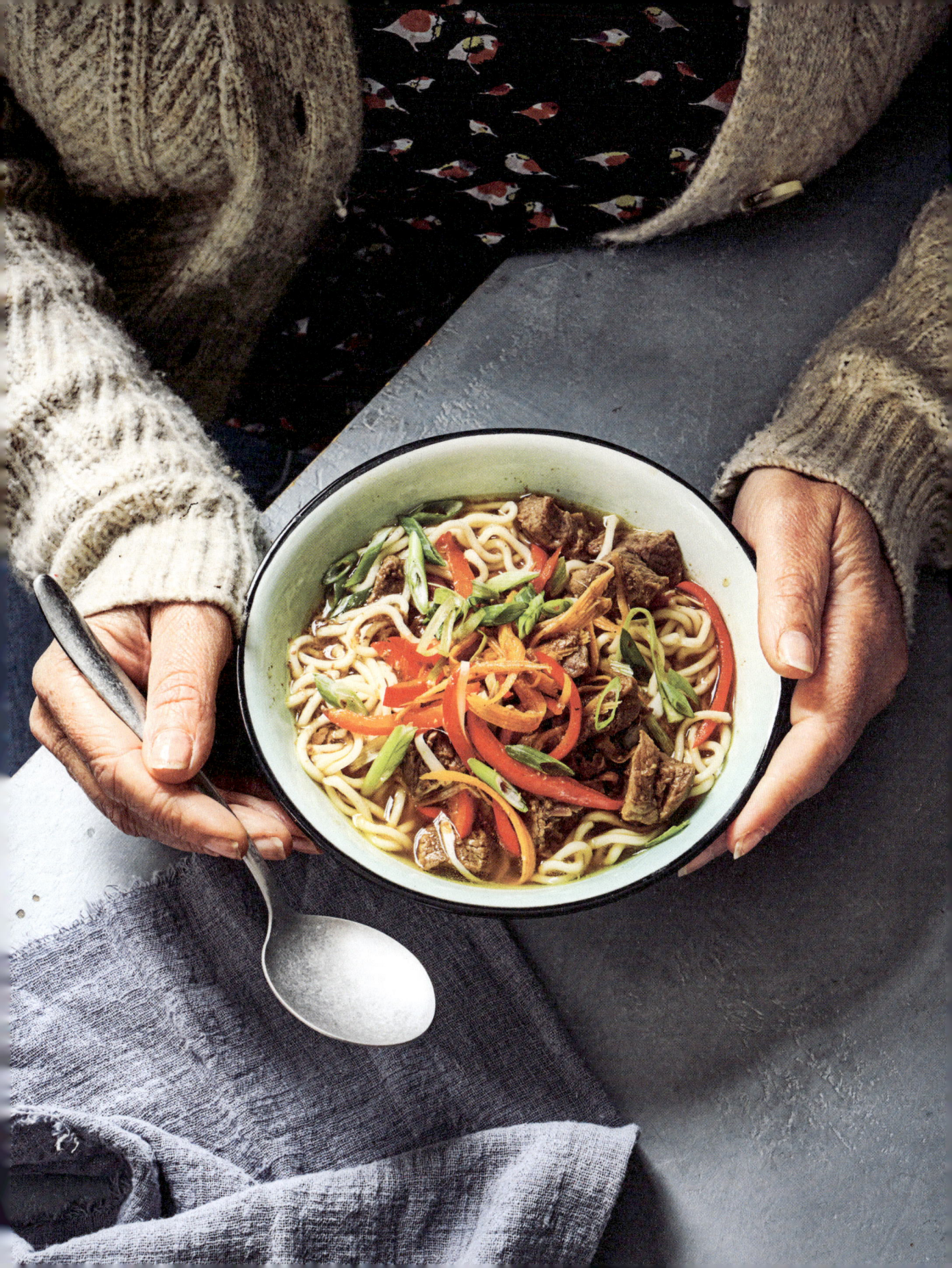

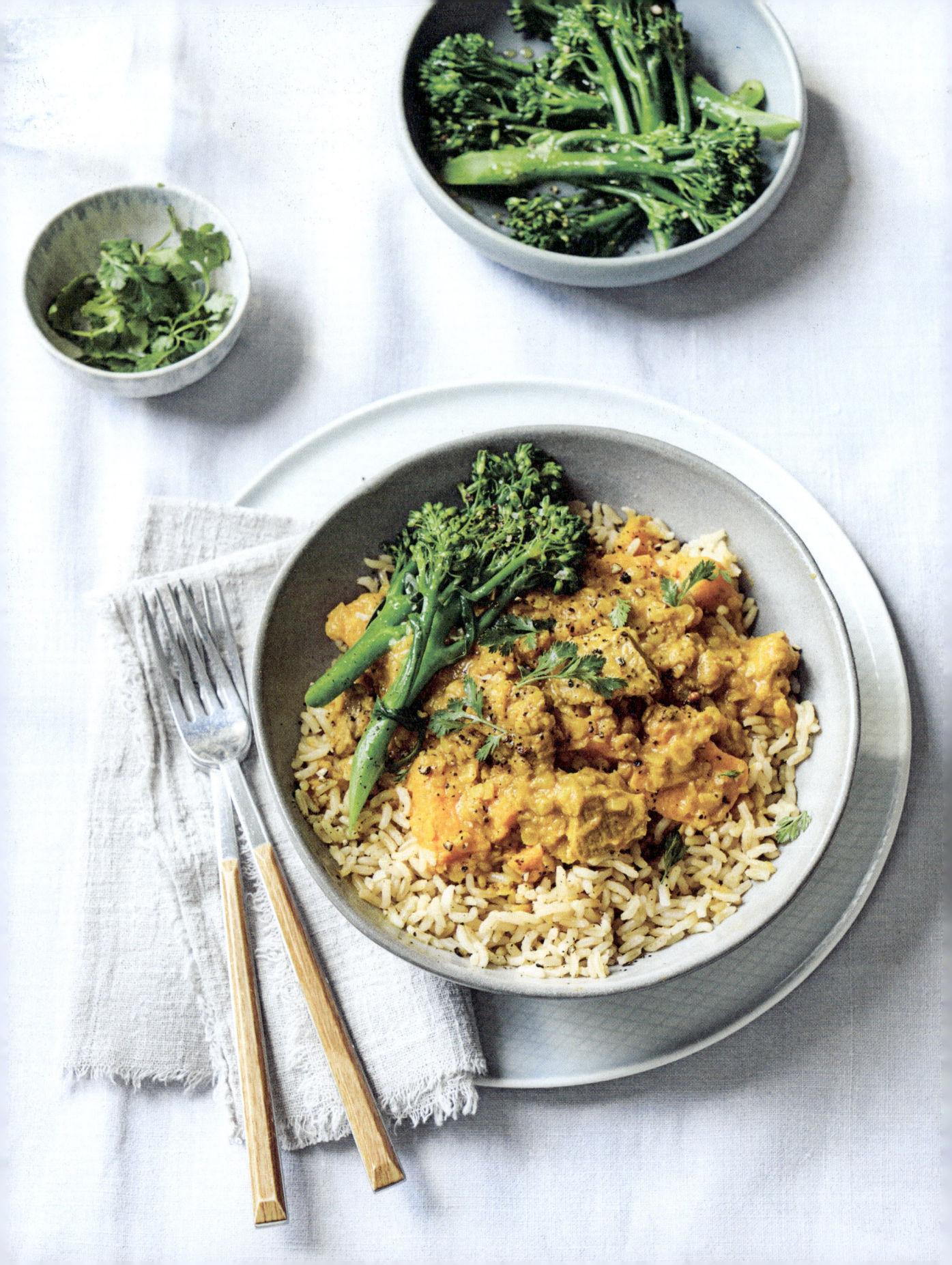

THAI-STYLE BEEF, SWEET POTATO & RED LENTIL CURRY

SERVES 6
PREP TIME 5 minutes
COOK TIME 5–6 hours (high);
7–8 hours (low)

400g (14oz) chopped lean braising beef

2 medium sweet potatoes (total weight 500g/1lb 2oz), peeled and chopped

300g (10½oz) red lentils

800ml (1 pint 8fl oz) hot beef stock

1 shallot, finely chopped

3 garlic cloves, crushed

4 tablespoons tomato purée

400g (14oz) can of light (reduced-fat) coconut milk

2 tablespoons red or green Thai curry paste (see note)

1 tablespoon garam masala

1 teaspoon ground turmeric

1 teaspoon ground ginger

1 teaspoon brown sugar

1 teaspoon coarse salt

Ready-made Thai curry paste makes a tasty base for this dish. Red lentils give the sauce a lovely thick texture as well as adding protein, fibre and other nutrients for great filling-power. I serve this with brown rice and Tenderstem broccoli.

1   Put all the ingredients into the slow-cooker bowl and cook on high for 5–6 hours, or low for 7–8 hours.

NOTE

There are so many different brands of Thai curry paste around and each can make a real difference to the flavour and spiciness of this dish. If you already have a favourite, that's great. If not, I have found that the supermarket own-brands don't seem to have half as much flavour as the more authentic tubs you can find in specialist supermarkets, or online. If you don't want it to be too spicy, you can always just add 1 tablespoon to start with, and, when the dish is cooked, give it a taste test to see how you feel about the strength of flavour. If you think it needs a bit more, then separately fry another 1 tablespoon of paste in 1 teaspoon of oil in a small frying pan for a couple of minutes, before stirring it through the curry.

PER SERVING

CALORIES	FAT	SAT FAT	CARBS	SUGARS	FIBRE	PROTEIN	SALT
412	10G	6.1G	43G	7.4G	14G	30G	1.4G

PORK GOULASH

SERVES 4
PREP TIME 10 minutes
COOK TIME 5–6 hours (high);
6–7 hours (low)

spray oil

1 large onion, halved and sliced

2 sweet peppers (red and yellow),
    deseeded and finely sliced

500g (1lb 2oz) lean pork, chopped

3 garlic cloves, crushed

400g (14oz) can of chopped
    tomatoes

3 tablespoons tomato purée

2 tablespoons red wine vinegar

2 teaspoons smoked paprika

1 teaspoon dried oregano

½ teaspoon cayenne pepper

100ml (3½fl oz) hot beef stock

2 bay leaves

1 teaspoon cornflour

salt and pepper

4 tablespoons reduced-fat crème
    fraîche, to serve

A classic comfort food dish, this Hungarian-inspired stew is seasoned with smoked paprika and, though the flavours are fairly simple, it's hearty, warming, comforting and satisfying. You can serve this up with rice or mashed potato, or Cannellini Bean Mash with Rosemary & Lemon (see page 198) and the green vegetables of your choice.

1   Spray a frying pan with oil and fry the onion for about 10 minutes while you prepare the rest of your ingredients.

2   Put all the ingredients apart from the crème fraîche, including the onion, into the slow-cooker bowl. Season with salt and pepper and mix everything together.

3   Cook on high for 5–6 hours, or low for 6–7 hours.

4   When you are ready to serve, stir the crème fraîche through the hot goulash.

NOTE

You can substitute the pork for beef, if you prefer, and customize the level of spiciness by adjusting the amount of cayenne pepper.

PER SERVING

CALORIES	FAT	SAT FAT	CARBS	SUGARS	FIBRE	PROTEIN	SALT
263	5.9G	2.6G	16G	13G	5.1G	32G	0.5G

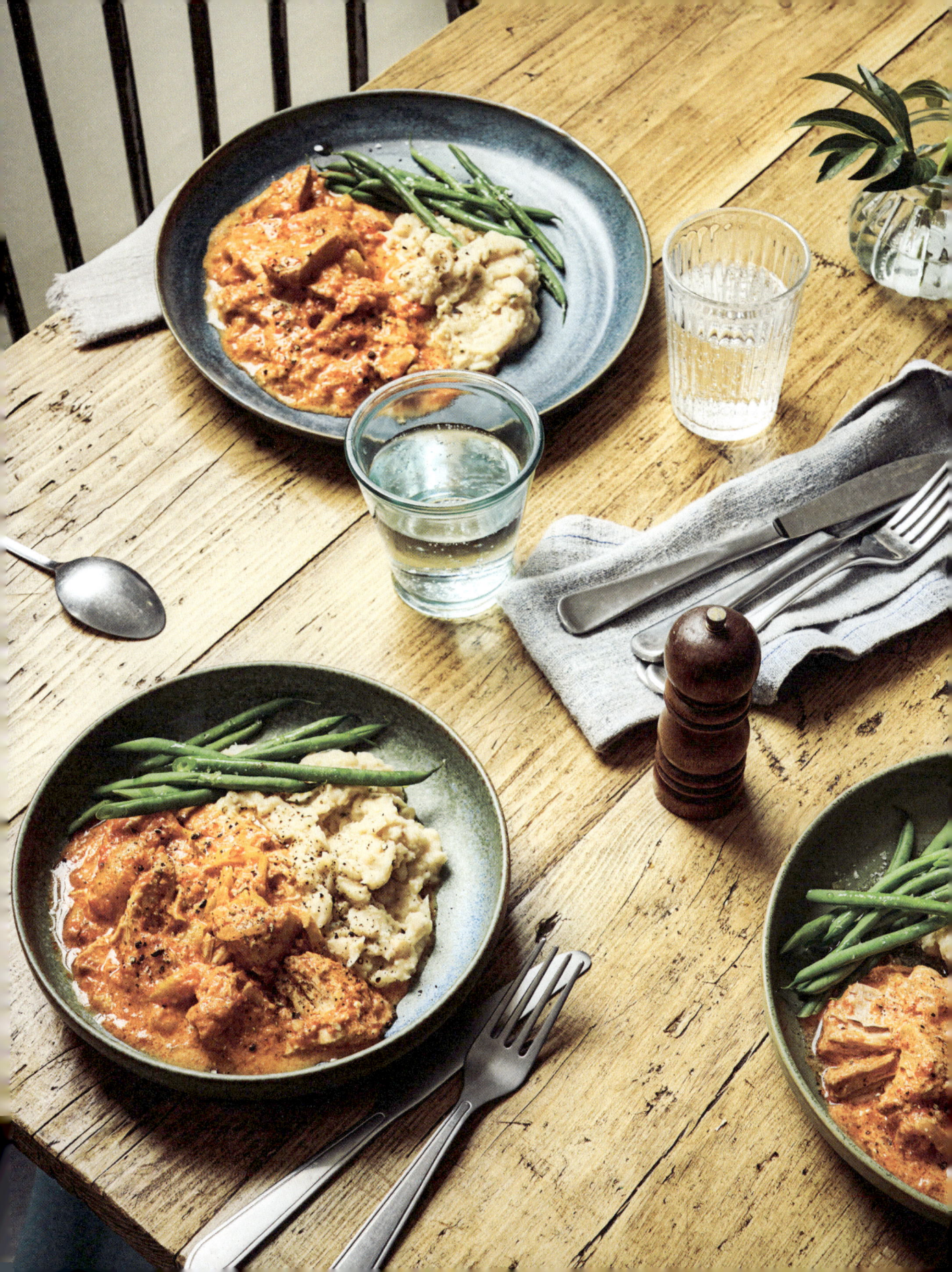

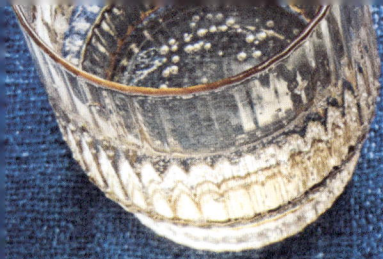

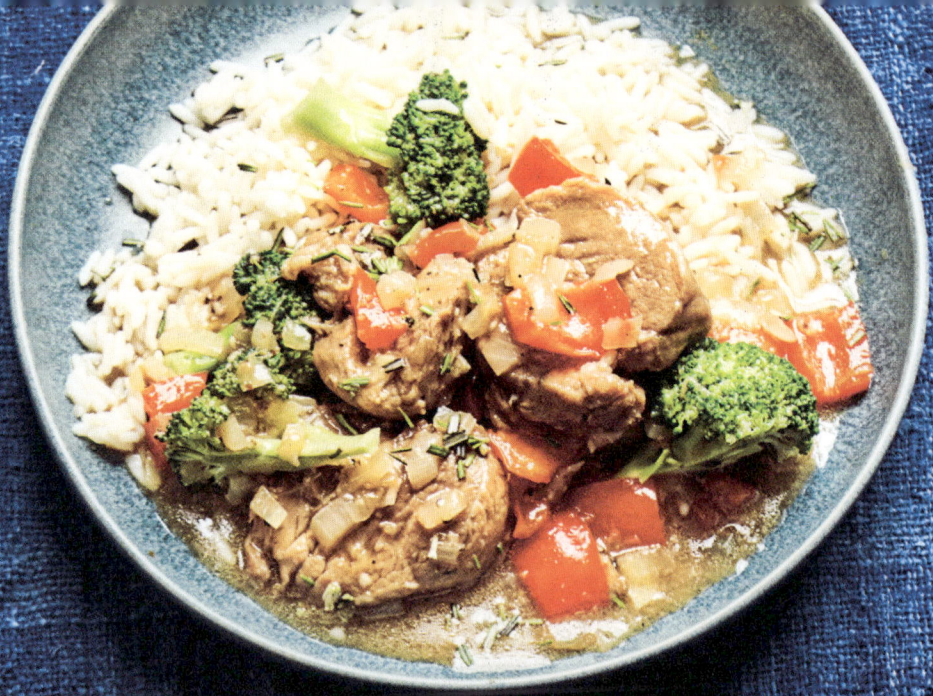

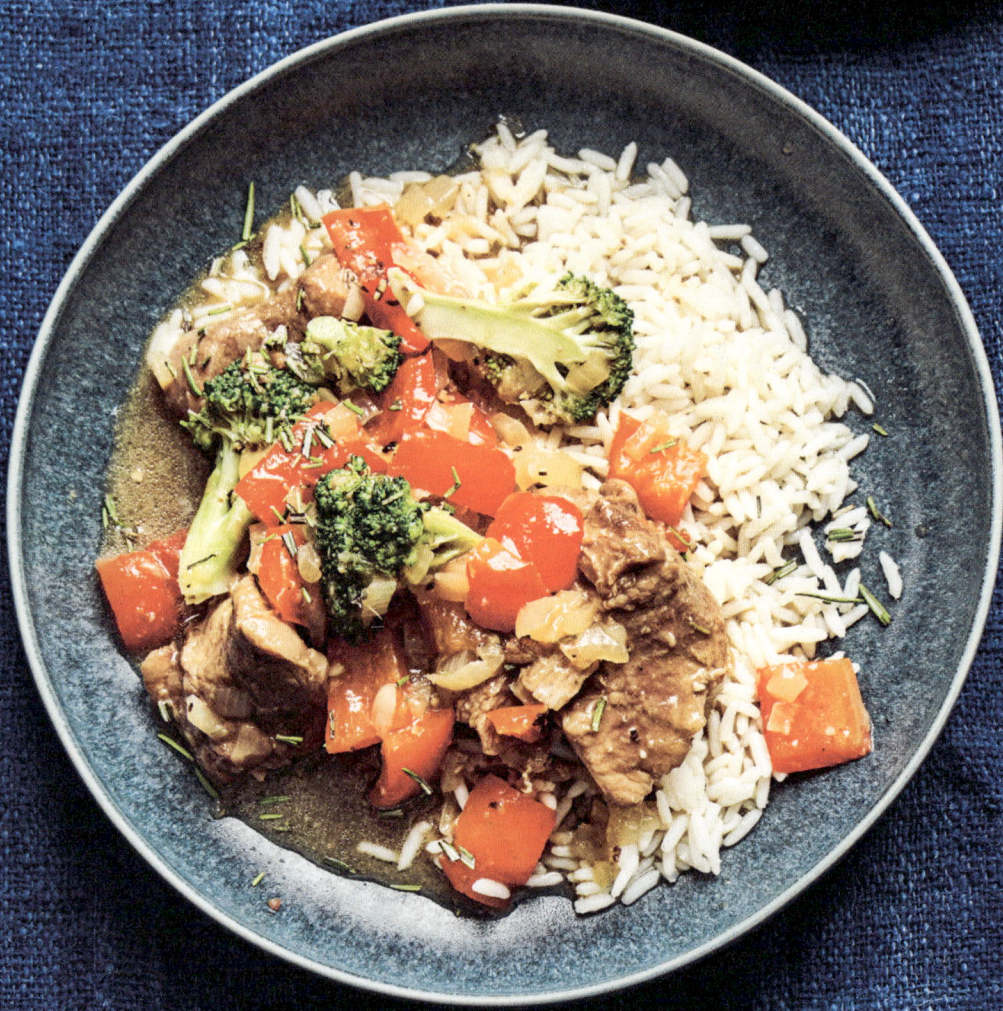

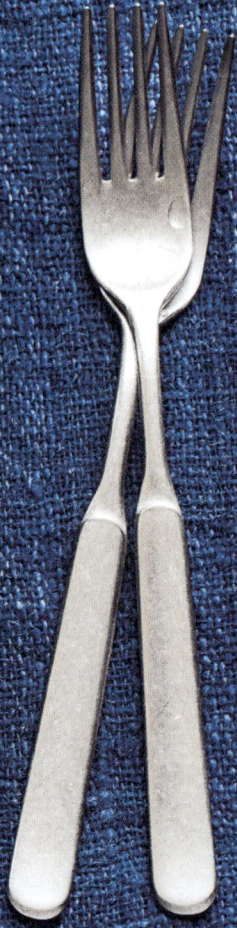

PEPPERY PORK

SERVES 4
PREP TIME 10 minutes
COOK TIME 2–3 hours (high);
4–5 hours (low)

1 pork tenderloin/fillet (total
   weight 500g/1lb 2oz)
3 sweet peppers, deseeded and
   chopped
2 onions, chopped
1 head of broccoli, cut into florets

FOR THE MARINADE
2 tablespoons dark soy sauce
2 tablespoons honey
1 tablespoon rice wine
1 tablespoon cornflour
2 teaspoons pepper
1 teaspoon ginger purée from a jar
1 teaspoon garlic purée from a jar
½ teaspoon dried rosemary

TO SERVE
sliced spring onions
sesame seeds

Tender pork with a flavourful marinade and a peppery kick.
Serve with white or wholegrain rice.

1   Make up the marinade by mixing all the ingredients in a bowl.

2   Slice the pork and mix with the marinade. Put the peppers, onions and pork mixture into the slow-cooker bowl and mix thoroughly.

3   Cook on high for 2–3 hours, or low for 4–5 hours, adding the broccoli 30 minutes before the end of cooking time.

4   Scatter with spring onions and sesame seeds, then serve.

NOTE

Fancy extra vegetables in this? Add 200g (7oz) button mushrooms or chopped carrots along with the onions and peppers.

CALORIES	FAT	SAT FAT	CARBS	SUGARS	FIBRE	PROTEIN	SALT
259	5.3G	2G	21G	16G	3.3G	30G	1.4G

PER SERVING

HONEY-LIME CHICKEN & BUTTERNUT SQUASH

SERVES 4
PREP TIME 5 minutes
COOK TIME 4–5 hours (high);
6–8 hours (low)

4 spring onions, sliced, reserve
   some for a garnish
750g (1lb 10oz) frozen butternut
   squash cubes
4 skinless chicken breasts
finely grated zest and juice of
   2 limes
2 garlic cloves, crushed
2 teaspoons peeled and finely
   grated root ginger, or ginger
   purée from a jar
2 tablespoons soy sauce
1 tablespoon apple cider vinegar
1 tablespoon honey
250ml (9fl oz) hot chicken stock
1 tablespoon cornflour
salt and pepper

Using frozen butternut squash chunks in this easy slow-cooker meal cuts down the prep time and means you can have this on and cooking in just 5 minutes! I serve this with rice.

1   Put the spring onions, butternut squash and chicken breasts into the slow-cooker bowl.

2   In a small bowl, mix the lime zest and juice, garlic, ginger, soy sauce, apple cider vinegar and honey. Pour this sauce into the slow-cooker bowl.

3   Pour in the hot stock. In a small bowl, mix the cornflour with a couple of tablespoons of cold water until there are no lumps, then pour this into the slow-cooker too and season with salt and pepper.

4   Mix everything together and cook on high for 4–5 hours, or low for 6–8 hours.

5   Use 2 forks to shred the chicken into the sauce before serving, scattered with the reserved spring onions.

NOTE

You can easily substitute fresh squash, if you prefer. Simply peel, deseed and cube the same weight (see page 70 for my method) before adding it to the slow-cooker. You can also add finely chopped red chilli, or chilli flakes, if you'd like a bit of heat in the dish.

PER SERVING

CALORIES	FAT	SAT FAT	CARBS	SUGARS	FIBRE	PROTEIN	SALT
326	2.5G	0.7G	26G	15G	4.6G	47G	2G

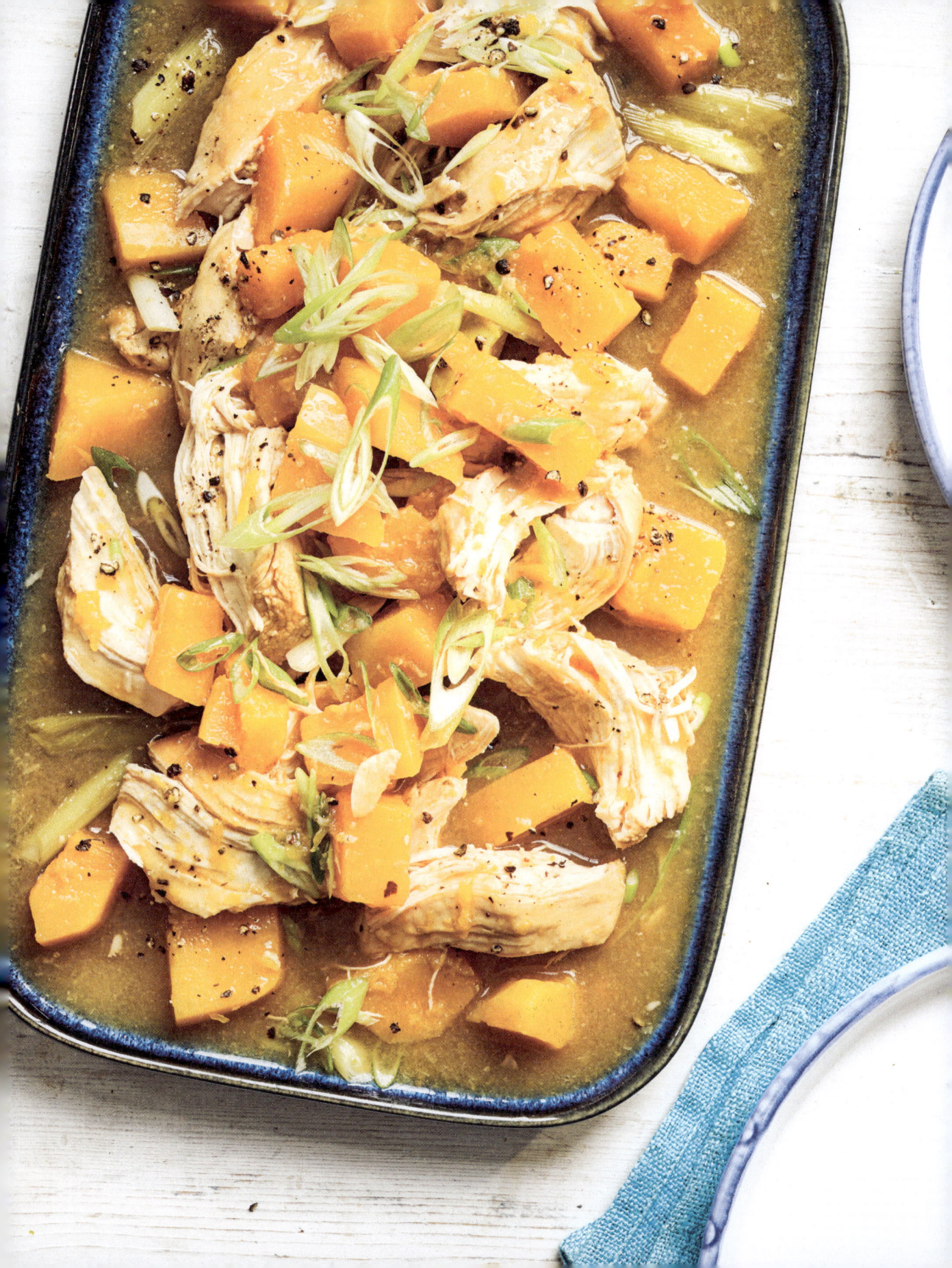

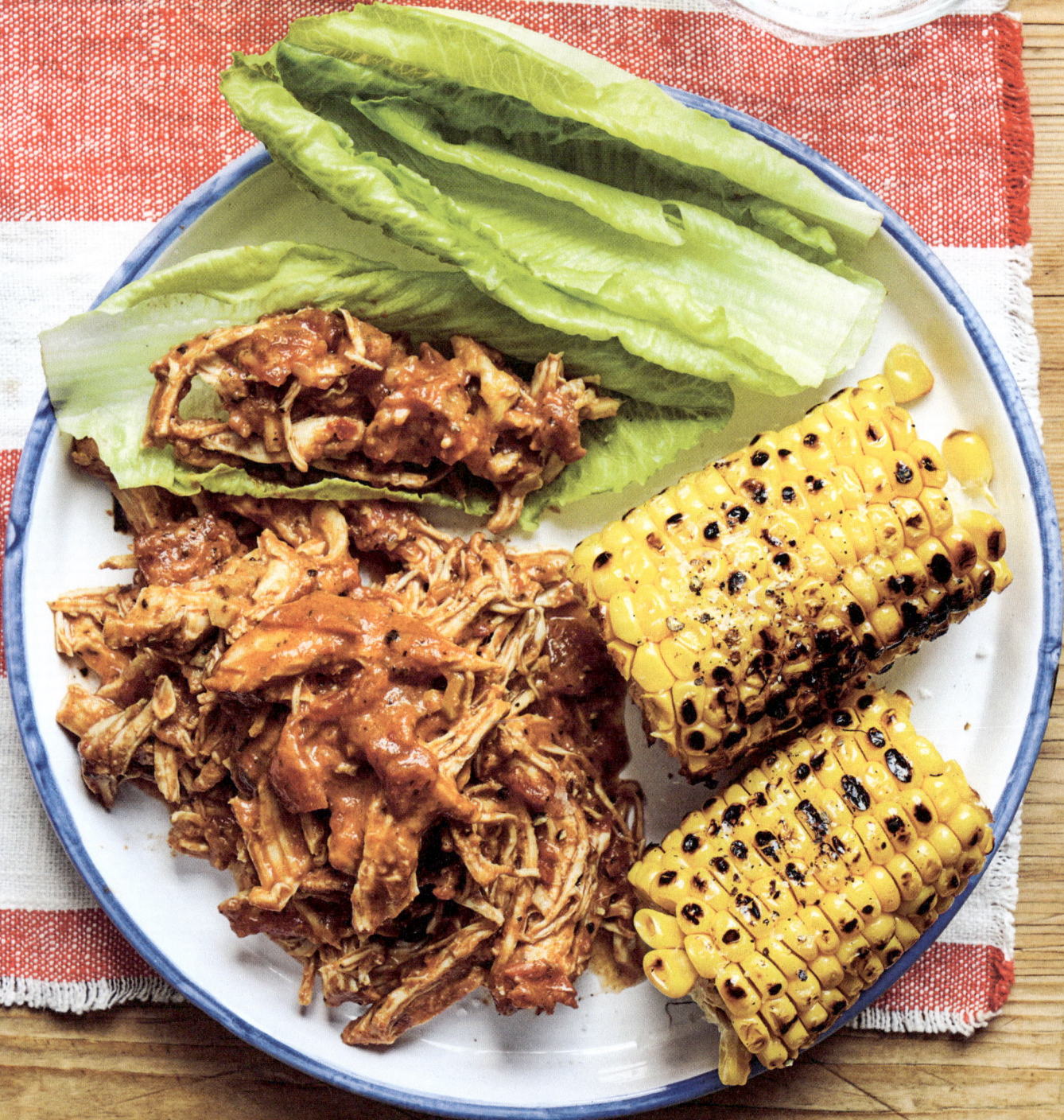

PULLED PERI-PERI CHICKEN

SERVES 4
PREP TIME 5 minutes
COOK TIME 4 hours (high);
6–8 hours (low)

4 skinless chicken breasts

1 tablespoon peri-peri seasoning

100ml (3½fl oz) peri-peri sauce,
  such as Nando's

400g (14oz) can of chopped
  tomatoes

1 chicken stock cube, crumbled

4 garlic cloves, crushed

50g (1¾oz) light (reduced-fat)
  cream cheese

salt and pepper

parsley leaves, or coriander,
  to serve

A fiery and flavour-packed pulled chicken, which has minimal prep but punchy flavour. This is perfect to serve with rice and vegetables, to add to wraps with crisp lettuce, or even to serve over homemade fries, to make 'dirty' fries.

1 Put the chicken breasts into the slow-cooker bowl and add the rest of the ingredients, except the herbs. Season with salt and pepper and give everything a good stir.

2 Cook on high for 4 hours, or low for 6–8 hours.

3 Use 2 forks to shred the chicken and mix it thoroughly with the sauce, scatter with the herbs and serve.

NOTE

To make pulled chicken in the oven, you need to cook it low and slow. Place all the ingredients except the herbs into a baking dish, cover tightly with foil and bake at 180°C/160°C fan (350°F), Gas Mark 4 for 1 hour. It should be tender enough to shred with 2 forks at this point, but if it's not, put it back in the oven and cook for another 10 minutes.

PER SERVING

CALORIES	FAT	SAT FAT	CARBS	SUGARS	FIBRE	PROTEIN	SALT
263	4.6G	1.6G	8.6G	6.7G	1.8G	45G	2.2G

BUTTER CHICKEN

SERVES 4
PREP TIME 10 minutes
COOK TIME 3–4 hours, plus 20 minutes (high); 6–7 hours, plus 20 minutes (low)

2 tablespoons (30g/1oz) butter

2 large, or 4 small onions, chopped

2 tablespoons tomato purée

1½ tablespoons garlic purée from a jar

1½ tablespoons ginger purée from a jar

2 tablespoons sweet (unsmoked) paprika

2 tablespoons garam masala

1½ teaspoon coarse salt

1 teaspoon ground cumin

1 teaspoon ground coriander

½ teaspoon cayenne pepper

½ teaspoon pepper

400g (14oz) can of chopped tomatoes

200ml (7fl oz) water

4 skinless chicken breasts, chopped into large chunks

250g (9oz) fat-free Greek yogurt

This slow-cooked butter chicken was a huge hit with my whole family. The recipe produces a flavoursome, rich curry sauce with tender chunks of chicken breast. I use a small amount of butter to fry the onions until they are soft and sweet, which then forms the tasty base for this sauce: this little bit of prep time is all you need before leaving the slow-cooker to do the rest of the work. There isn't any cream used, just fat-free yogurt, but there is still a real sense of indulgence to this meal. I like to serve this with basmati rice.

1   Melt the butter in a saucepan and fry the onions over a medium heat for 15 minutes, stirring regularly to prevent burning. You want them to be soft, sweet, and golden.

2   Add the tomato, garlic and ginger purées plus the paprika, garam masala, salt, cumin, coriander, cayenne and regular pepper and stir-fry for about 2 minutes. Tip in the chopped tomatoes and measured water, then stir everything together.

3   Use a stick blender to blend the tomato mixture into a smooth sauce, or alternatively transfer to a blender.

4   Pour the sauce into the slow cooker bowl, then add the chicken and give it a stir. Leave to cook on high for 3-4 hours, or low for 6-7 hours.

5   Before serving, scoop the yogurt on top of the curry and leave it in the slow-cooker bowl, lid on, for 10 minutes. This allows the yogurt to warm up before you stir it in, which helps to prevent it from splitting in the sauce.

6   Stir the yogurt into the sauce, then serve.

NOTE

The key to this tasty sauce is having the patience to cook the onions for the full 15 minutes in butter to get them lovely and sweet. You can swap out the butter if you wish, but that will affect the overall flavour.

PER SERVING

CALORIES	FAT	SAT FAT	CARBS	SUGARS	FIBRE	PROTEIN	SALT
387	10G	4.6G	18G	16G	5.7G	5.2G	2.9G

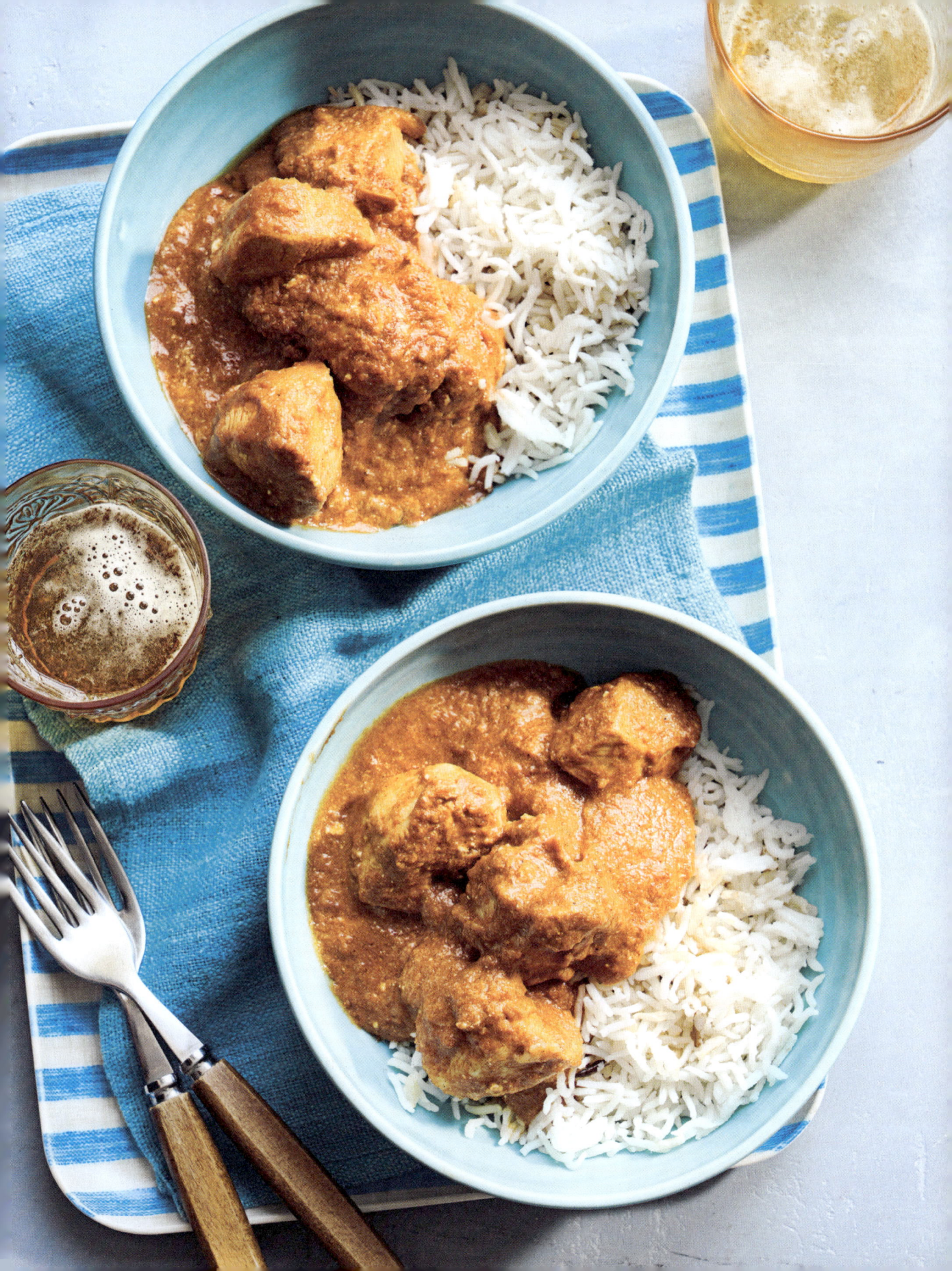

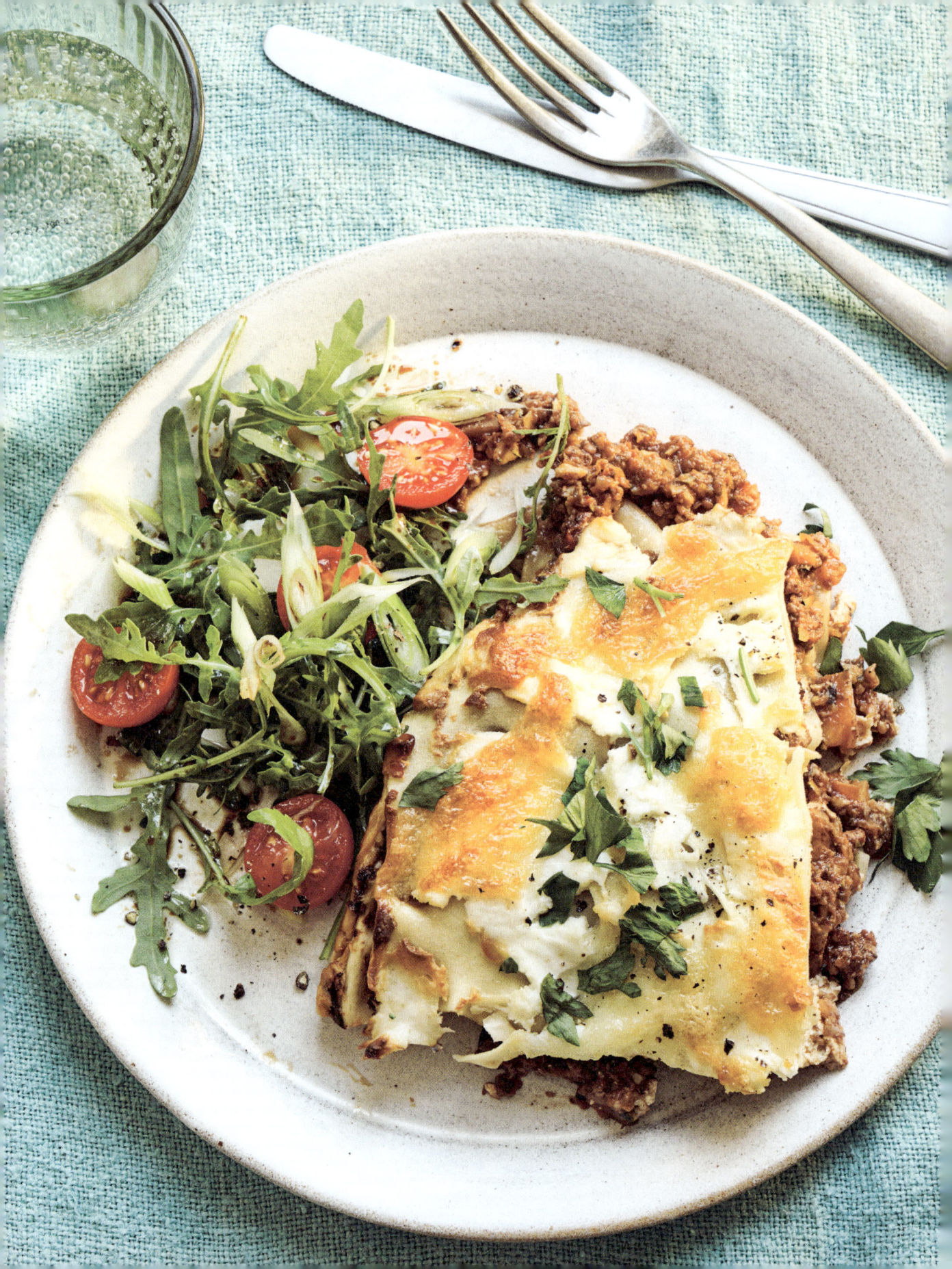

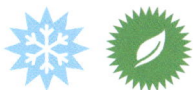

SCRUMMY VEGGIE LASAGNE

SERVES 4
PREP TIME 10 minutes
COOK TIME 2–3 hours (high);
5–6 hours (low)

2 carrots (total weight about 150g/5½oz), peeled and roughly chopped

250g (9oz) chestnut mushrooms, roughly chopped

1 courgette (about 250g/9oz), roughly chopped

50g (1¾oz) walnuts

400g (14oz) can of chopped tomatoes

2 tablespoons tomato purée

2 tablespoons pesto

1 teaspoon dried mixed herbs, plus more to sprinkle

1 teaspoon garlic granules

1 teaspoon coarse salt

½ teaspoon pepper

250g (9oz) ricotta cheese

100g (3½oz) fat-free cottage cheese

50ml (1¾fl oz) semi-skimmed milk

6–8 dried lasagne sheets

75g (2¾oz) mozzarella balls, torn into small pieces

A flavoursome, ragu-style vegetable sauce is layered with pasta sheets and ricotta to make this tasty lasagne. It is so easy to make, as you just blend everything together to make the sauce, so very little chopping! It's also great for fussy eaters, as the vegetables are well blended in so you can enjoy their flavours without any of the chunks or lumps that children might pick out. I like to serve this with a side salad.

1 Put the carrots, mushrooms, courgette and walnuts into the food processor and pulse a few times to chop them up a bit more finely.

2 Add the tomatoes, tomato purée, pesto, herbs, garlic granules, salt and pepper, then blend again. You want to chop everything finely, but keep a little texture in there, so don't go too far and blend it into a paste.

3 In a separate bowl, combine the ricotta, cottage cheese and milk, stirring together to make a creamy cheese sauce.

4 Spoon one-third of the vegetable mixture into the slow-cooker bowl and spread it into an even layer. Break up 2 lasagne sheets to go over the top, getting the best coverage you can. Spoon over one-third of the cheese sauce and spread carefully over the pasta to form another even layer.

5 Repeat each layer twice more, finishing with the cheese sauce, then top with the mozzarella dotted around evenly and a sprinkling of mixed herbs.

6 Cook on high for 2–3 hours, or low for 5–6 hours.

7 If you want a browned top, you can pop the slow-cooker bowl under a hot grill for a few minutes at the end of cooking.

NOTE

You can add different vegetables to this depending on what needs using up: sweet peppers, aubergines, sweet potatoes and butternut squash all work well. If you're adding onion or leek, fry these until they are soft before blending with the other ingredients.

PER SERVING

CALORIES	FAT	SAT FAT	CARBS	SUGARS	FIBRE	PROTEIN	SALT
455	25G	9.3G	31G	13G	5.1G	22G	1.9G

FEASTS WITH FRIENDS

7

CREAMY SWEET POTATO & CHICKEN CURRY

SERVES 8
PREP TIME 15 minutes
COOK TIME 50 minutes

spray oil
2 onions, chopped
6 skinless chicken breasts, chopped
2 teaspoons garlic purée from a jar, or 4 garlic cloves, crushed
2 teaspoons ginger purée from a jar, or 5cm (2 inches) root ginger, peeled and finely grated
2 tablespoons tomato purée
500g (1lb 2oz) tomato passata
400g (14oz) can of light (reduced-fat) coconut milk
600ml (20fl oz) hot chicken stock
200g (7oz) red lentils
3 medium sweet potatoes (total weight about 600g/1lb 5oz), peeled and chopped into 1cm (½ inch) cubes

FOR THE SPICE MIX
1 tablespoon mild curry powder
1 tablespoon cumin seeds
1 tablespoon ground coriander
1 teaspoon ground turmeric
1 teaspoon coarse salt
½ teaspoon ground cinnamon
½ teaspoon pepper

A crowd-pleasing curry, perfect for feeding a group, with a mild and creamy sauce thickened with red lentils and full of tender chicken and sweet potato. If I'm cooking curry for a big group, I tend to keep the heat levels low to accommodate most palates, then offer finely chopped chilli or chilli sauce on the side for anyone who prefers it a little more fiery. Please note that you'll need a large cooking pot for this... I only just squeezed it into my 30cm (12 inch) shallow cast-iron casserole dish! I serve it with basmati rice, mango chutney, lime pickle and/or aubergine pickle and sometimes mini naans on the side, another curried vegetable dish, such as saag aloo, or my Aloo Tikki (see page 214).

1 Make up the spice mix in a small bowl by mixing all the ingredients together.

2 Choose a large flameproof casserole dish with a capacity of at least 3.65 litres (6¼ pints), Spray it with oil and fry the onions for 5 minutes.

3 Add the chicken pieces and stir-fry for another 5 minutes.

4 Now add the garlic, ginger and tomato purées, tip in the spice mix and stir-fry for 2 minutes. Add the passata, coconut milk and hot stock to the pan and bring to a gentle simmer.

5 Add the lentils and sweet potatoes to the pan and return to a simmer. Gently simmer for 40 minutes, stirring occasionally, by which time the sauce should have thickened. If it's still a bit watery, simmer it for a little longer until you have a creamy consistency.

NOTE

A few handfuls of baby spinach, or frozen spinach, stirred through in the last few minutes add extra nutrients and colour to this curry. You can change out the sweet potato for butternut squash, if you prefer. To really speed up the prep time, you can use frozen chopped onion, sweet potato and even pre-chopped chicken.

PER SERVING

CALORIES	FAT	SAT FAT	CARBS	SUGARS	FIBRE	PROTEIN	SALT
402	7.3G	3.8G	37G	12G	5.7G	41G	1.8G

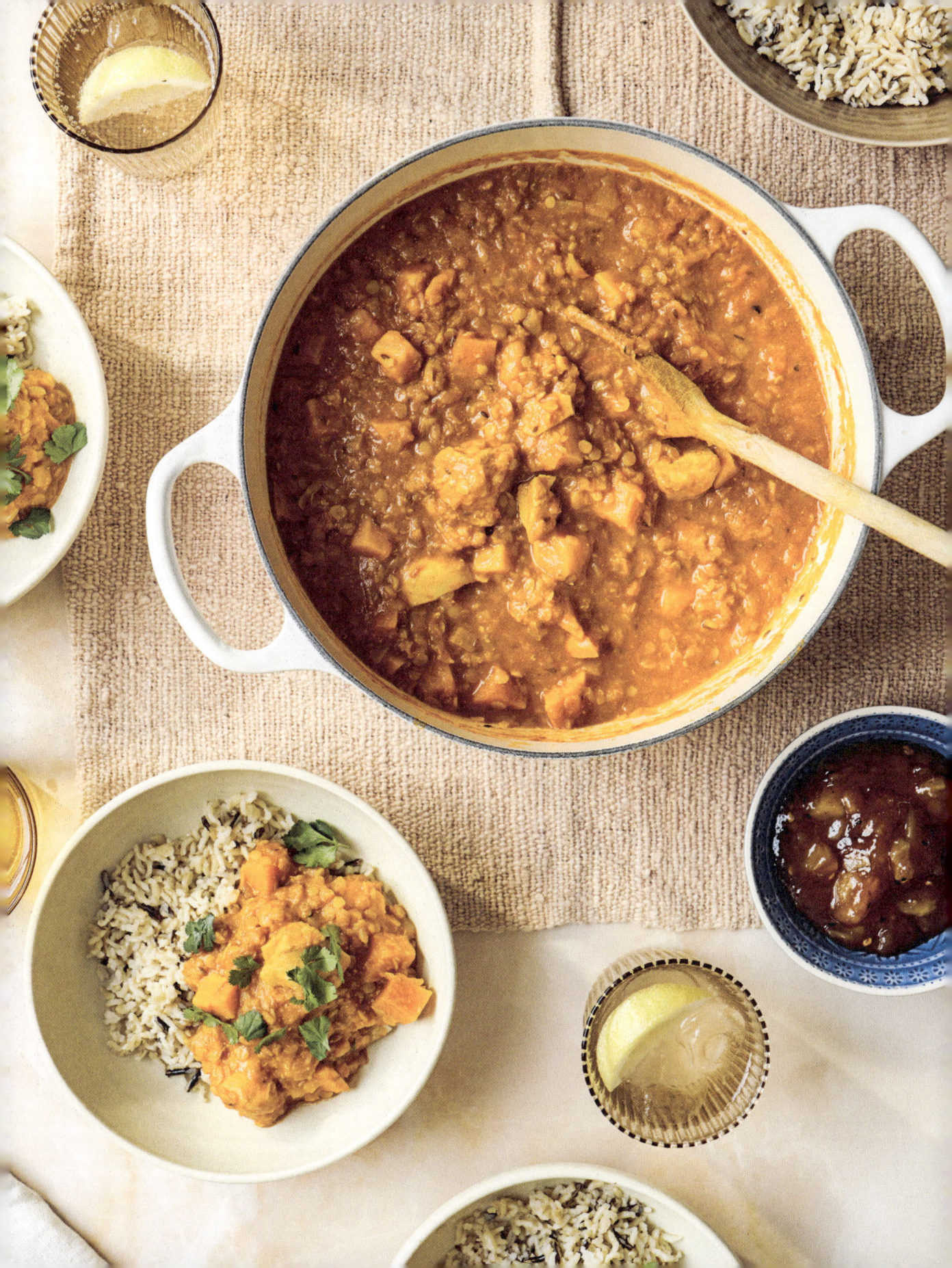

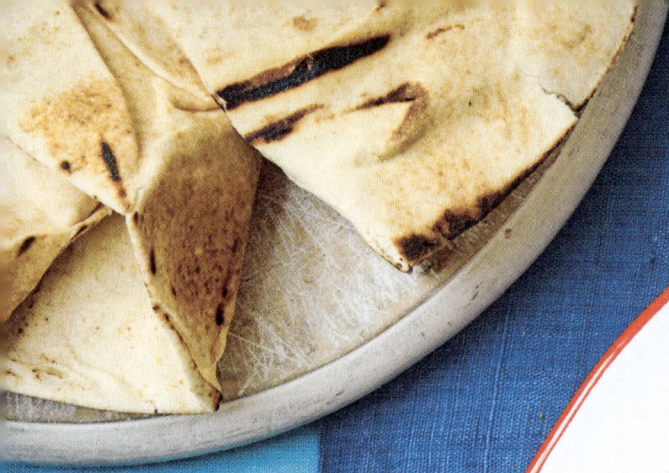

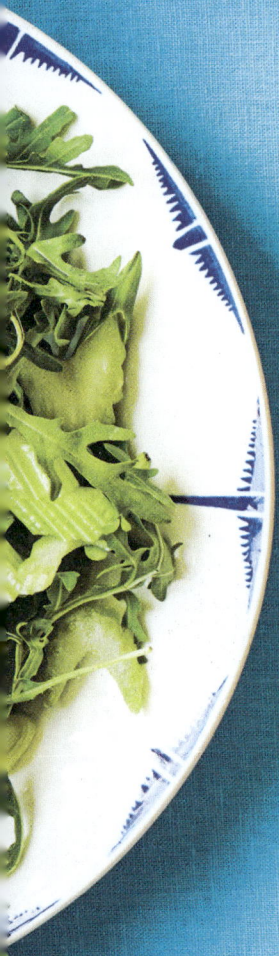

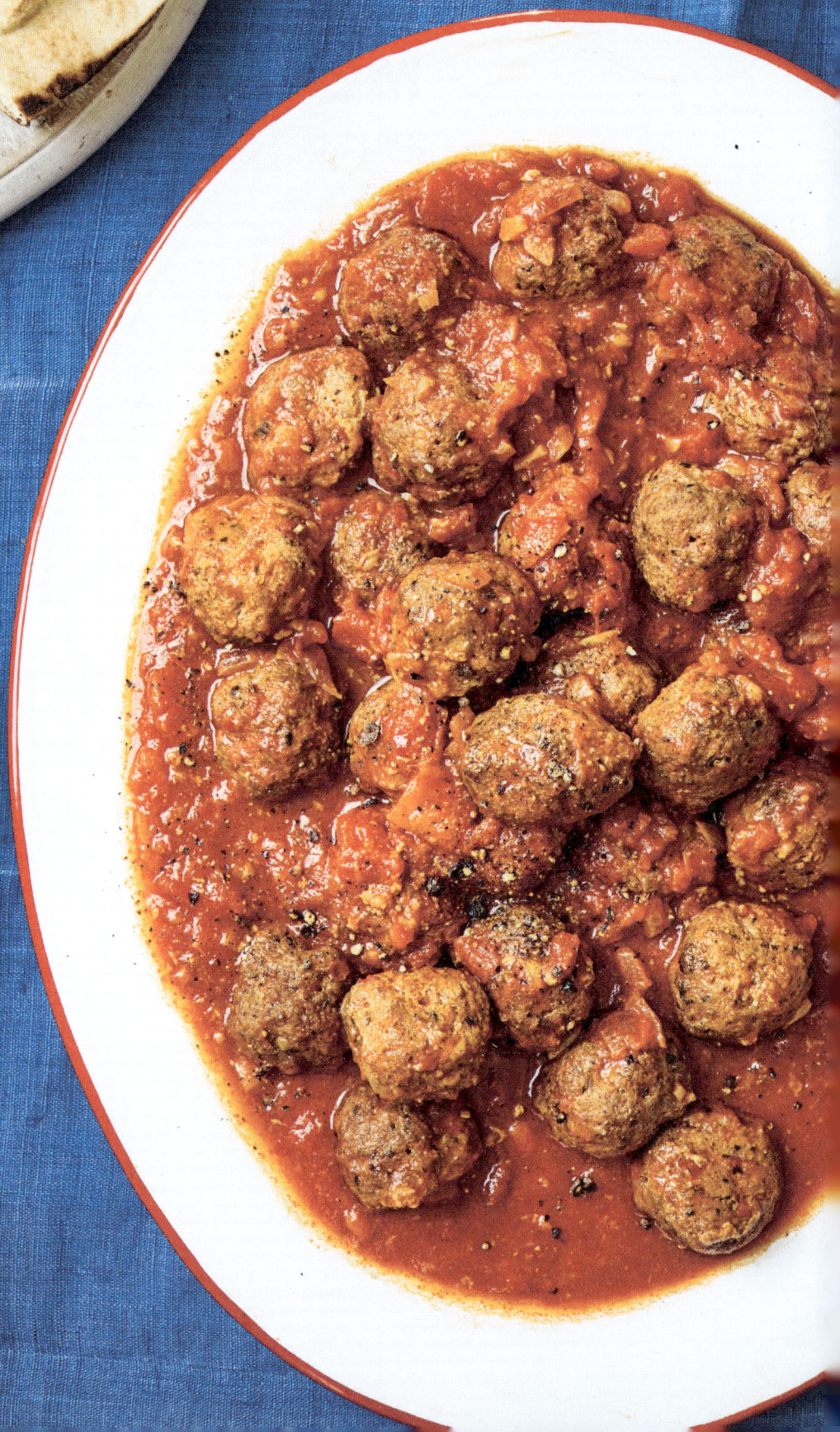

SERVES 8
PREP TIME 15 minutes
COOK TIME 35 minutes

KOFTA-STYLE MEATBALLS IN HARISSA SAUCE

FOR THE MEATBALLS

500g (1lb 2oz) minced lamb

500g (1lb 2oz) lean minced beef (less than 5 per cent fat)

2 tablespoons dried oregano

2 tablespoons sweet (unsmoked) paprika

1 tablespoon garlic granules

1 tablespoon onion granules

1 teaspoon mild chilli powder

1 egg, lightly beaten

salt and pepper

FOR THE SAUCE

spray oil

1 large onion, finely chopped

1 tablespoon garlic purée from a jar, or 4 garlic cloves, crushed

2 x 400g (14oz) cans of chopped tomatoes

400ml (14fl oz) water

2 tablespoons harissa paste

2 tablespoons tomato purée

1 tablespoon honey

TO SERVE

large handful of parsley leaves, finely chopped

large handful of mint leaves, finely chopped

juice of 1 lemon

These tasty meatballs, a mixture of minced lamb and beef, are served up in a rich and mildly spiced harissa sauce to make a meal perfect for a big family get-together. They work really well with brown or white rice, a bulgur wheat salad (see page 188), or couscous. Depending on how many people I'm feeding, I might add flatbreads and green salad on the side.

1 Preheat the oven to 220°C/200°C fan (425°F), Gas Mark 7.

2 Combine all the meatball ingredients in a large bowl, season well and use a wooden spoon to thoroughly mix everything together. Use your hands to shape meatballs 2.5–3cm (1–1¼ inches) in diameter and place them on an extra-large baking tray, leaving a little space between each (use 2 baking trays if necessary).

3 Put the tray of meatballs into the oven and bake for 15 minutes.

4 Meanwhile, make the sauce. Spray a large, deep saucepan with oil and stir-fry the onion for 8 minutes until softened, then stir in the garlic.

5 Add the tomatoes, measured water, harissa, tomato purée and honey, season with salt and pepper, stir together and leave simmering while the meatballs are cooking.

6 When the meatballs are ready, remove the tray from the oven and use a slotted spoon to lift them into the pan of sauce (leave behind any fat that has drained out of them). Once all the meatballs have been added to the pan, leave to simmer for 20 minutes, stirring every now and again.

7 After 20 minutes of simmering, the sauce should have thickened and reduced. Stir in the herbs and lemon juice, then serve.

NOTE

To make this into a more substantial meal, or to feed more people, you can add 2 x 400g (14oz) cans of drained chickpeas to the sauce at the same time as the meatballs. Some spinach stirred through for the last few minutes also makes a great addition. If you are serving this with brown rice, try adding some toasted sunflower and pumpkin seeds to it, as well as a handful of chopped herb leaves, to make it look a bit more special.

PER SERVING

CALORIES	FAT	SAT FAT	CARBS	SUGARS	FIBRE	PROTEIN	SALT
308	16G	6.8G	11G	9.2G	1.8G	28G	0.5G

SUMAC ROAST CHICKEN, POTATO & CARROT TRAYBAKE

SERVES 8
PREP TIME 15 minutes
COOK TIME 45 minutes

16 skinless chicken thigh fillets, excess fat trimmed away

1.5kg (3lb 5oz) baby potatoes, halved if large

750g (1lb 10oz) carrots, peeled, halved lengthways, then sliced on the diagonal into 3–4cm (1¼–1½ inch) pieces

2 tablespoons olive oil

salt

FOR THE MARINADE

2 tablespoons sumac

2 tablespoons tomato purée

2 tablespoons red wine vinegar

1 tablespoon garlic purée from a jar, or 4 garlic cloves, crushed

2 teaspoons dried thyme, or fresh thyme leaves

1 teaspoon chilli flakes

1 teaspoon coarse salt

1 teaspoon olive oil

½ teaspoon ground cinnamon

finely grated zest and juice of 1 lemon

TO SERVE (OPTIONAL)

chopped parsley leaves

pomegranate seeds

shelled unsalted pistachios

Sumac has an amazing tangy flavour, which pairs perfectly with chicken in this easy traybake that both adults and children will enjoy. There is very little preparation involved, and it looks and tastes great. Serve it with either fresh green vegetables (asparagus, broccoli, green beans or courgette ribbons) or a crunchy green salad. For a larger group, serve with flatbreads, and a side such as Big Bold Bulgur Salad (see page 188). You will need two large baking trays to accommodate everything here – just make sure all the ingredients are in a single layer, to ensure that everything cooks evenly.

1   Preheat the oven to 220°C/200°C fan (425°F), Gas Mark 7.

2   Make the marinade by mixing all the ingredients together in a bowl, then pour it over the chicken thighs and mix thoroughly to coat. Set aside while you get the vegetables on to roast.

3   Divide the potatoes and carrots equally between 2 large baking trays. Drizzle 1 tablespoon of the oil into each baking tray and mix around to make sure everything is coated in oil. Spread out the potatoes and carrots on each tray and make sure everything is in a single layer, then sprinkle some salt over each tray.

4   Put both trays into the oven and roast for 15 minutes.

5   After 15 minutes, remove the trays from the oven, give them a stir, then place 8 chicken thigh fillets on each tray, spaced apart among the vegetables. I always face up the 'rougher' side of the chicken, as this way you will get some nice little charred edges as it cooks.

6   Return to the oven and roast for 30 minutes. Halfway through the cooking time, swap each tray's position, so each gets a turn at the hottest part of the oven (usually at the top). The chicken should be cooked through with some charred edges, the carrots softly roasted and the potatoes golden and tender – if you think it needs a bit longer, then just put it back into the oven for a few minutes longer.

7   I serve these in the trays on the table. If I want it to look a bit more fancy, I scatter it with parsley, pomegranate seeds and pistachios.

PER SERVING (EXCLUDING OPTIONAL SERVING SUGGESTIONS)

CALORIES	FAT	SAT FAT	CARBS	SUGARS	FIBRE	PROTEIN	SALT
434	11G	2.5G	34G	9.3G	5.6G	46G	1.3G

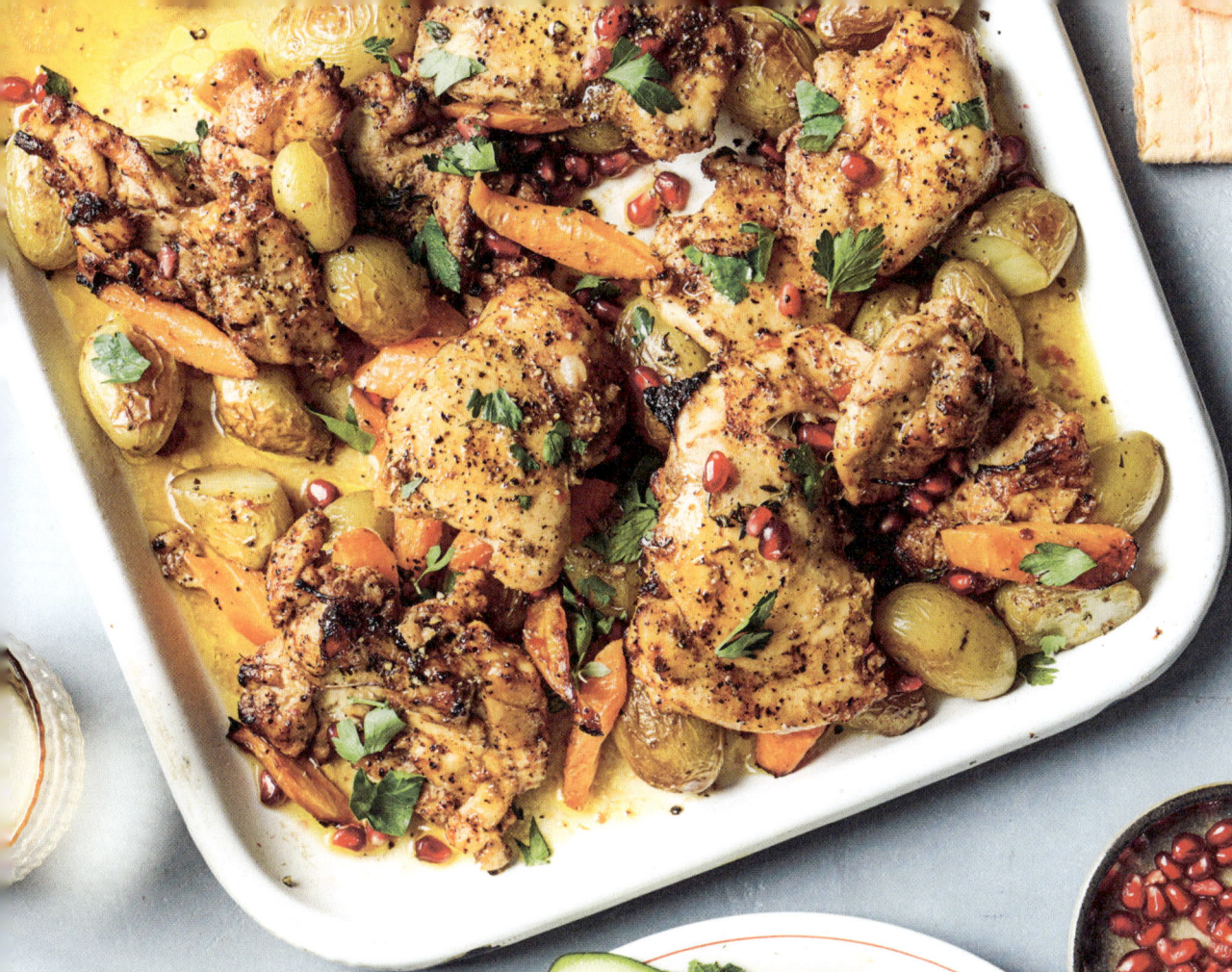

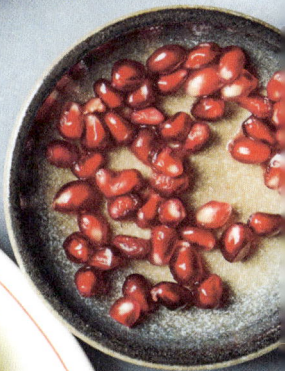

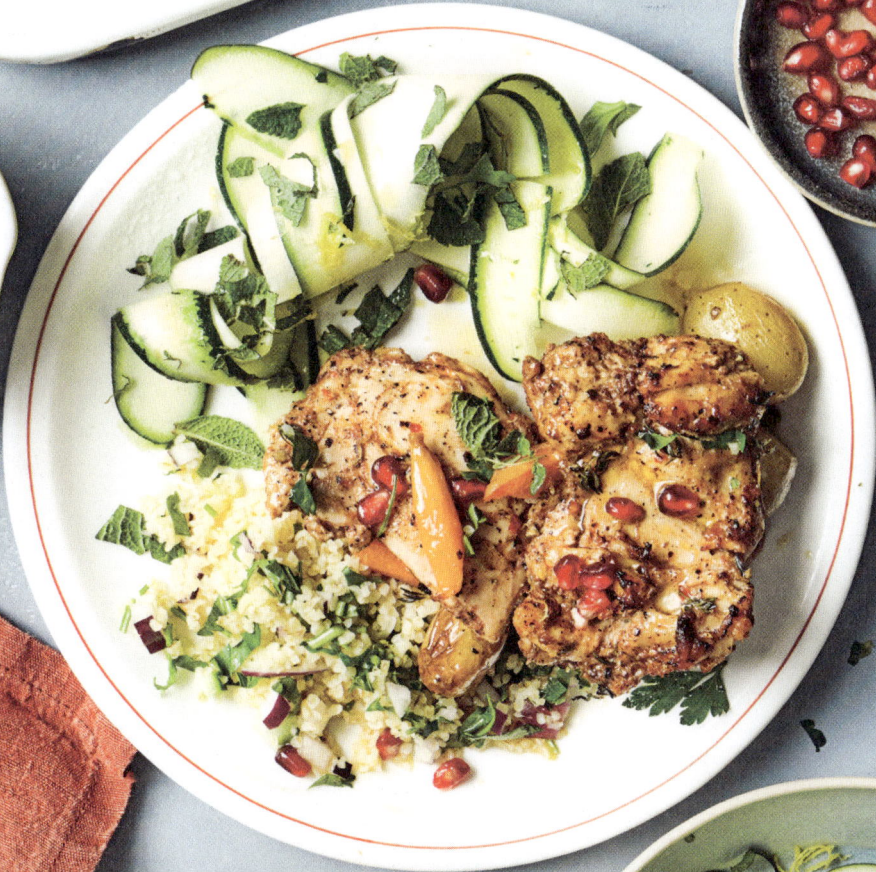

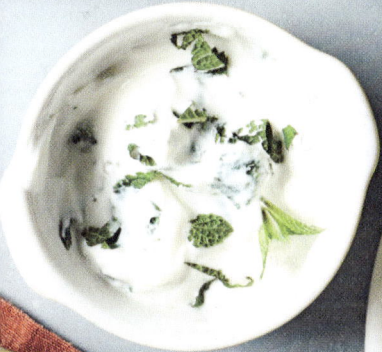

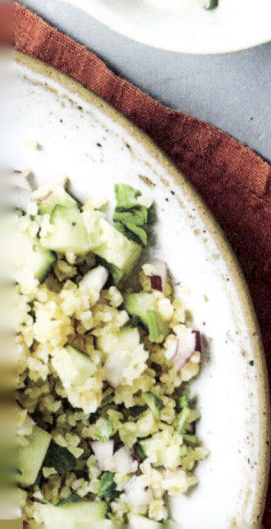

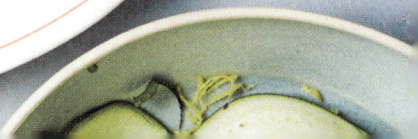

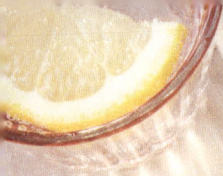

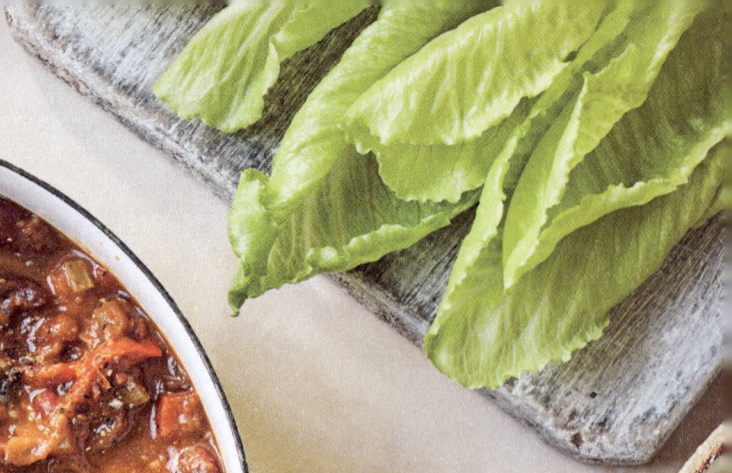

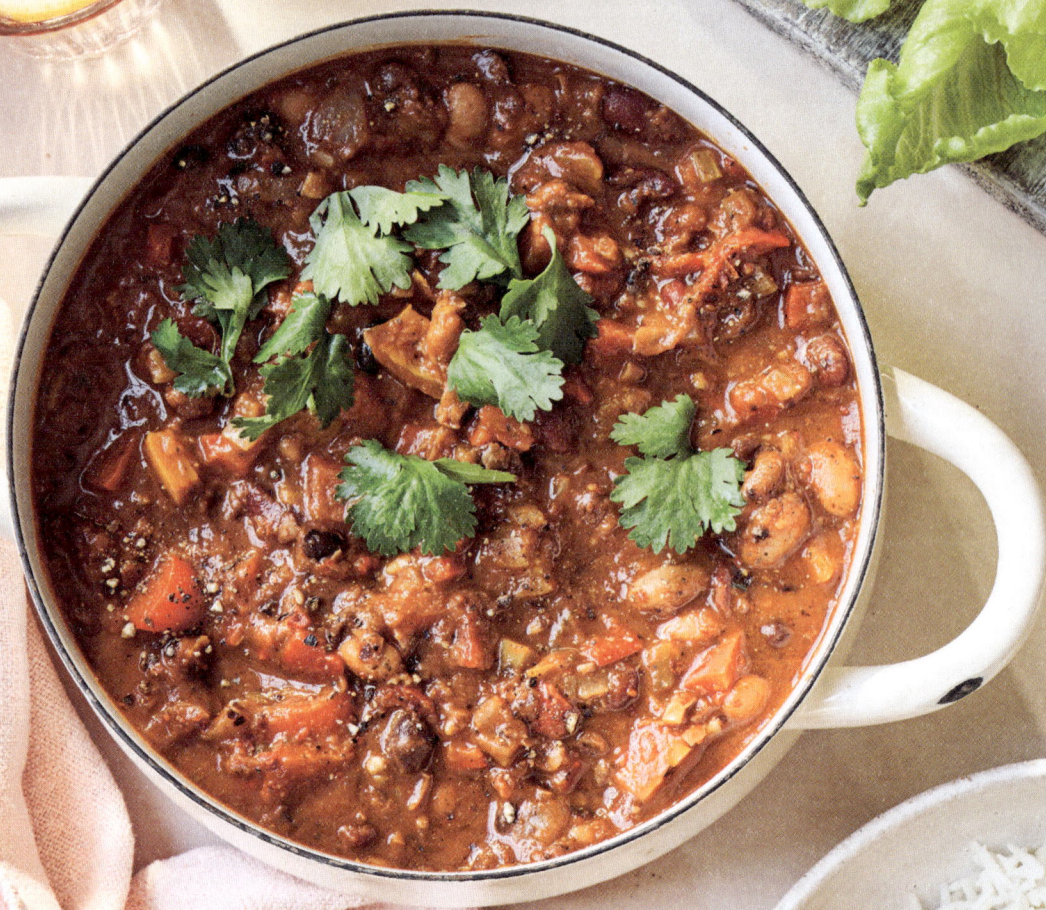

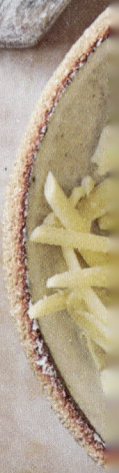

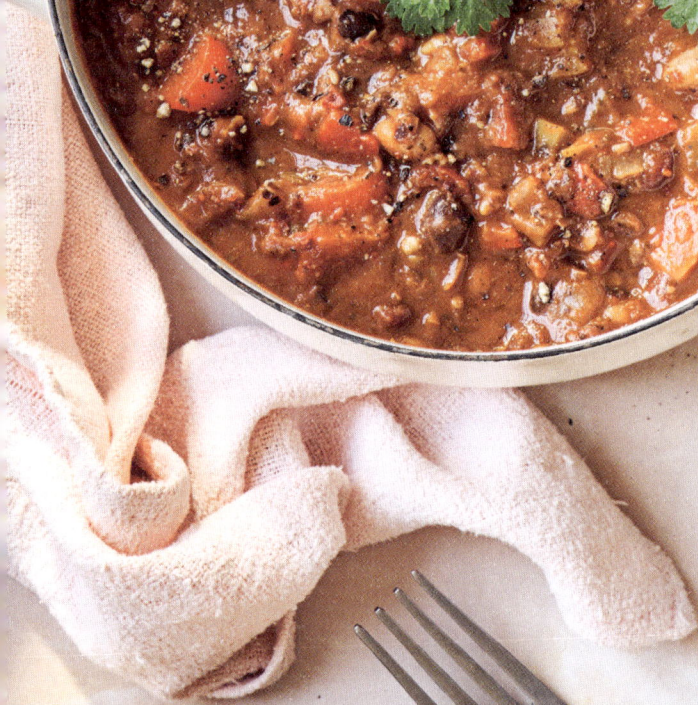

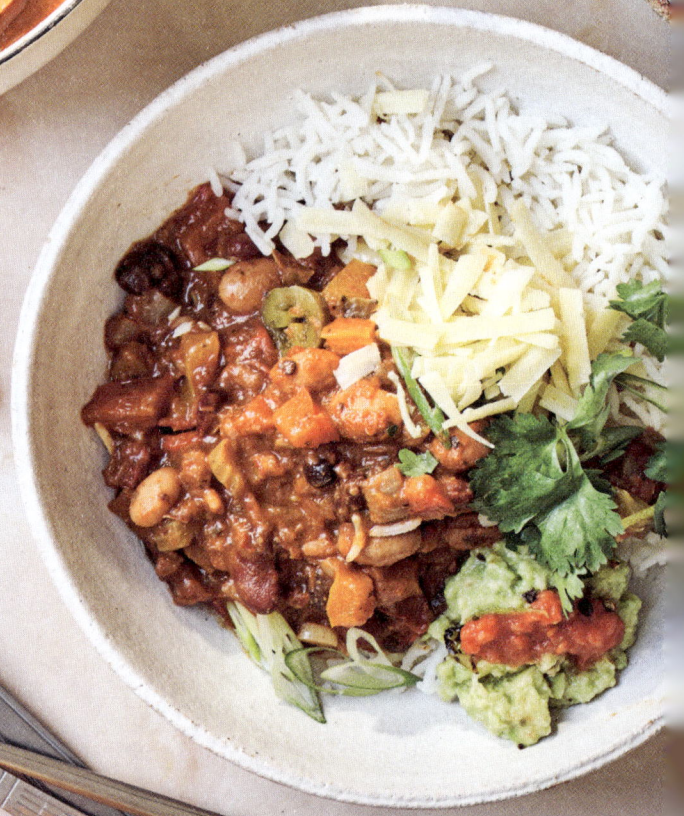

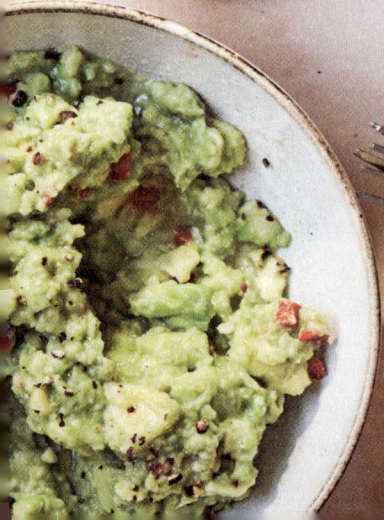

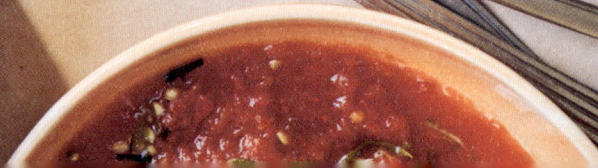

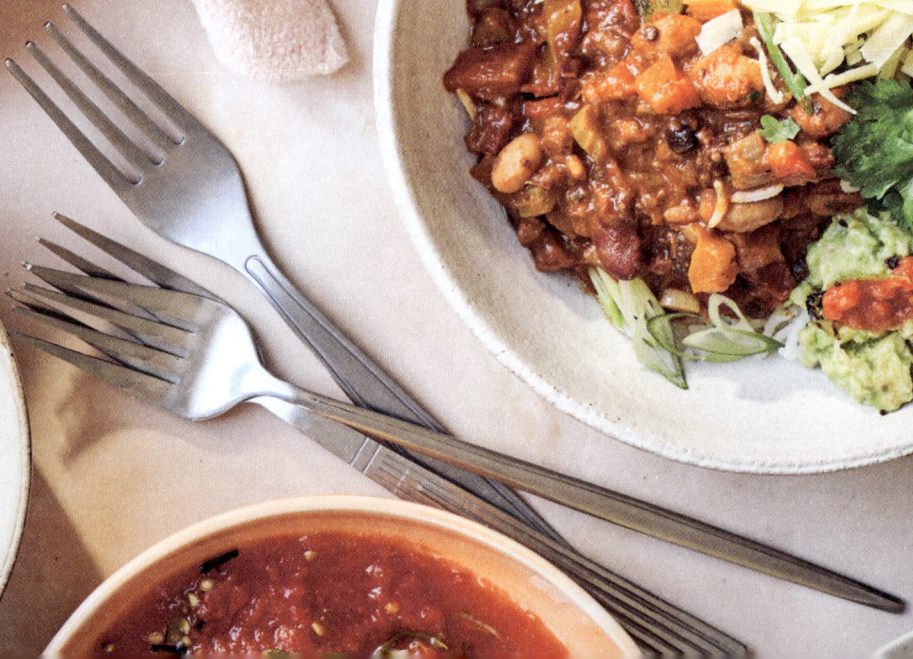

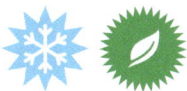

SWEET PEPPER THREE-BEAN CHILLI

SERVES 8
PREP TIME 20 minutes
COOK TIME 1 hour

FOR THE REFRIED BEANS

400g (14oz) can of pinto beans

2 tablespoons pickled jalapeños

4 garlic cloves

2 tablespoons red wine vinegar

finely grated zest and juice of 1 lime

1 tablespoon smoked paprika

1 tablespoon ground cumin

½ teaspoon ground cinnamon

FOR THE CHILLI

1 tablespoon olive oil

2 onions, chopped

2 celery sticks, chopped

4 sweet peppers (red, orange or yellow), deseeded and chopped

2 roast peppers (from a jar), chopped

2 x 400g (14oz) cans of chopped tomatoes

400ml (14fl oz) water

4 tablespoons tomato purée

1 tablespoon dried oregano

1 tablespoon cocoa powder

1 tablespoon maple syrup, or honey

2 teaspoons chipotle chilli flakes, or chipotle chilli paste

400g (14oz) can of pinto beans

400g (14oz) can of black beans

400g (14oz) can of kidney beans

salt and pepper

My mission here was to make a veggie chilli that I would enjoy eating as much as the meat-based version! Quite often, if you are cooking for a bigger group of friends, there will be a vegetarian in the mix and this recipe is perfect to have up your sleeve for that scenario. I make a refried bean mix to add to the sauce, which helps make it thick, rich and flavoursome. Serve with all of the usual favourite chilli additions: brown or white rice, guacamole, tortilla chips, salsa (try my Two-Minute Salsa on page 209), grated cheese, coriander leaves... whatever you fancy, really. This can make a great spread for a group of people, or simply a nice big batch of chilli so you can stash a few portions in the freezer.

1   To make the refried bean mix, put all the ingredients in a mini chopper and blend until smooth.

2   For the chilli, heat the oil in your biggest pot (or you may have to split between 2 pans) and stir-fry the onions and celery for 8 minutes, until they have softened. Add the raw peppers and stir-fry for another 5 minutes.

3   Add the refried bean mix and stir-fry for about 2 minutes.

4   Add the roast peppers, chopped tomatoes, measured water, tomato purée, oregano, cocoa, maple syrup or honey and chipotle chilli and mix well. Bring to a simmer and cook for 20 minutes, stirring occasionally.

5   Drain the 3 cans of beans of their liquid, then add the beans to the pot and stir well. Season with salt and pepper and simmer gently for another 25 minutes, stirring occasionally. At the end of the cooking time, you should have a thick, rich luxurious chilli.

6   Sprinkle with chopped coriander before serving with the sides of your choice (see recipe introduction).

NOTE

When I'm cooking for friends, I like to make something that I have mainly prepped in advance, so I don't miss out on all the chat by spending most of the time in the kitchen! This meal is perfect for this, as you can make it in advance and just reheat it when you need it, plus most of the accompaniments can be put into bowls and covered until needed. The only thing that really needs attending to just before serving is the rice, if you're serving it.

PER SERVING

CALORIES	FAT	SAT FAT	CARBS	SUGARS	FIBRE	PROTEIN	SALT
211	3.2G	0.5G	27G	16G	12G	11G	0.4G

CHICKEN PROVENÇAL WITH CRISPY LEMON SMASHED POTATOES

SERVES 8
PREP TIME 15 minutes
COOK TIME 55 minutes

An easy oven-baked all-in-one-tray option that is really packed with flavour and ideal for a big group. I serve with crispy smashed potatoes cooked alongside it in the oven and they are always a big hit, then add rocket leaves.

1kg (2lb 4oz) cherry tomatoes

8 garlic cloves, crushed

130g (4¾oz) pitted black olives, halved

50g (1¾oz) canned anchovies, drained and finely chopped

500g (1lb 2oz) tomato passata

250ml (9fl oz) red wine

200ml (7fl oz) chicken stock

finely grated zest and juice of 2 lemons

1 tablespoon dried rosemary

1 tablespoon dried thyme

2 large red onions, cut into wedges

16 skinless chicken thigh fillets (total weight about 2kg/4lb 8oz), excess fat removed

spray oil

2kg (4lb 8oz) baby potatoes

3 tablespoons olive oil

120g (4¼oz) rocket

salt and pepper

chopped herb leaves, such as basil, parsley, rosemary, thyme or oregano, to serve

1   Preheat the oven to 210°C/190°C fan (410°F), Gas Mark 6½.

2   Put the tomatoes in a large, deep roasting tray (see note) with the garlic, olives, anchovies, passata, red wine, stock, lemon juice (reserve the zest for now) rosemary and thyme and mix everything together.

3   Lay the onion wedges and chicken thighs over the top, season everything generously with salt and pepper and spray with oil. Bake the tray on the top shelf of the oven for 25 minutes.

4   Meanwhile, put the potatoes into a large pan of boiling water and simmer for 20 minutes. After 20 minutes, drain and let them steam off for a couple of minutes.

5   Remove the chicken from the oven, stir everything together thoroughly, then return to the oven, this time on the middle shelf to keep cooking alongside the potatoes.

6   Place the potatoes into another large roasting tray, drizzle with 1 tablespoon of the olive oil and shake them to spread out the oil. Use a potato masher to partially squash the potatoes: you want them to burst and flatten slightly, but not completely mash. Drizzle over the remaining oil, scatter over the lemon zest and stir well to distribute. Season with salt and pepper and place on the top shelf of the oven to roast for 30 minutes, until they are golden brown with crisp edges.

7   I either serve these straight from the roasting trays, with the rocket in a separate bowl, or transfer into large dishes to go on the table for everyone to help themselves. Either way, scatter with herbs to serve.

NOTE

I have 2 large roasting trays with grill racks from IKEA, which are especially useful for meals like this. They are 40 x 32cm (16 x 13 inches) and made from stainless steel, which I find really easy to clean.

PER SERVING

CALORIES	FAT	SAT FAT	CARBS	SUGARS	FIBRE	PROTEIN	SALT
590	15G	3.1G	47G	14G	9G	52G	2.3G

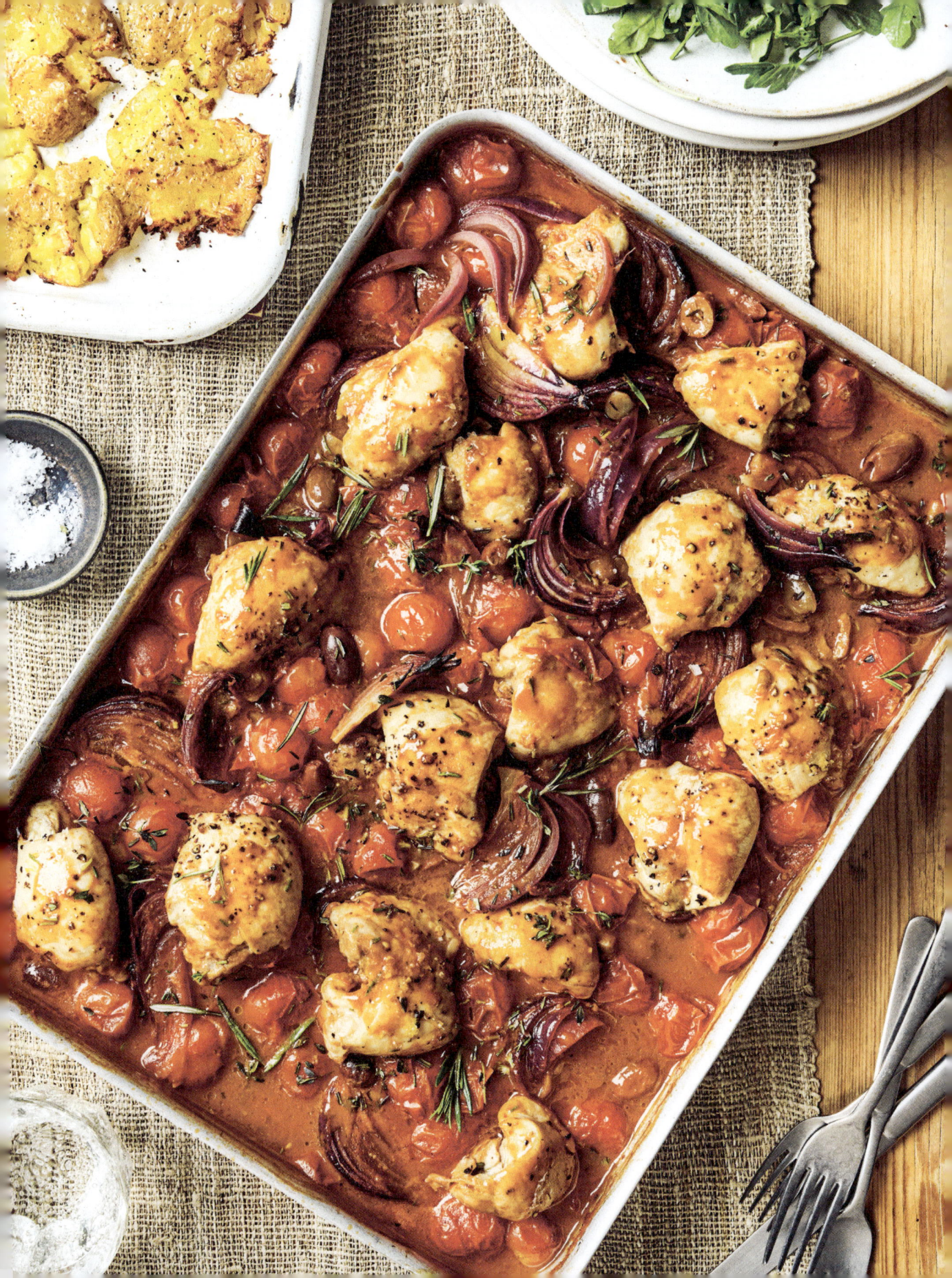

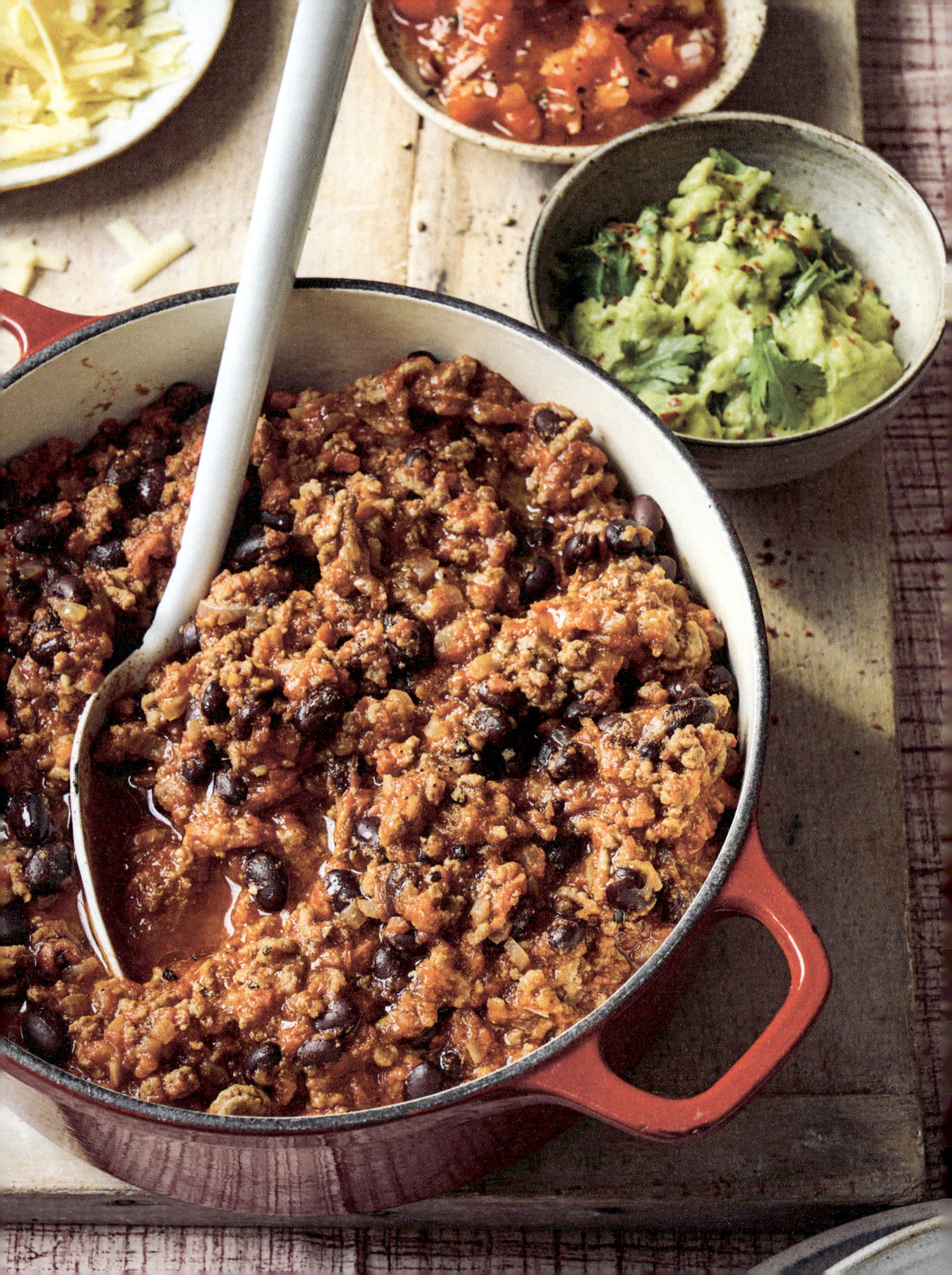

CHILLI CON CARNE

SERVES 8
PREP TIME 15 minutes
COOK TIME 40-60 minutes

spray oil

3 onions, finely chopped

6 garlic cloves, crushed

1kg (2lb 4oz) lean minced beef (less than 5 per cent fat)

4 x 400g (14oz) cans of chopped tomatoes

4 tablespoons tomato purée

1 beef stock cube or pot

1 tablespoon Worcestershire sauce

1 tablespoon dried oregano

2 teaspoons smoked paprika

2 teaspoons ground cumin

2 teaspoons onion granules

2 teaspoons chilli powder

2 x 400g (14oz) cans of black beans, drained and rinsed

salt and pepper

A classic for a reason: it's uncomplicated comfort food which hits the spot every time. This is a brilliant dish to make for a big group because you can prepare it in advance and it's easy to dress up with sides and toppings to make a feast. If you know your guests aren't keen on spicy food, simply leave out the actual chilli and instead offer chilli sauce, finely chopped fresh chilli and pickled jalapeños on the side. Black beans are my favourite for chilli con carne, but you can use a mix of black beans, kidney beans and pinto beans depending on your preference. Adding extra beans is also a great way to pad this out cheaply to feed more people! This recipe is perfect when you're making a larger batch of chilli, but if you're after a quicker option, check out my 15-Minute Chilli Con Carne (see page 21).

1   Spray a large flameproof casserole dish with oil and fry the onions for about 5 minutes, then add the garlic and stir through for another minute.

2   Add the minced beef and stir-fry, breaking it up as you go, until browned (about 5 minutes).

3   Now tip in the chopped tomatoes and tomato purée and stir to combine. Add the beef stock cube or pot, Worcestershire sauce, oregano, spices and black beans.

4   Season well, stir everything together thoroughly and leave on a low simmer for 40 minutes, stirring occasionally. (If I have time, I will leave it simmering for up to 1 hour.)

NOTE

When I am cooking this for a large group, I add a big batch of rice (allow 75g/2¾oz per person), with other dishes on the side. You could try:

baked potatoes
grated cheese
soured cream
Guacamole (see page 210)
pickled jalapeños
Two-Minute Salsa (see page 209)
green salad

PER SERVING

CALORIES	FAT	SAT FAT	CARBS	SUGARS	FIBRE	PROTEIN	SALT
321	6.6G	2.8G	22G	16G	9.4	36G	1.1G

THE ULTIMATE SALAD

SERVES 8
PREP TIME 25 minutes
COOK TIME 35 minutes

2 large (total weight 1kg/2lb 4oz) sweet potatoes, peeled and chopped into small cubes

1 tablespoon olive oil

1 teaspoon coarse salt

1 large cauliflower, chopped into florets

spray oil

100g (3½oz) shelled, unsalted pistachios

100g (3½oz) cashew nuts

1 head of broccoli, finely chopped (see note)

300g (10½oz) fine green beans, topped and tailed and cut into 2cm (¾ inch) pieces

100g (3½oz) edamame beans (if using frozen beans, blanch them with the broccoli)

150–180g (5½–6oz) rocket

250g (9oz) cooked beluga lentils, or Puy lentils (see note)

160g (5¾oz) sugar snap peas

400g (14oz) feta cheese, finely chopped, and/or mozzarella balls

salt and pepper

FOR THE DRESSING

2 tablespoons balsamic vinegar

1 tablespoon Dijon mustard

juice of 1 lemon

2 teaspoons olive oil

This is how to make a salad the main event: it is packed full of flavour, texture and goodness and it's a great crowd-pleaser. Because this is filling and hearty, any leftovers are great for lunches. If I'm making this for a group of friends, I'd add a couple of sliced baguettes on the side.

1   Preheat the oven to 220°C/200°C fan (425°F), Gas Mark 7.

2   Put the sweet potato cubes into a roasting tin, drizzle over the olive oil and sprinkle with the salt, then stir well to distribute the oil. Spread the cauliflower over another baking tray and spray with oil. Put both trays into the oven to roast.

3   Roast for 20 minutes, then give both trays a shake to help them to cook evenly and add the pistachios and cashews to the cauliflower tray. Roast the cauliflower and nuts for 5 more minutes, then remove the tray from the oven and leave to cool. Roast the sweet potato cubes for 15 minutes more, until they are soft and a little charred on the edges.

4   Meanwhile, blanch the broccoli and fine beans (and the edamame if you are using frozen.) To do this, bring a large pan of water to the boil, add the chopped broccoli and fine beans, simmer for 2 minutes, then drain and immediately transfer to a large bowl of cold water (add a couple of ice cubes if you have them). Leave for a few minutes to fully cool, then drain again.

5   Make up the dressing by mixing all the ingredients together until fully combined (you can just shake this up in a jam jar).

6   Now it is time to build the salad. You need a really big bowl for this, or 2–3 large bowls. If I'm splitting the salad across a few bowls, I just make sure that I put a roughly even amount of ingredients in each. Add the rocket, lentils, sweet potatoes, cauliflower and nuts, blanched broccoli, fine green beans and edamame, raw sugar snap peas and feta. Pour over the dressing and use salad servers or your hands to gently mix up the ingredients and make sure everything is well distributed, then serve.

PER SERVING

CALORIES	FAT	SAT FAT	CARBS	SUGARS	FIBRE	PROTEIN	SALT
547	28G	9.7G	43G	14G	13G	24G	2G

NOTE

To finely chop broccoli start by using a large, sharp knife. Begin at the florets (the flowery part of the head) and slice through the broccoli in the same manner as you would an onion. Continue slicing until you reach the thicker stem. Chop the stem finely.

You can buy packets of pre-cooked beluga and Puy lentils, often from the Merchant Gourmet brand in the UK. These are both lovely additions to this salad as they look great as well as having a lovely texture and flavour. For a more budget-friendly option, you could use canned green lentils, or cook your own.

CUSTOMIZATION IDEAS

1. Proteins:

Cooked, chopped skinless chicken
(leftovers from a roast are great here)

Sliced rare steak strips

Pan-seared tofu

Canned chickpeas or black beans

Smoked salmon or cooked prawns

2. Seasonal vegetables:

Chopped roast beetroot, or julienned carrot

Grilled asparagus or courgette

Fresh or roasted cherry tomatoes

Sliced radishes or cucumber

Shredded Brussels sprouts or kale

Chopped avocado

3. Nuts and seeds:

Swap pistachios and cashews for almonds, pecans or walnuts

Add pumpkin seeds, sunflower seeds or sesame seeds

4. Cheese variations:

Replace feta or mozzarella with crumbled goat's cheese, blue cheese or shaved Parmesan

Add chopped, fried halloumi

Use vegan cheese alternatives for a dairy-free option

5. Herbs and spices:

Add fresh herbs, such as basil, parsley or mint leaves

Sprinkle with chilli flakes or black pepper for a touch of heat

Add dried herbs, such as oregano, thyme or rosemary

6. Grains and legumes:

Cooked quinoa or pearl barley

Cooked brown rice or wild rice

Lentils other than beluga or Puy lentils, such as green or red lentils

Pearl couscous or orzo pasta

7. Dressing variations:

Swap balsamic vinegar for red wine vinegar or apple cider vinegar

Add a touch of honey or maple syrup for sweetness

Experiment with different mustard varieties, such as wholegrain or spicy mustard

Incorporate tahini or fat-free Greek yogurt

8. Finishing touches:

Toasted coconut flakes or sesame seeds

Sliced spring onions or chives

Crispy bacon bits or prosciutto

Dried fruit, such as cranberries, or chopped dried apricots, for a hint of sweetness

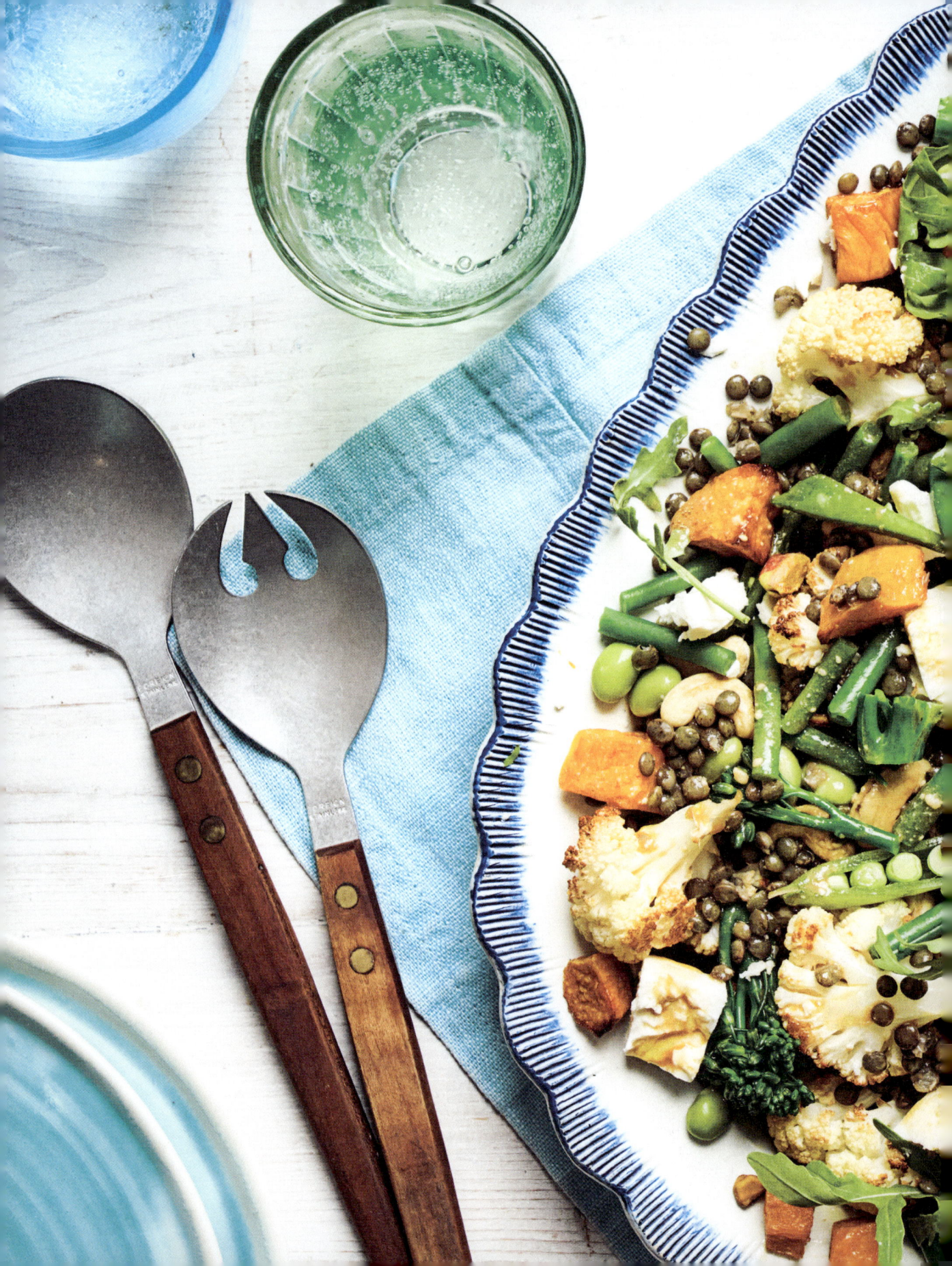

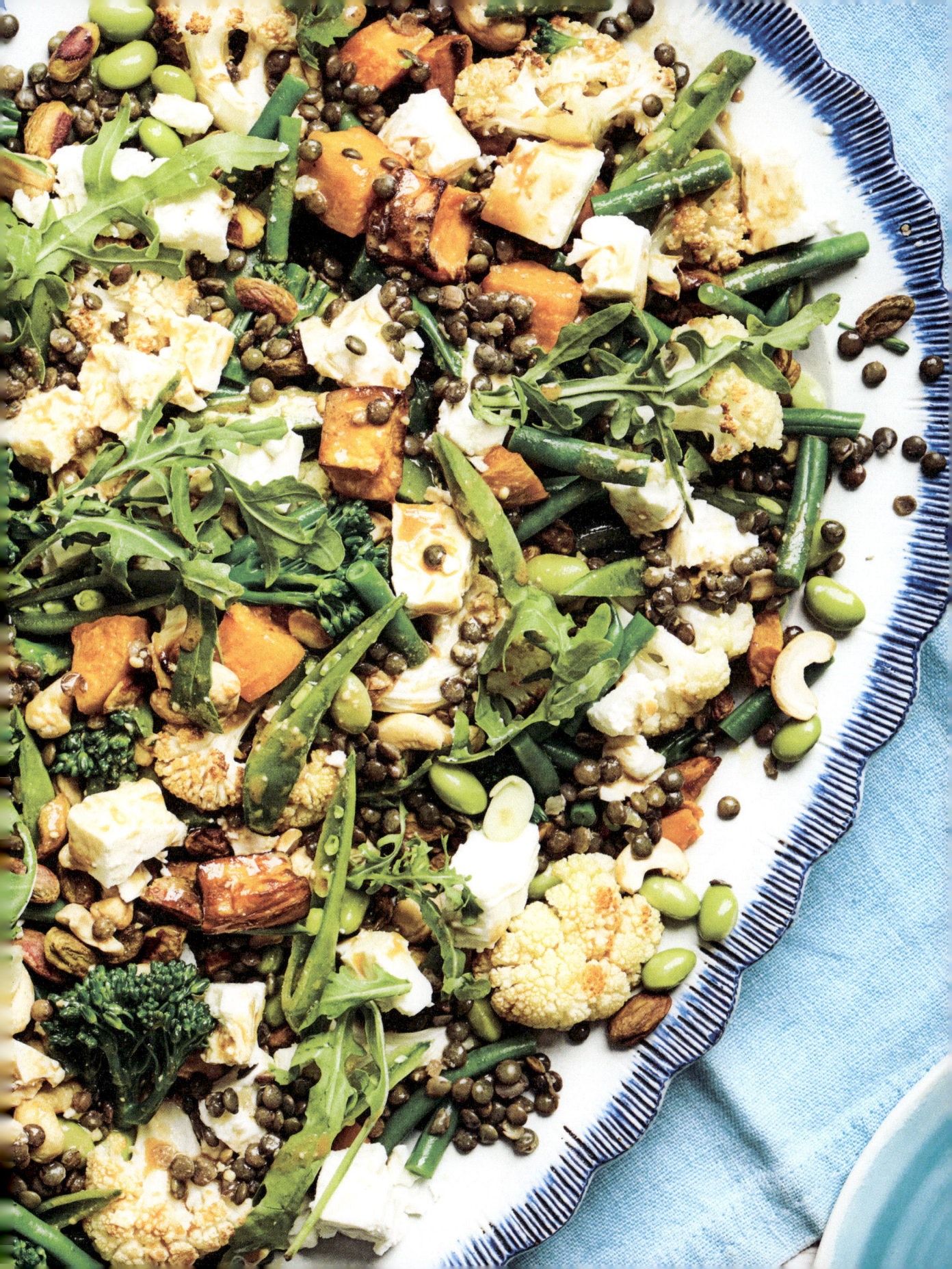

BIG BOLD BULGUR SALAD

SERVES 8 (as a side dish)
PREP TIME 10 minutes
COOK TIME 15 minutes

400g (14oz) uncooked bulgur
  wheat
100g (3½oz) flaked almonds
1 sweet green pepper, finely
  chopped
1 red onion, finely chopped
½ cucumber, finely chopped
1 large carrot, grated
large handful of mint leaves,
  finely chopped
large handful of parsley leaves,
  finely chopped
150g (5½oz) pomegranate seeds
finely grated zest and juice of
  1 lemon
1½ teaspoons coarse salt

If I'm cooking for a big group, I nearly always have a grain salad on the side that complements my main dish. It's a great, cost-effective way of padding out a meal and very easy to tweak so it goes with whatever you are eating. I have used bulgur wheat here, but I'll often mix different grains, such as quinoa and buckwheat or couscous. This recipe goes well with my Kofta-Style Meatballs in Harissa Sauce (see page 175), but see below for more ideas!

1 Put the bulgur wheat into a large pan of boiling water and cook according to the packet instructions (usually around 15 minutes).

2 Meanwhile, pop the flaked almonds into a dry frying pan and stir-fry them over a high heat for a few minutes. You want them to turn a light golden brown and have that delicious toasty smell, but you need to keep an eye on them to make sure they don't burn. As soon as they are done, pop them aside in a bowl ready for assembling the salad.

3 Prepare all the vegetables and herbs and place into a large bowl.

4 Once the bulgur wheat is cooked, you can either leave it to cool (if you have time) or tip it into a large sieve and place it under cold running water from the tap.

5 Once the bulgur wheat has cooled, add it to the bowl of vegetables and herbs. When you are ready to serve the salad, stir through the pomegranate seeds, toasted almonds, lemon zest and juice and salt.

NOTE

Here are some more ideas for things you could add to this salad:

Raw veg Chopped courgettes, sweet peppers, sugar snap peas, fine green beans, baby tomatoes, spring onions.

Cooked vegetables Sweetcorn, peas, broccoli, runner beans, asparagus, mushrooms, cauliflower, aubergine.

Garlic-lemon dressing Crushed garlic cloves, honey and lemon juice.

Balsamic vinaigrette Mix together balsamic vinegar, olive oil, Dijon mustard, very finely chopped shallots, honey and a pinch of dried Italian seasoning.

Lemon-dill dressing Lemon juice, olive oil, finely chopped dill, finely grated lemon zest, minced garlic, salt and pepper.

Sriracha-lime dressing Whisk together sriracha sauce, lime juice, rice vinegar, soy sauce (or tamari for a gluten-free option), peeled and finely grated root ginger and a drizzle of sesame oil.

PER SERVING

CALORIES	FAT	SAT FAT	CARBS	SUGARS	FIBRE	PROTEIN	SALT
293	8.3G	0.8G	42G	6.1G	6.5G	9G	0.95G

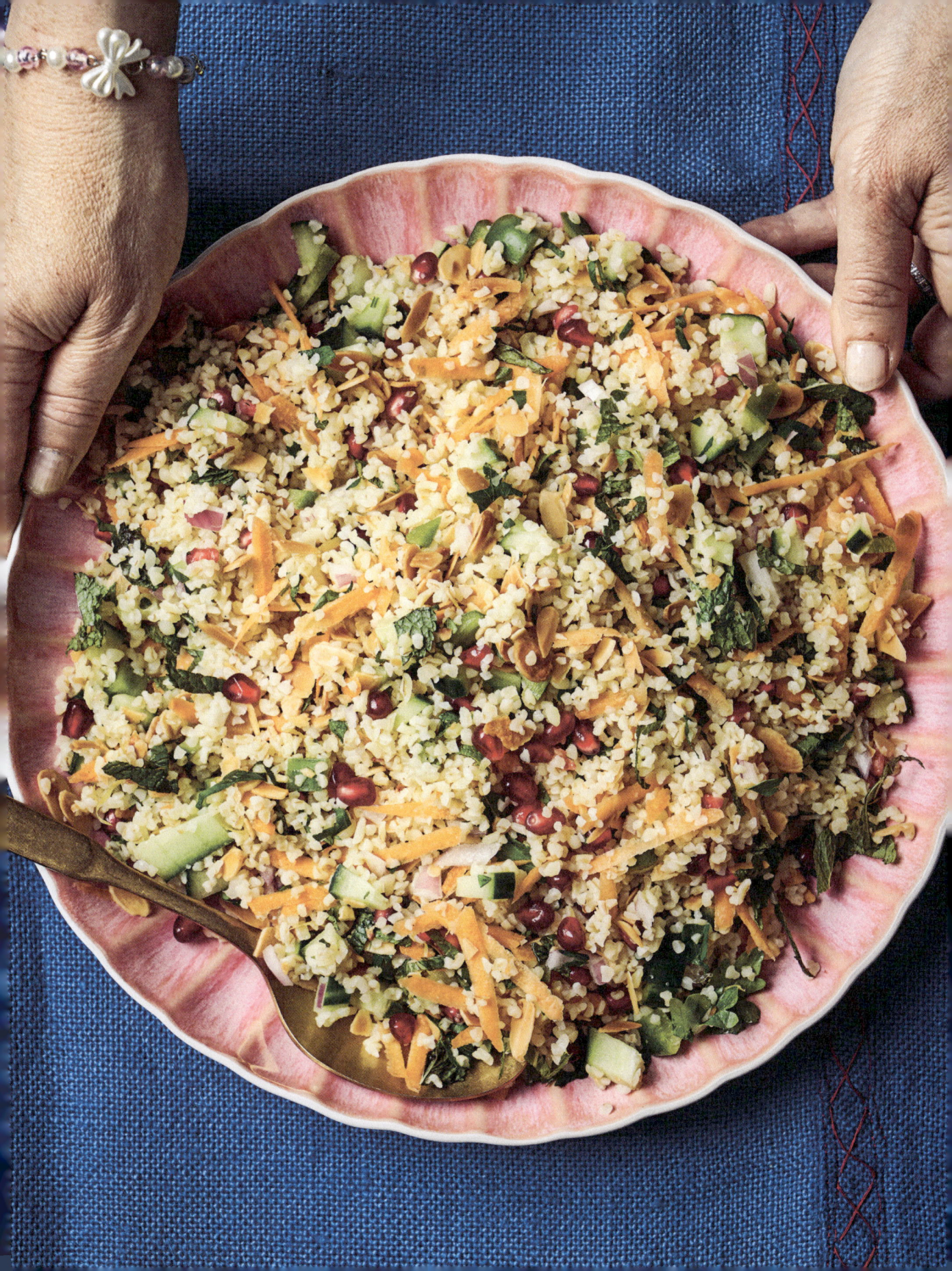

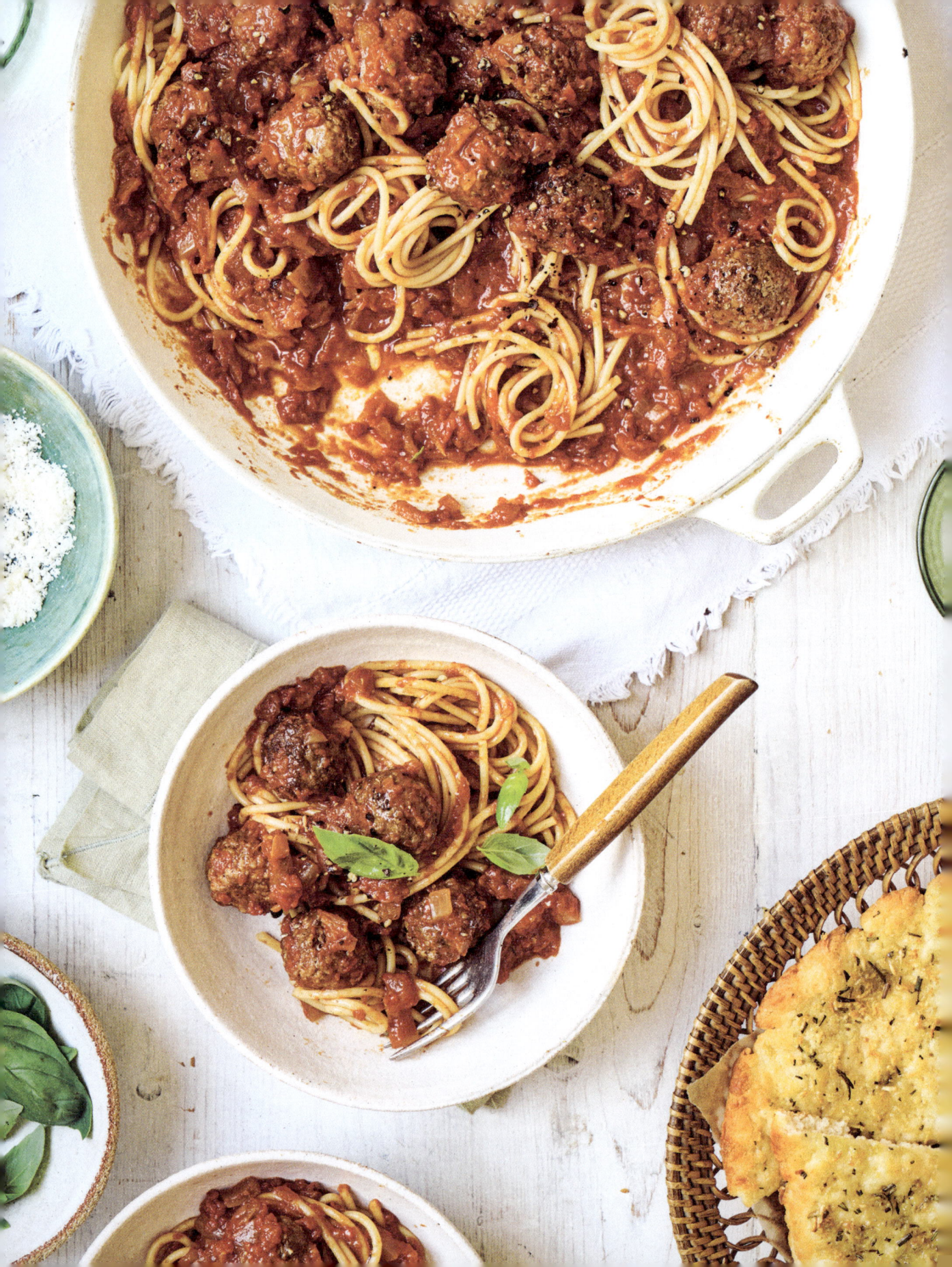

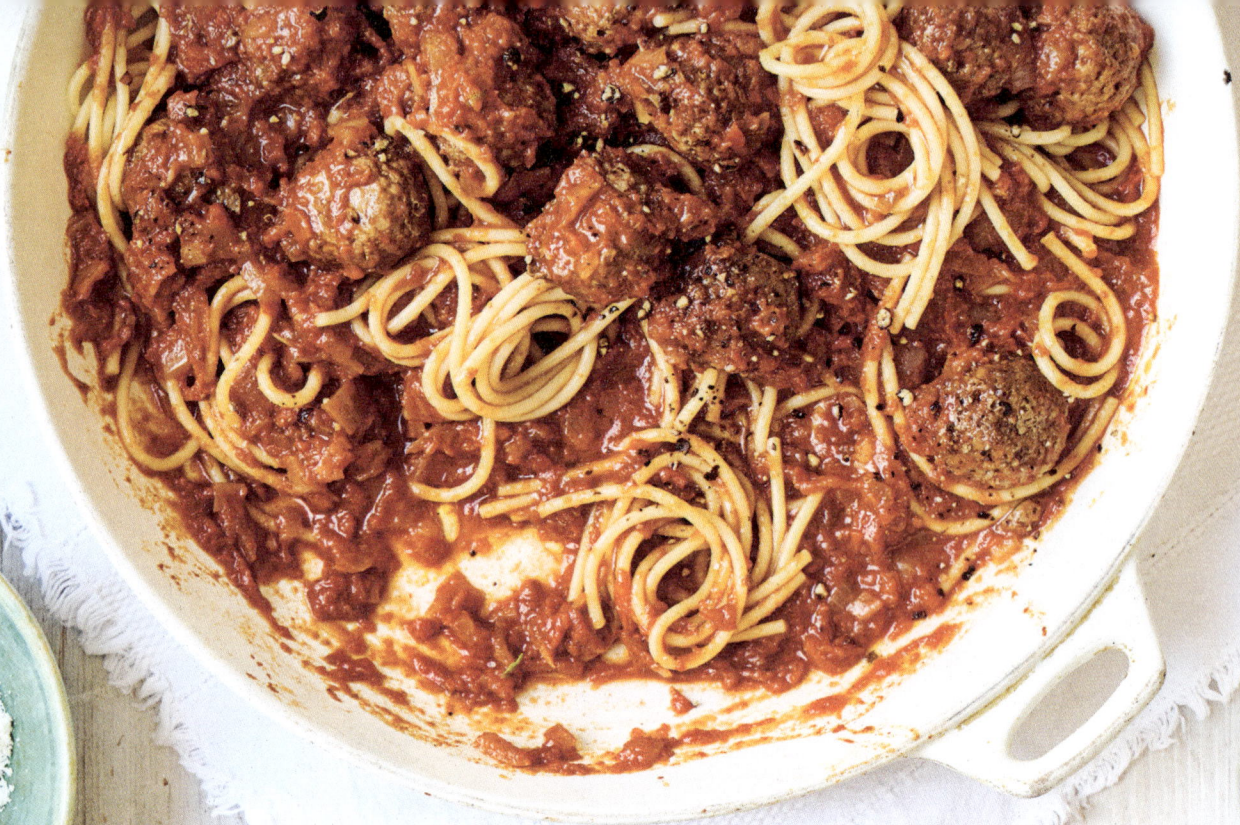

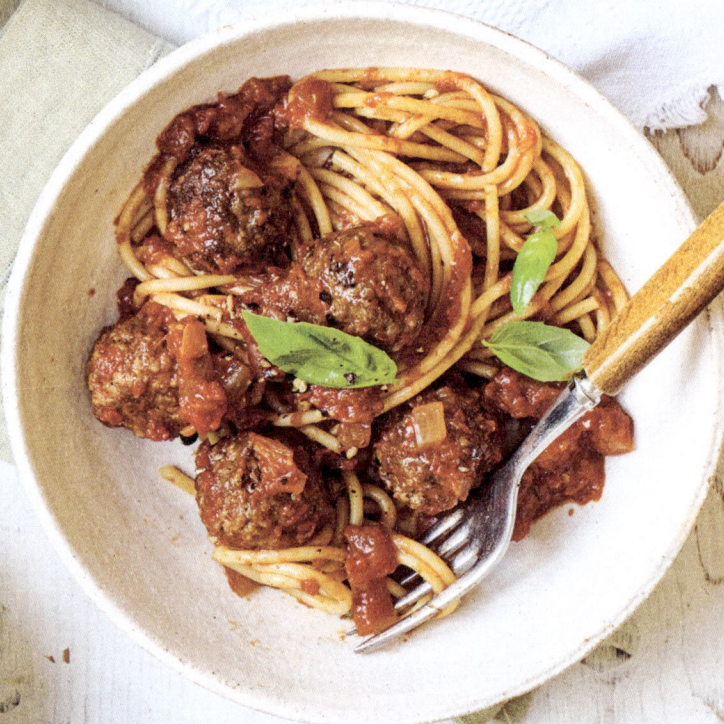

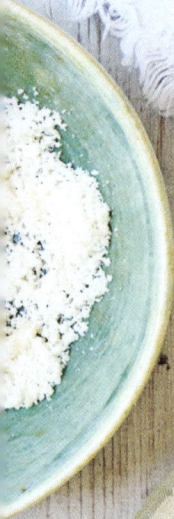

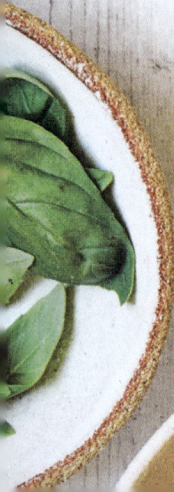

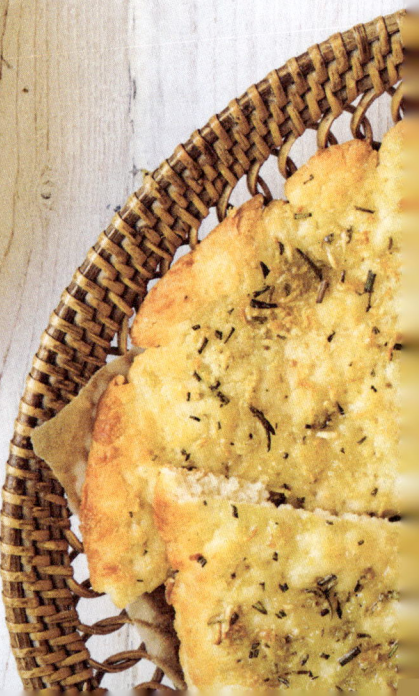

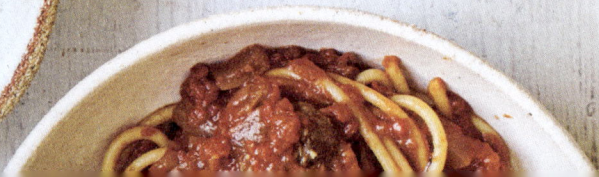

THE MEATBALL CLUB SPECIAL

SERVES 8
PREP TIME 20 minutes
COOK TIME 55 minutes

1 tablespoon olive oil

3 onions, finely chopped

750g (1lb 10oz) lean minced beef (less than 5 per cent fat)

6 garlic cloves, crushed

1 tablespoon dark muscovado sugar

3 x 400g (14oz) cans of chopped tomatoes

350ml (12fl oz) water

2 tablespoons balsamic vinegar

2 tablespoons tomato purée

1 tablespoon cocoa powder

1 beef stock cube or stock pot

1–2 teaspoons chilli powder, to taste

1½ teaspoons coarse salt

1 teaspoon coarsely ground black pepper

600g (1lb 5oz) spaghetti

TO SERVE
parsley or basil leaves
grated Parmesan cheese

This was my signature dish during my years of living with friends in London. It is such an easy meal to scale up for larger numbers, and you can serve it up with extras, such as Easiest Ever Rustic Garlic Bread (see page 213), or rocket salad. I have always kept the meatballs in this completely basic, with nothing added at all, as there is plenty of flavour in the sauce, but you can add herbs, seasoning and breadcrumbs if you wish.

1 Preheat the oven to 220°C/200°C fan (425°F), Gas Mark 7.

2 Heat the oil in a frying pan and fry the onions gently for 15 minutes, stirring regularly, to soften and slightly caramelize them.

3 Meanwhile, make the meatballs. Simply roll the minced beef with your hands into small meatballs (2–2.5cm/1 inch in diameter) and place them on a baking tray (or 2) as you make them, giving them some space. Put the meatballs in the oven to bake for 15 minutes. When they are cooked, you can just remove them from the oven until you are ready to add them to the sauce.

4 After the onions have cooked for 15 minutes, stir through the garlic for a minute, then add the dark muscovado sugar, chopped tomatoes, the water, balsamic vinegar, tomato purée, cocoa powder, beef stock cube, chilli powder, salt and pepper to the pan, then simmer for 30 minutes.

5 Use a stick blender to blend the sauce until smooth. Add the meatballs to the sauce and simmer while you cook the spaghetti.

6 Bring a large pan of water (or use 2 pans) to a simmer and add the spaghetti. Simmer according to the packet instructions (usually 9–12 minutes) until al dente. If I'm cooking a large amount of spaghetti like this, I make sure I shuffle it with a fork a few times during cooking, to prevent clumping.

7 For large meals like this I put the food in the middle of the table and let everyone help themselves. Scatter with herbs and offer Parmesan on the side for grating over.

NOTE

You can make the meatballs and sauce well in advance for this, as it's one of those dishes that tastes even better the next day! If you have it ready, then all you need to do is reheat it and cook the spaghetti when needed.

PER SERVING

CALORIES	FAT	SAT FAT	CARBS	SUGARS	FIBRE	PROTEIN	SALT
470	7.1G	2.4G	65G	14G	5.8G	32G	1.4G

SIDES, SPICE MIXES, DIPS & NIBBLES

8

SESAME ROAST POTATOES

SERVES 4
PREP TIME 5 minutes
COOK TIME 55 minutes

1kg (2lb 4oz) potatoes (I usually use Maris Piper), peeled and cut into even-sized chunks
2 tablespoons sesame oil
1 teaspoon coarse salt
¼ teaspoon pepper
1 tablespoon sesame seeds

I am a big fan of mixing up a traditional roast dinner with some new combinations: I think it keeps things interesting, and it's also a great way to introduce children to novel flavours in a familiar meal. I made these once to go alongside my Peking-Inspired Roast Chicken (see page 104) and they went down a storm with my family.

1   Preheat the oven to 200°C/180°C fan (400°F), Gas Mark 6.

2   Place the potato chunks into a large saucepan of cold water (I add the chunks to the water as I peel and cut them), bring to a gentle simmer and simmer for 10 minutes.

3   Pour the sesame oil into a medium-sized roasting tin and pop in the oven for a few minutes to get it hot and sizzling.

4   Drain the potatoes, allow them to steam off for a couple of minutes, then shake them up in the colander or pan to roughen up the outsides, ready to become nice and crispy!

5   Carefully transfer the potatoes to the hot sesame oil in the roasting tin (be cautious as hot oil can spit, so don't lean over the tray and use oven gloves to move it), then use tongs to turn them to ensure they are evenly covered in oil. You need the potatoes to be in a single layer, with space between them to ensure a good crispy edge.

6   Put the tray into the oven and roast for 45 minutes, turning them every 15 minutes.

7   When the potatoes have 5 minutes of cooking time remaining, season them with the salt and pepper and sprinkle over the sesame seeds. After 45 minutes the potatoes should be golden and crisp, but if you think they need a bit longer, leave them in the oven and check on them every 5 minutes.

NOTE

For alternative flavour combinations, try using different oils and seasonings. You could experiment with olive oil, crushed garlic and finely chopped rosemary leaves for a more traditional flavour. Add the garlic and rosemary during the final 15 minutes of roasting, to prevent burning. Alternatively, for a different twist, you could use coconut oil and curry powder, adding the curry powder when shaking up the potatoes in step 4. Simply swap in the alternative oil in step 3 and ensure it evenly coats the potatoes before roasting.

PER SERVING

CALORIES	FAT	SAT FAT	CARBS	SUGARS	FIBRE	PROTEIN	SALT
263	8.1G	1.3G	40G	2G	4.9G	4.7G	1.3G

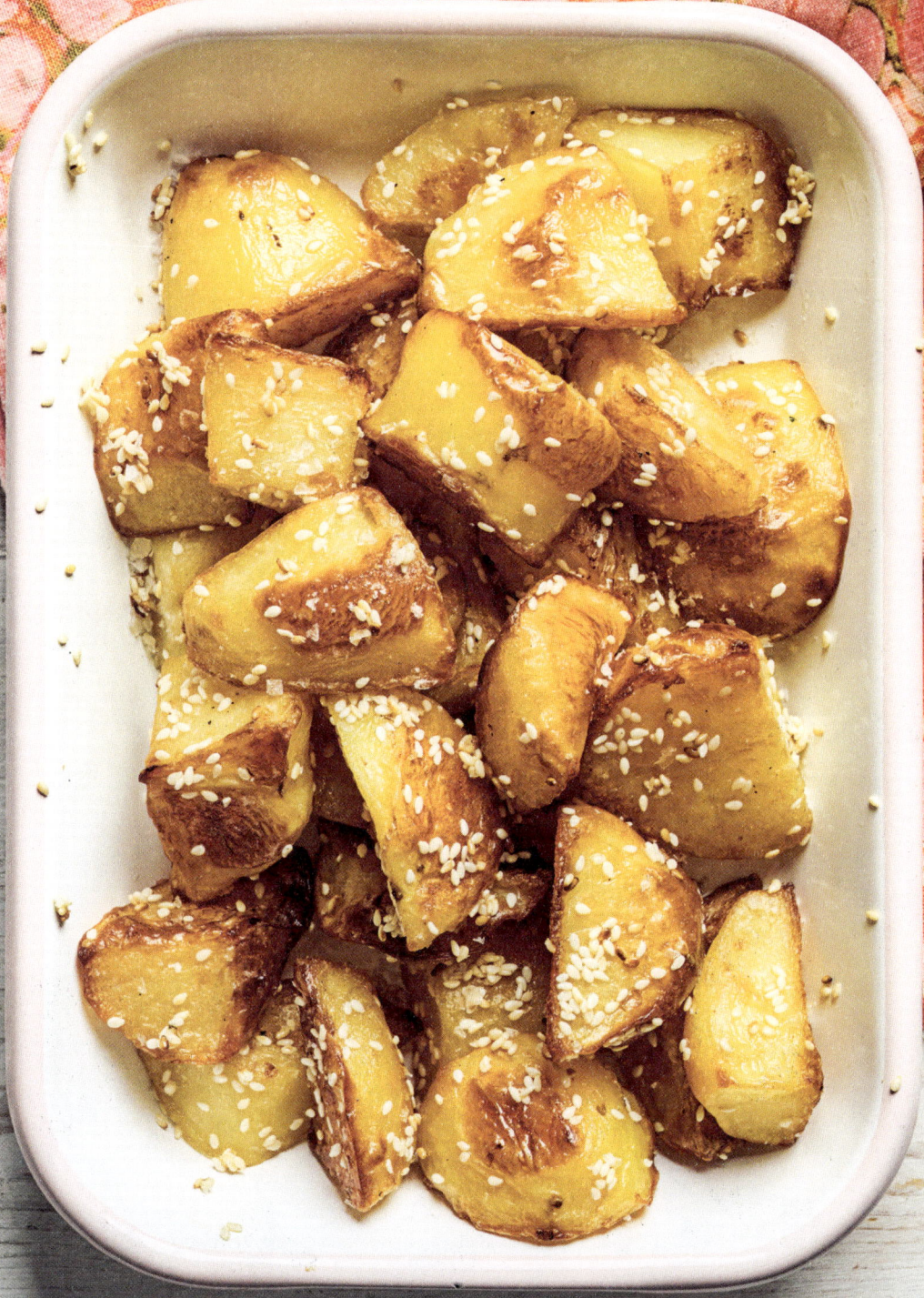

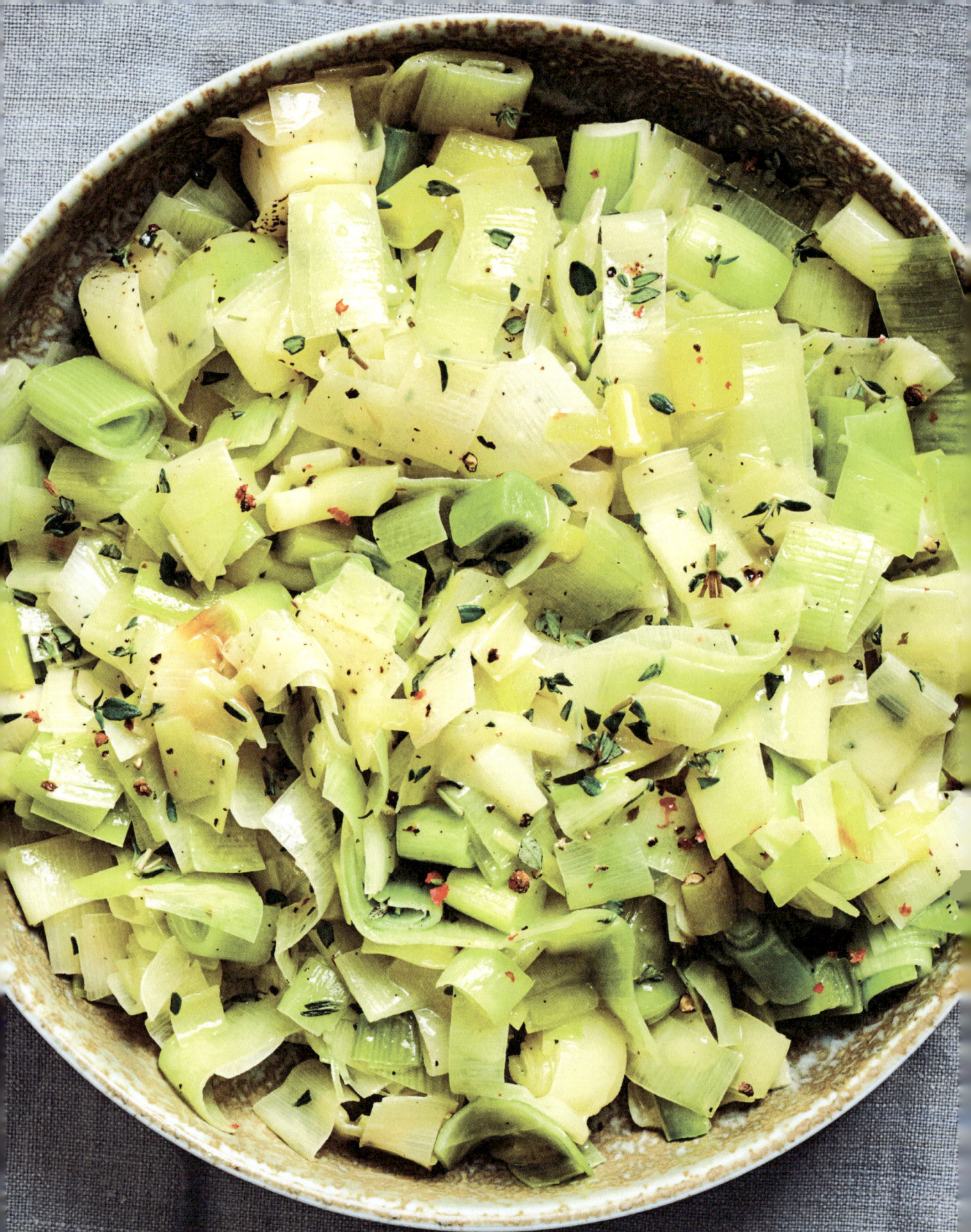

BRAISED LEEKS

SERVES 4
PREP TIME 5 minutes
COOK TIME 15 minutes

4 leeks
2 teaspoons (10g/¼oz) butter
½ teaspoon dried thyme
150ml (¼ pint) hot chicken stock
salt and pepper

Leeks are so flavoursome, and, if you buy them in season, they are great value and work with so many different dishes. I often use this simple recipe as a side dish to a roast dinner.

1   Trim the leeks, pull away the tough outer layers, slice them in half lengthways and rinse any dirt out of them. Slice them into 1cm (½ inch) thick pieces.

2   Melt the butter in a sauté pan, add the leeks and stir-fry them for 5 minutes.

3   Sprinkle the thyme over the leeks and stir-fry them for another minute.

4   Pour in the hot stock, cover the pan and braise them over a gentle heat for 10 minutes until tender. Season, then serve.

NOTE

To make these vegetarian, swap the chicken stock for vegetable stock. For added depth of flavour, add a splash of white wine with the stock. If you would prefer a creamier dish, stir in a couple of tablespoons of light (reduced-fat) crème fraîche before serving.

PER SERVING

CALORIES	FAT	SAT FAT	CARBS	SUGARS	FIBRE	PROTEIN	SALT
78	2.5G	1.4G	7.3G	6.8G	5.1G	4G	0.27G

CANNELLINI BEAN MASH WITH ROSEMARY & LEMON

SERVES 4
PREP TIME 5 minutes
COOK TIME 12 minutes

1 tablespoon olive oil

1 shallot, finely chopped

2 garlic cloves, crushed

2 x 400g (14oz) cans of cannellini beans, drained and rinsed

50ml (1¾fl oz) hot water, chicken stock or vegetable stock, plus more if needed

½ teaspoon dried rosemary

juice of ¼ lemon

salt and pepper

This makes a brilliant alternative to mashed potato, it's also super-quick and easy to make and you can adjust the flavours to suit whatever it accompanies. Try it with grilled sausages and fried onions, or with Pork Goulash (see page 158).

1   Heat the oil in a saucepan, which has a lid, and fry the shallot for 5 minutes, then stir through the garlic and fry gently for 2 more minutes.

2   Add the cannellini beans, measured hot water or stock and rosemary, pop the lid on the pan and simmer over a low heat for 5 minutes.

3   Season with salt and pepper, squeeze in the lemon juice and use a potato masher to mash the beans to your desired consistency: you can mash them until smooth, if you like, or keep a bit of texture. If you think they look too dry, just splash in a little extra water or stock.

NOTE

You can vary the flavours in this to complement the meal you are serving. Try different dried or fresh herbs, such as parsley, thyme, sage, or basil. You can also add grated Parmesan cheese, roast garlic (see page 206) or caramelized onions for extra depth and richness.

PER SERVING

CALORIES	FAT	SAT FAT	CARBS	SUGARS	FIBRE	PROTEIN	SALT
173	5.1G	0.8G	18G	1.2G	8.5G	9.4G	0.15G

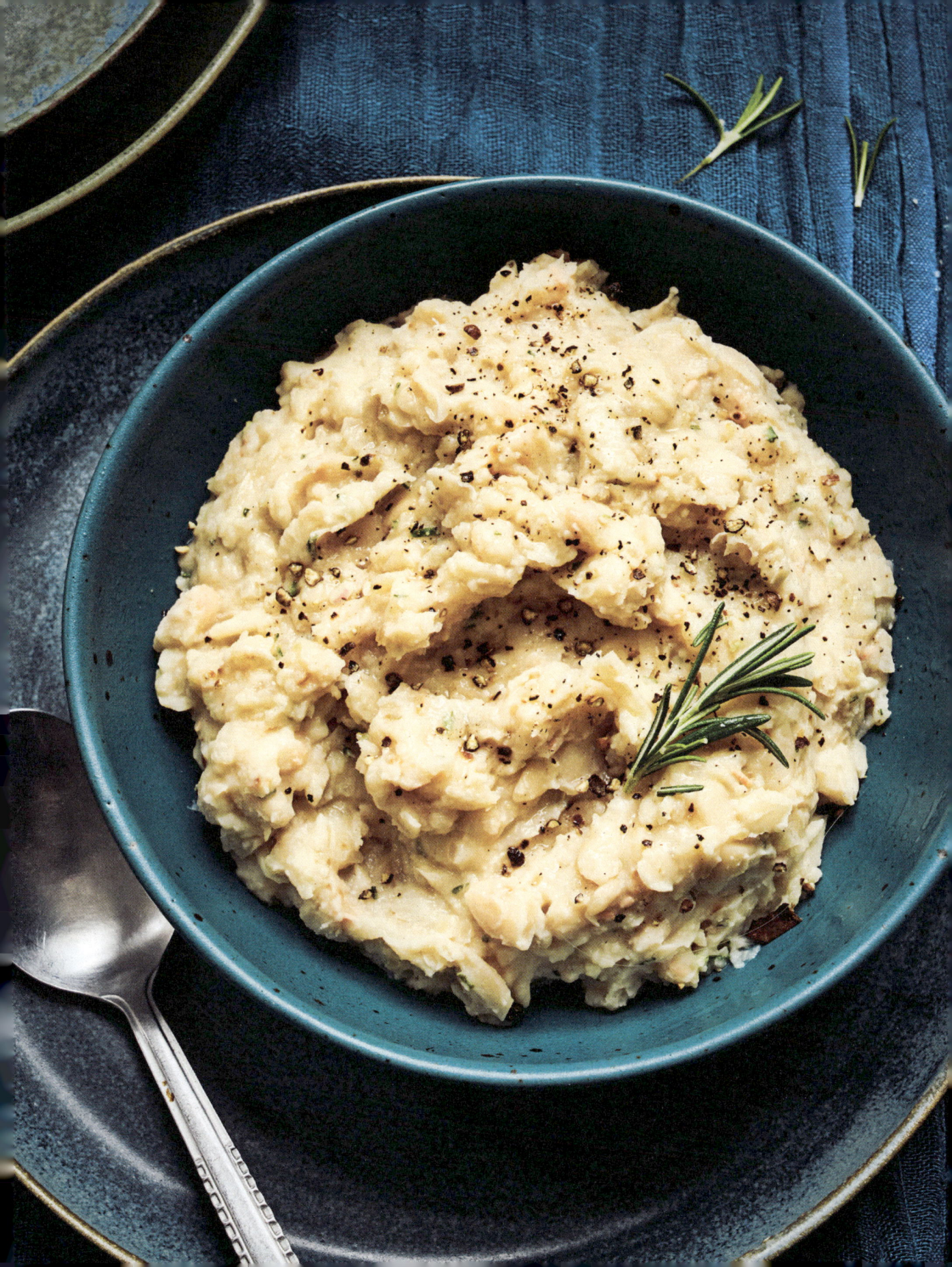

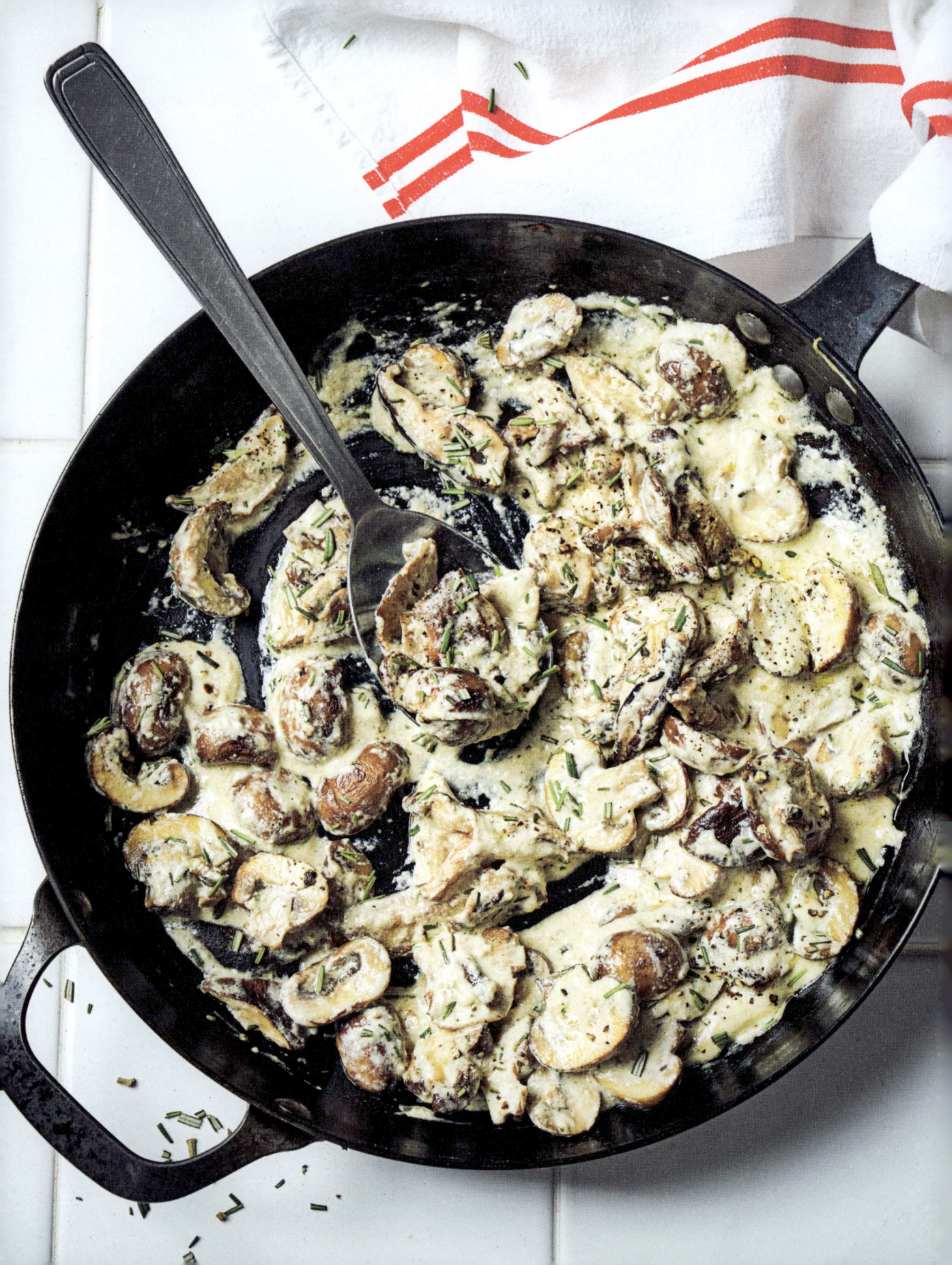

GARLIC MUSHROOM SAUCE

SERVES 4
PREP TIME 5 minutes
COOK TIME 10 minutes

spray oil

3 garlic cloves, crushed

250g (9oz) chestnut mushrooms, sliced

120g (4¼oz) shiitake mushrooms, sliced

leaves from 1 rosemary sprig, finely chopped

4 tablespoons chicken stock

4 tablespoons crème fraîche

salt and pepper

A good garlic mushroom sauce is a fantastic and versatile recipe to have up your sleeve. In this recipe, shiitake mushrooms really get extra flavour in. It makes a great steak or chicken sauce, or it works well on toast, with a jacket potato and even makes a tasty pasta sauce!

1 Spray a frying pan with oil and fry the garlic for 1 minute, then add the sliced mushrooms and rosemary and stir-fry for 7 minutes.

2 Add the chicken stock and crème fraîche and stir-fry for another 2 minutes. Finally, season with salt and pepper and serve.

NOTE

Swap the chicken stock for vegetable stock for a vegetarian version.

PER SERVING

CALORIES	FAT	SAT FAT	CARBS	SUGARS	FIBRE	PROTEIN	SALT
116	8.5G	5.5G	4.6G	2.6G	2G	4.4G	0.24G

BAHARAT SPICE MIX

MAKES 3 tablespoons
(enough for 3 meals)
PREP TIME 2 minutes
COOK TIME none

2 teaspoons sweet (unsmoked)
 paprika
2 teaspoons ground cumin
1 teaspoon ground coriander
1 teaspoon pepper
½ teaspoon ground cinnamon
½ teaspoon ground nutmeg
¼ teaspoon ground cloves

Baharat is a Middle Eastern blend which can vary between regions, but always consists of warming, aromatic spices. My version is made from ingredients which can be easily found in the UK. It is a quick way to add real depth of flavour to meals. Try it in Chicken Kofta (see page 47).

1   Simply put all the ingredients into a clean, dry jar and shake them up together.

NOTE

How to use:

As a dry rub for meat Before grilling or barbecuing.

For stews, tagines or casseroles Baharat pairs especially well with chicken and lamb, as well as with ingredients, such as chickpeas, root vegetables and tomato-based sauces.

Sprinkle it Over grain dishes, such as rice, couscous, quinoa and bulgur wheat.

Add to soups for warm and spicy flavour This works especially well with lentil-, chickpea- and tomato-based soups.

Add to hummus For a Middle Eastern twist.

PER 1 TABLESPOON

CALORIES	FAT	SAT FAT	CARBS	SUGARS	FIBRE	PROTEIN	SALT
16	0.9G	0.2G	0.6G	0.5G	1.6G	0.8G	TRACE

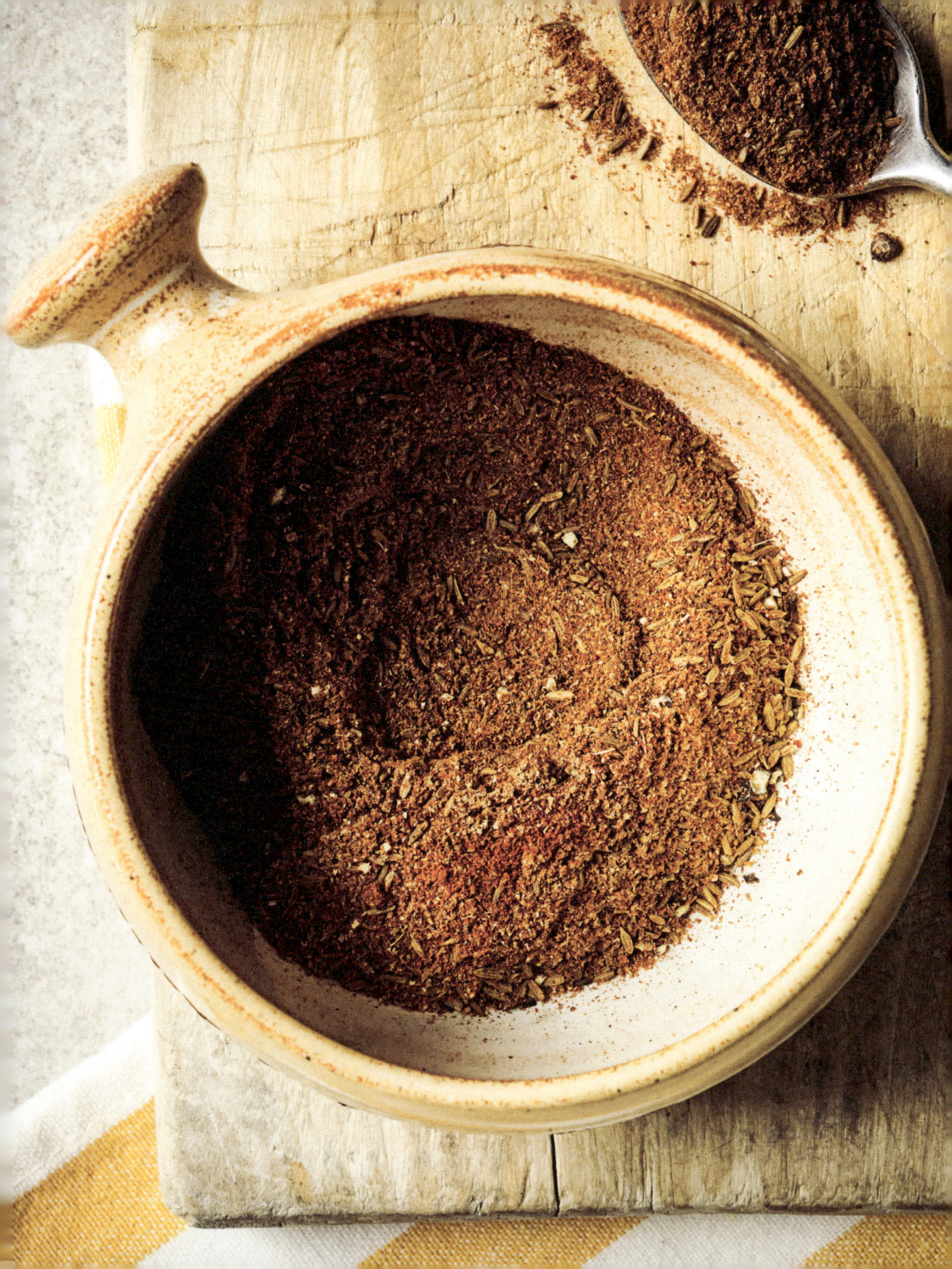

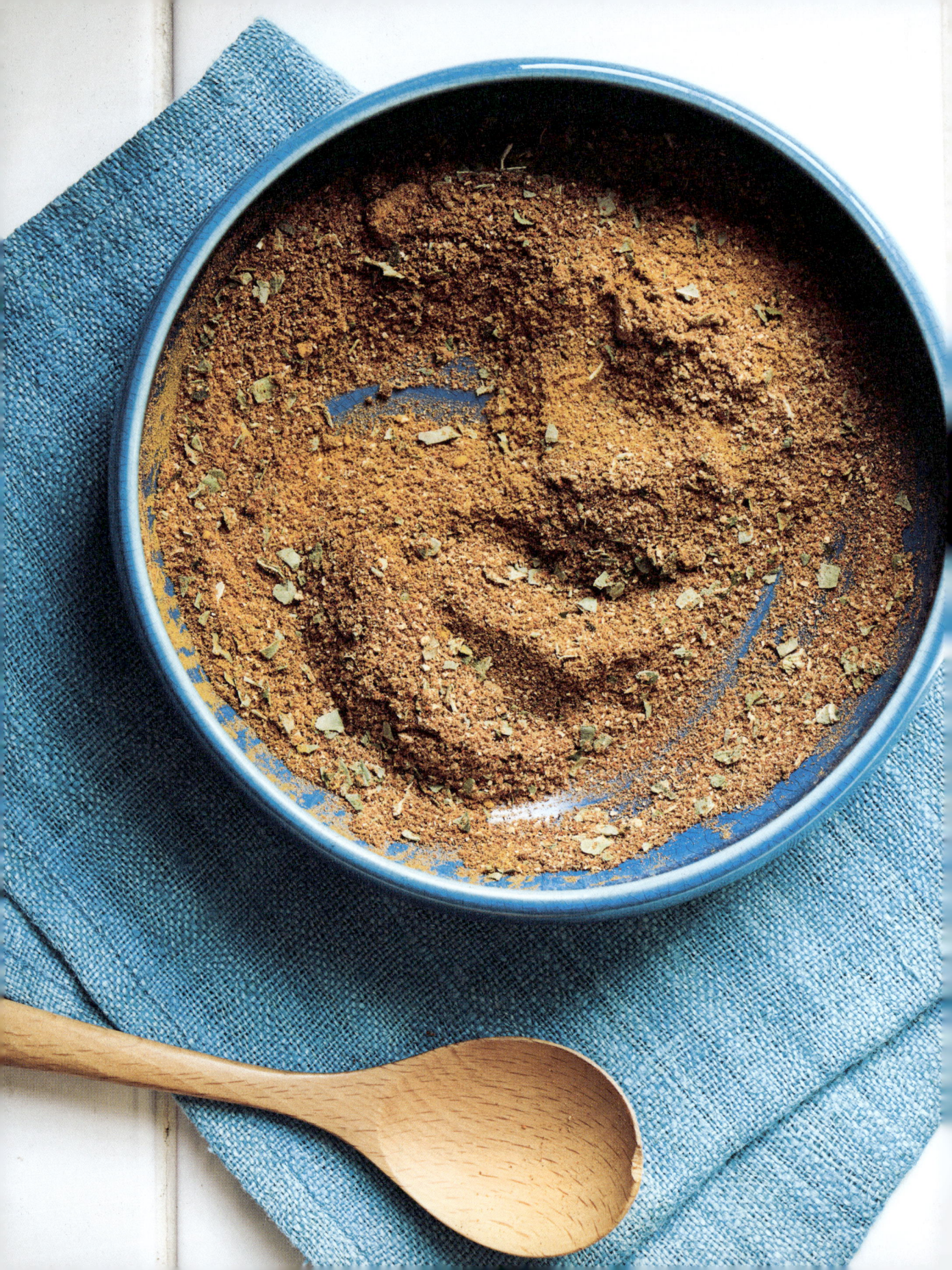

CHERMOULA SPICE BLEND

MAKES 7 tablespoons
PREP TIME 2 minutes
COOK TIME none

2 tablespoons ground cumin

1 tablespoon ground coriander

1 tablespoon dried parsley

2 teaspoons chilli powder

2 teaspoons sweet (unsmoked)
   paprika

1½ teaspoons ground cinnamon

1½ teaspoons dried ginger

1 teaspoon ground allspice

1 teaspoon garlic granules

1 teaspoon ground turmeric

This is my take on the popular North African spice blend.
Try it in Kofta-Style Meatballs in Harissa Sauce (see page 175).

1   Measure all the spices into a clean, dry jar and shake up to blend.

NOTE

This spice blend is incredibly versatile and can be used in a variety of
dishes. Try it as a rub for grilled chicken or fish for a fragrant, spiced kick.
You can also mix it with olive oil and lemon juice to make a marinade
for vegetables, or stir it into couscous or quinoa for a tasty side dish.
It's a great way to add depth to salads, soups or stews as well.

PER 1 TABLESPOON

CALORIES	FAT	SAT FAT	CARBS	SUGARS	FIBRE	PROTEIN	SALT
18	0.8G	0	1.2G	0.5G	1.6G	0.8G	TRACE

ROASTED GARLIC & RED PEPPER HUMMUS

SERVES 8
PREP TIME 2 minutes
COOK TIME 6–45 minutes
(depending on how you cook the garlic)

2 x 400g (14oz) cans of chickpeas, drained and rinsed
1 large garlic bulb, roasted (see note)
juice of 1 lemon
6 tablespoons fat-free Greek yogurt
1 roasted red pepper (from a jar)
1 teaspoon coarse salt
¼ teaspoon cayenne pepper

Hummus is a such a versatile dish to make, because it works well both as a dip and a side dish. I usually make a batch if I'm going to a friend's house for dinner and take along crudités as well as toasted pitta fingers for dipping. I also like having it in the refrigerator to go with lunchtime salads, pitta breads or falafel. Roasted garlic has a sweet, mild flavour.

1   Put all the ingredients into a food processor and blend until you have a smooth hummus.

NOTE

To roast the garlic, cut about 1cm (½ inch) from the top of the bulb with a sharp knife, just enough to expose the top of the garlic cloves. Remove any of the loose outer layers of papery skin.

Put the garlic cut side up on a piece of foil big enough to wrap it in, spray the top of the cloves with oil, completely wrap in the foil, place on a baking tray and roast in an oven preheated to 220°C/200°C fan (425°F), Gas Mark 7 for 45 minutes. Allow to cool enough to handle before squeezing the soft garlic from the cloves.

Microwave method Place the trimmed garlic bulb into a microwave-safe bowl and add 2 tablespoons of water. Spray the exposed top of the cloves with oil. Cover the dish with a microwave-safe lid. Microwave for 3 minutes, then carefully remove the lid and check it by poking with a fork: if the cloves are still hard, then pop it back into the microwave, cook for another 2 minutes, then check again. If the cloves still aren't soft, microwave for 1 minute at a time until the cloves are very soft and can be pierced easily with a fork. Leave it until cool enough to handle, then squeeze the garlic out of the cloves.

Air-fryer method Follow the oven instructions for preparation, then pop the foil-wrapped garlic into the air fryer for 16–20 minutes at 190°C (375°F) until the cloves are soft.

PER SERVING

CALORIES	FAT	SAT FAT	CARBS	SUGARS	FIBRE	PROTEIN	SALT
108	1.9G	0.2G	12G	2.3G	4.6G	7.8G	0.65G

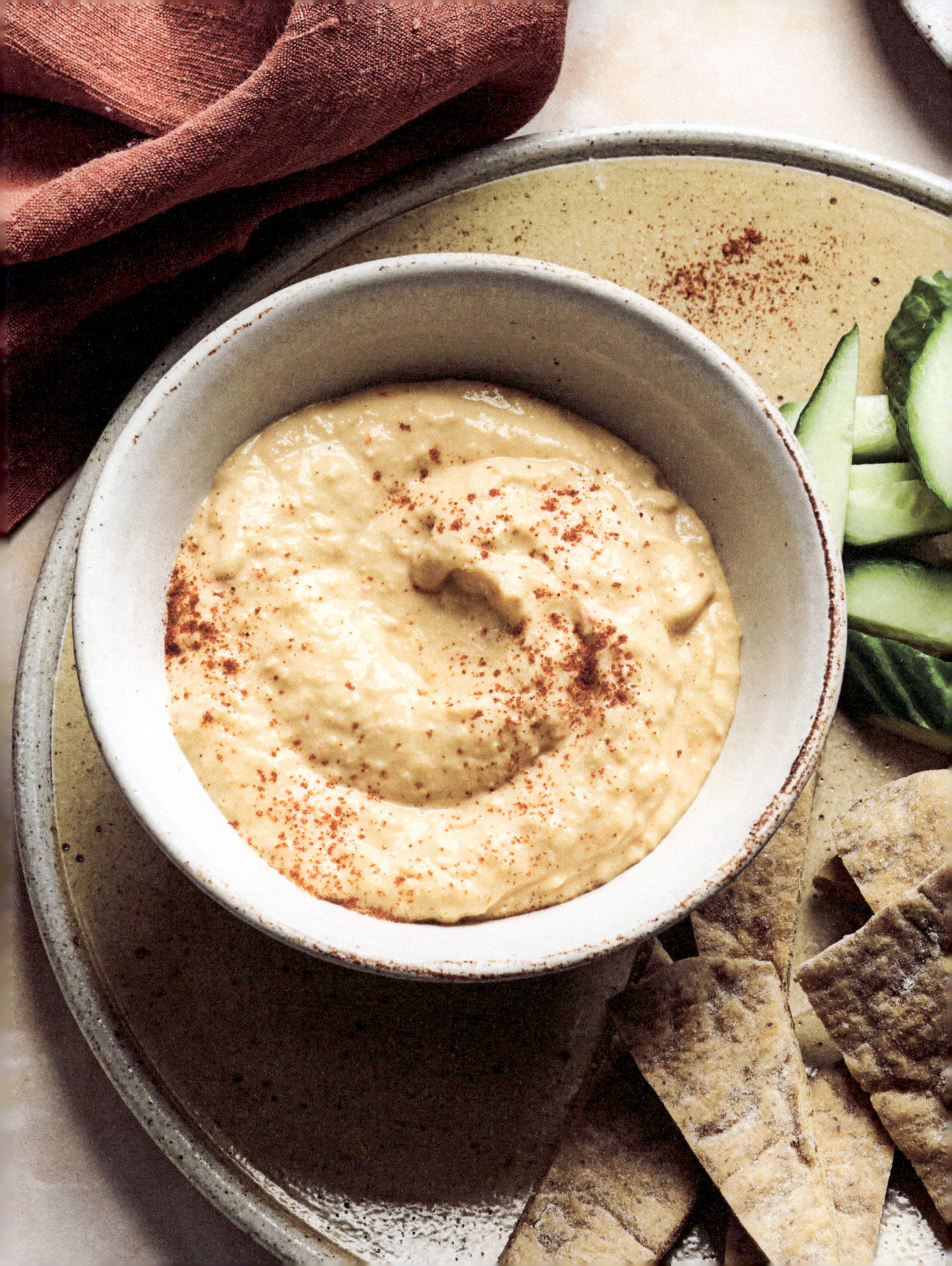

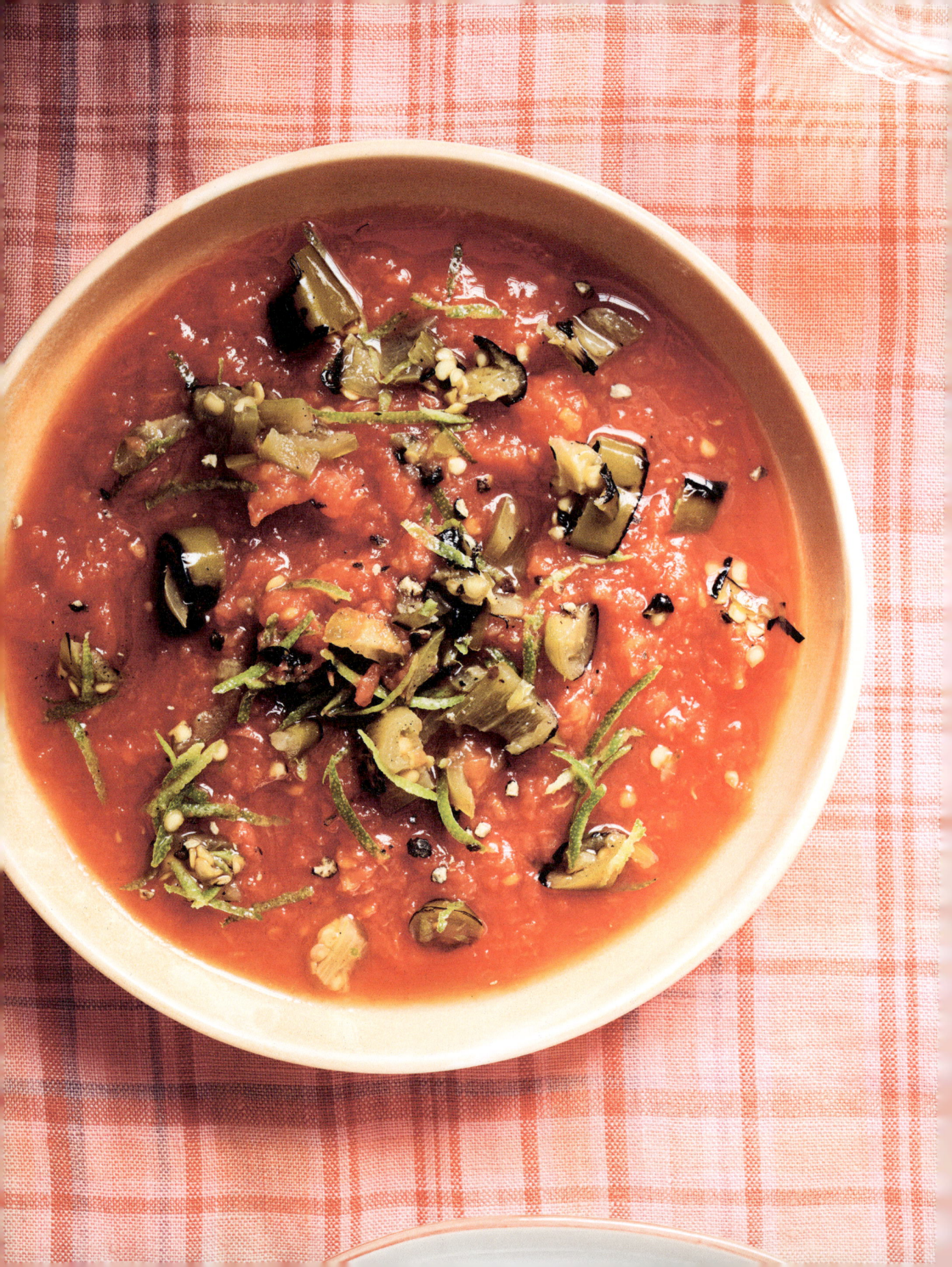

TWO-MINUTE SALSA

SERVES 4
PREP TIME 2 minutes
COOK TIME none

400g (14oz) can of chopped
   tomatoes (a good-quality
   can will improve the flavour,
   see note)
1 tablespoon pickled jalapeños
finely grated zest and juice of
   1 lime
couple of pinches of coarse salt

I whip this up when I need a super-quick salsa to go with a chilli, or to use as a dip. Usually if I make salsa, I will add onions and cook them first, but this is my 'emergency' recipe and I find I use it a lot as it's great with Mexican-inspired meals.

1   Put all the ingredients in a mini chopper and blend until the jalapeños are chopped up.

2   Taste it and add a little more salt if necessary.

NOTE

What do I mean by 'good-quality' chopped tomatoes? I always used to buy only supermarket own-brand chopped tomatoes, as they are markedly cheaper. In recent years, however, I tend to keep the more expensive variety in my cupboards, too. The cheap tomatoes are great and will still work well in a recipe, but there is a definite flavour difference from the pricier sort, and I think that if you are making something like this salsa without cooking the tomatoes – or if you are using them as a pizza sauce – it's worth spending the extra for the quality product. I love the Mutti-branded Polpa cans, because the tomatoes in those are much more finely chopped than the regular variety, so don't involve the 'cooking down' that chunkier chopped tomatoes usually require.

PER SERVING

CALORIES	FAT	SAT FAT	CARBS	SUGARS	FIBRE	PROTEIN	SALT
30	0	0	4.1G	3.9G	1G	1.2G	0.44G

GUACAMOLE

SERVES 4
PREP TIME 5 minutes
COOK TIME none

2 ripe avocados, halved and pitted
1 red chilli, deseeded and finely
    chopped
juice of 1 lime
½ teaspoon coarse salt

Guacamole is a classic, and homemade guacamole is far superior to those little pots you can buy in the supermarket; you can't beat it freshly made and it really is so quick to do. Personally, I prefer guacamole without tomatoes, but add chopped fresh tomatoes, if you like.

1   Scoop the flesh from the avocados into a bowl and add the chilli, lime juice and salt.

2   Mash with a fork until it's your desired consistency: some prefer it chunky, others like it smooth!

3   Cover the bowl tightly with clingfilm (or transfer to a plastic container with a lid) and keep it in the refrigerator until it's time to serve. Storing it with an airtight seal will prevent it from turning brown if you're not going to eat it straight away.

NOTE

If your avocado is not ripe enough, you will not be able to mash it or achieve a nice consistency for your guacamole. To test, give the avocado a gentle squeeze: if you feel the flesh underneath the skin give a little and it feels soft (but not mushy), it is perfect.

PER SERVING

CALORIES	FAT	SAT FAT	CARBS	SUGARS	FIBRE	PROTEIN	SALT
128	12G	2.9G	1.5G	0.6G	2.3G	1.4G	0.63G

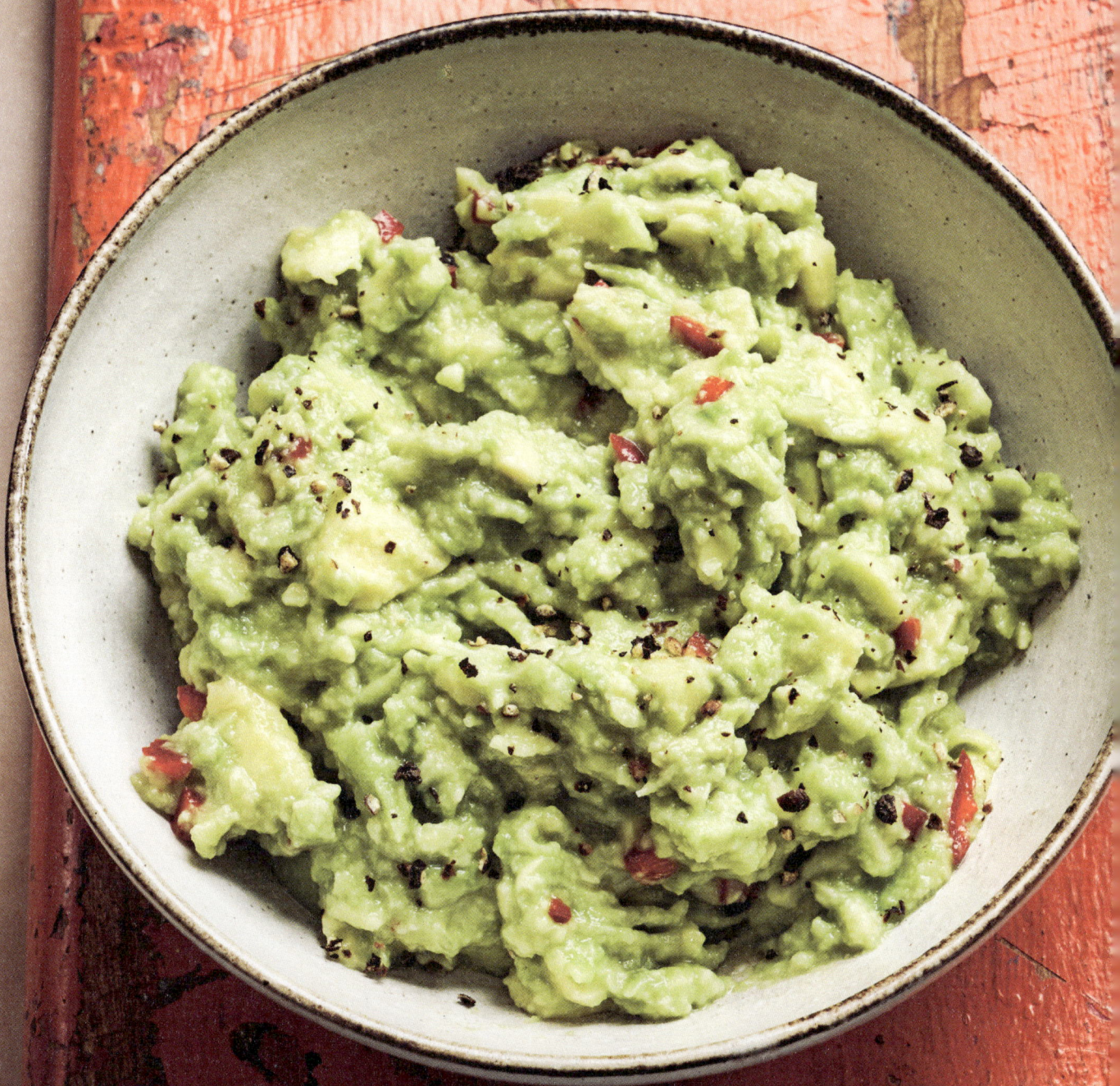

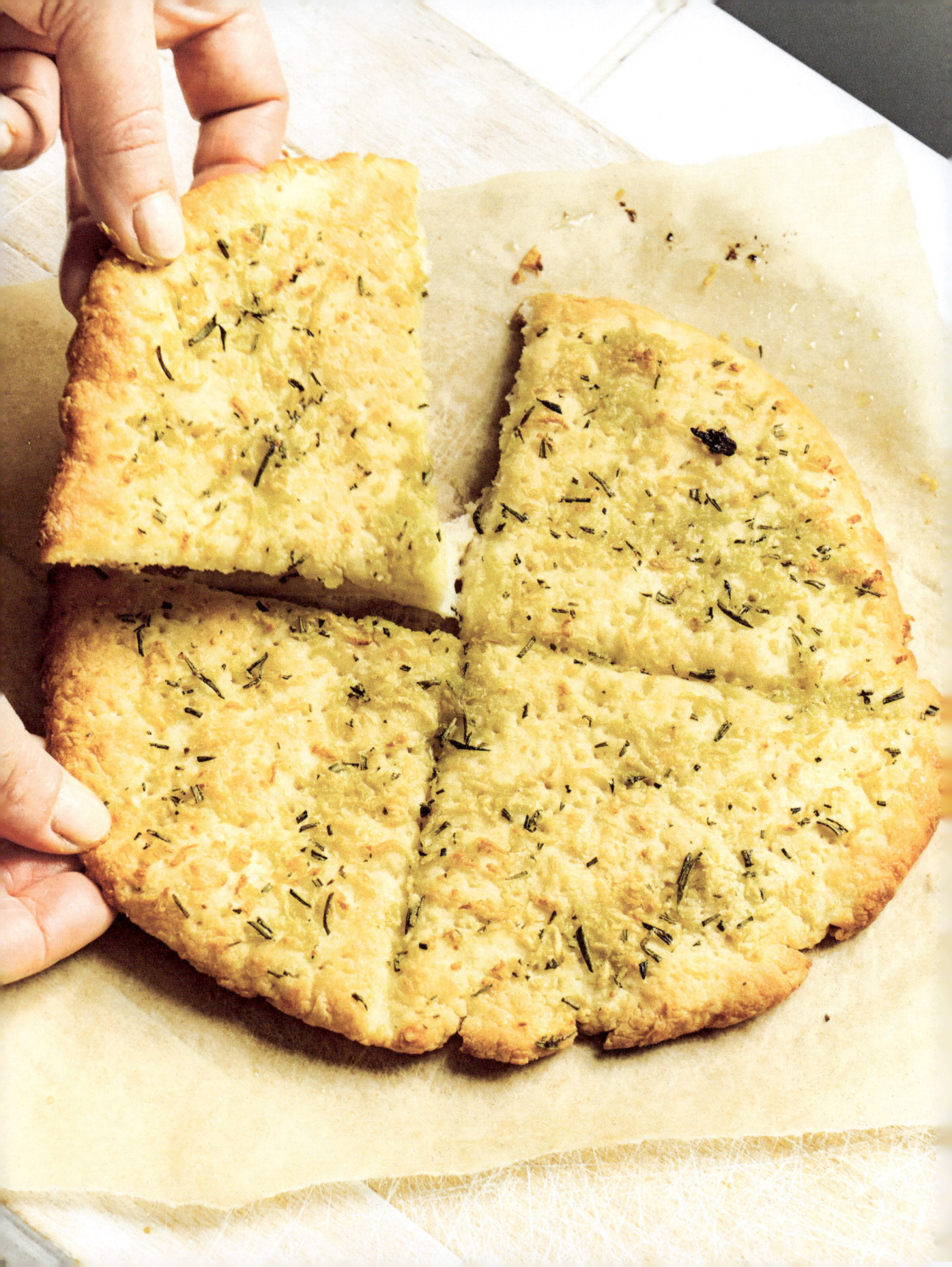

EASIEST EVER RUSTIC GARLIC BREAD

SERVES 4
PREP TIME 10 minutes
COOK TIME 10 minutes

100g (3½oz) self-raising flour, plus more if needed and to dust
100g (3½oz) fat-free Greek yogurt
1 tablespoon (15g/½oz) butter
2 garlic cloves, crushed
½ teaspoon chopped rosemary, fresh or dried
pinch of salt

Who doesn't love garlic bread? If you're going to indulge in it, you can't beat a homemade version.

1   Preheat the oven to 220°C/200°C fan (425°F), Gas Mark 7.

2   Put the flour and yogurt into a mixing bowl, use a table knife to mix them together, and, once they are starting to form a dough, use your hands to bring into a ball. If the dough is a little too sticky to handle, just add a bit more flour: the outcome depends on the consistency of the yogurt.

3   Roll the dough out on a lightly floured work surface into a circle around 15cm (6 inches) across. Use a fork to dot it all over with little indents. Move the dough onto a baking tray.

4   Put the butter into a microwave-safe bowl with the garlic, rosemary and salt and microwave for around 30 seconds, or until the butter has melted.

5   Give the melted butter a stir with a teaspoon, then spread it over the dough, covering all the way to the edges.

6   Place the garlic bread in the oven for 8–10 minutes until golden brown.

7   Use a pizza cutter to cut the bread into 4 pieces to serve.

NOTE

For a cheesy addition, sprinkle grated Parmesan or mozzarella cheese over the garlic butter before baking. You can also tailor the herbs to your preference by using parsley, thyme or oregano instead of rosemary. Enjoy this with your favourite pasta dish, or alongside soup.

PER SERVING

CALORIES	FAT	SAT FAT	CARBS	SUGARS	FIBRE	PROTEIN	SALT
131	3.4G	2G	19G	1.2G	1.1G	5.2G	0.45G

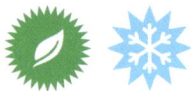

ALOO TIKKI (INDIAN-STYLE POTATO PATTIES)

MAKES 15
PREP TIME 10 minutes
COOK TIME 25 minutes

1 sweet potato (weight about 200g/7oz)

1 onion

2 carrots (total weight 200g/7oz)

1 potato, peeled

2.5cm (1 inch) piece of root ginger, peeled

1 garlic clove

1 tablespoon mild curry powder

½ teaspoon cumin seeds

½ teaspoon chilli powder

75g (2¾oz) frozen peas

1 egg

spray oil

salt and pepper

This recipe is loosely based on a North Indian snack of crispy potato patties. My version is baked rather than fried, and I have grated regular potato and used mashed sweet potato to help bind them. These make a great side dish to an Indian meal, or keep them in the refrigerator for tasty, nutritious snacks.

1   Preheat the oven to 220°C/200°C fan (425°F), Gas Mark 7.

2   Prick the sweet potato, place it on a microwave-safe plate and microwave it for 5 minutes, or until the flesh is tender.

3   Cut the sweet potato in half to allow it to cool a little while you prepare the rest of the ingredients.

4   Grate the onion, carrots, regular potato, ginger and garlic into a bowl, then stir in the curry powder, cumin seeds and chilli powder. Scoop the flesh from the sweet potato and add it to the mix with the frozen peas, then season with salt and pepper.

5   Crack the egg into the bowl, then mix everything together to thoroughly combine, making sure the sweet potato does not clump together, but spreads throughout the mixture.

6   Line a baking tray with nonstick baking paper and use your hands to form 15 balls; I make these a size which sits comfortably in my palms, about 3cm (1¼ inches) in diameter. Place each ball on the prepared tray. If there are any peas poking out, then just use your fingers to pop them into the patties so they don't burn. Spray the patties with oil, then pop them into the oven to bake for 20 minutes.

7   After 20 minutes they should be golden on the outside, with some little areas of char. Allow them to cool for a few minutes before removing from the tray.

NOTE

If you have mashed potato left over from another meal, this is a great way to use it up. You can mix up the flavours in these if you wish. Herb leaves, such as mint and coriander work well, as does finely grated lemon zest.

PER PATTY

CALORIES	FAT	SAT FAT	CARBS	SUGARS	FIBRE	PROTEIN	SALT
46	0.8G	0.2G	7.3G	2.5G	1.6G	1.4G	TRACE

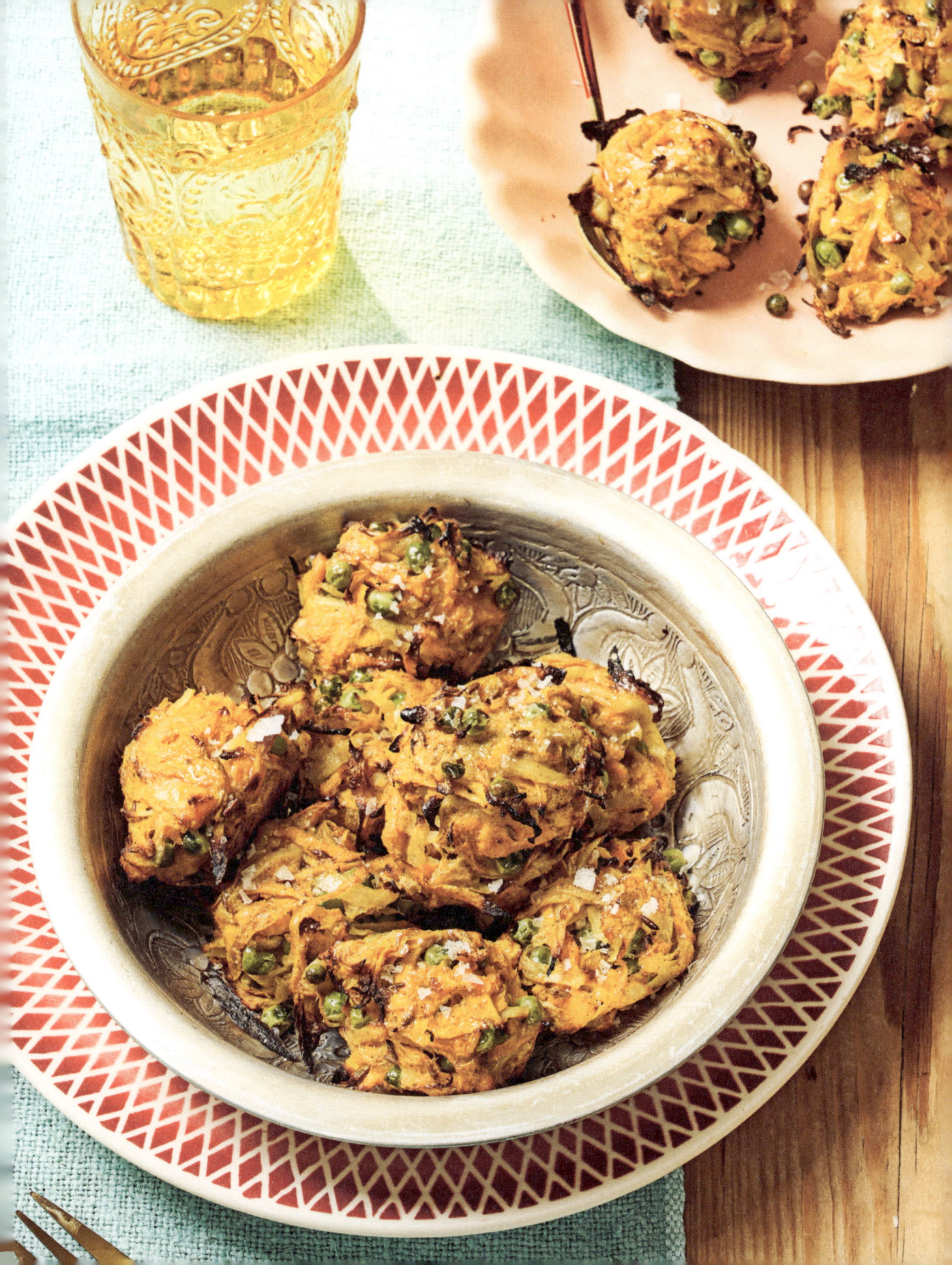

SWEET TREATS

9

MINI CINNAMON BUNS

MAKES 10
PREP TIME 10 minutes
COOK TIME 10 minutes

100g (3½oz) self-raising flour, plus more if needed and to dust
1 teaspoon baking powder
100g (3½oz) fat-free Greek yogurt
1 teaspoon vanilla extract
75g (2¾oz) pitted dates
25g (1oz) butter, melted
1 teaspoon ground cinnamon
pinch of salt
1 egg, lightly beaten

My daughter Marlie's favourite thing in the world is a cinnamon bun (it's a very close tie with pizza!) but I rarely have the patience for proving dough to make them from scratch. These little buns are a great quick solution, plus they are so cute that kids love them! Instead of sugar, I use dates to make that dark, sticky-sweet paste for the middle. I usually use fat-free Greek yogurt in the dough because it's something I always have in the refrigerator, but you can swap this out for full-fat Greek yogurt, if you prefer.

1   Preheat the oven to 200°C/180°C fan (400°F), Gas Mark 6.

2   Put the flour, baking powder, yogurt and vanilla into a mixing bowl and use a table knife to mix the ingredients and start to bring them together. Once they are well mixed, use your hands to form a ball of dough. If it is a bit too sticky, just add a little more flour (it will depend on the consistency of your yogurt).

3   Use your hands to shape the dough into a sausage shape, then place it on a floured work surface and roll it out with a rolling pin into a rectangle, about 25 x 15cm (10 x 6 inches).

4   Now neaten the edges; I just use my fingers to fold over the edges, then press those into the dough to make the shape a bit more uniform.

5   Place the dates, melted butter, cinnamon and pinch of salt into a mini chopper and blend into a smooth paste. Fill a mug with freshly boiled water and place the blade of a table knife into the water. Use the hot blade to spread the cinnamon paste evenly over the top of the dough.

6   Now carefully roll up the dough, starting at the top, long edge, so you have a long log. Use a sharp knife to slice this up into 10 mini buns.

7   Line a baking tray with nonstick baking paper and place the cinnamon buns on the tray with a little distance between each. Use your fingers to make sure they are a nice round shape, if they got a little squashed when you cut them up. Brush each with beaten egg, then place on the middle shelf of the oven and bake for 10 minutes.

NOTE

For an extra treat, you can make some icing to drizzle over the buns once they are cooked. Simply mix 2 tablespoons icing sugar with 1 tablespoon milk, then drizzle it over the buns with a spoon.

PER BUN

CALORIES	FAT	SAT FAT	CARBS	SUGARS	FIBRE	PROTEIN	SALT
93	2.7G	1.5G	13G	5.5G	1G	2.9G	0.37G

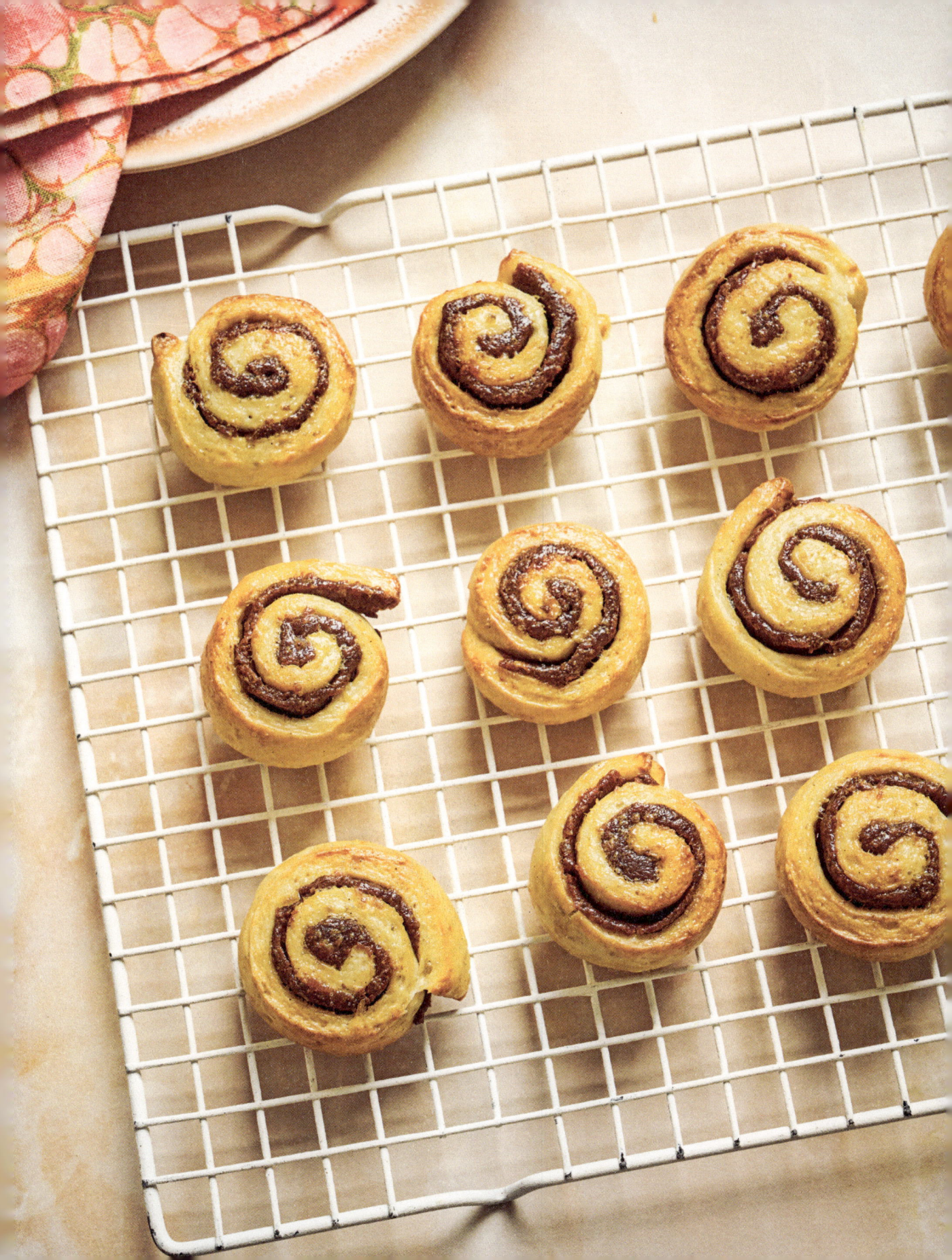

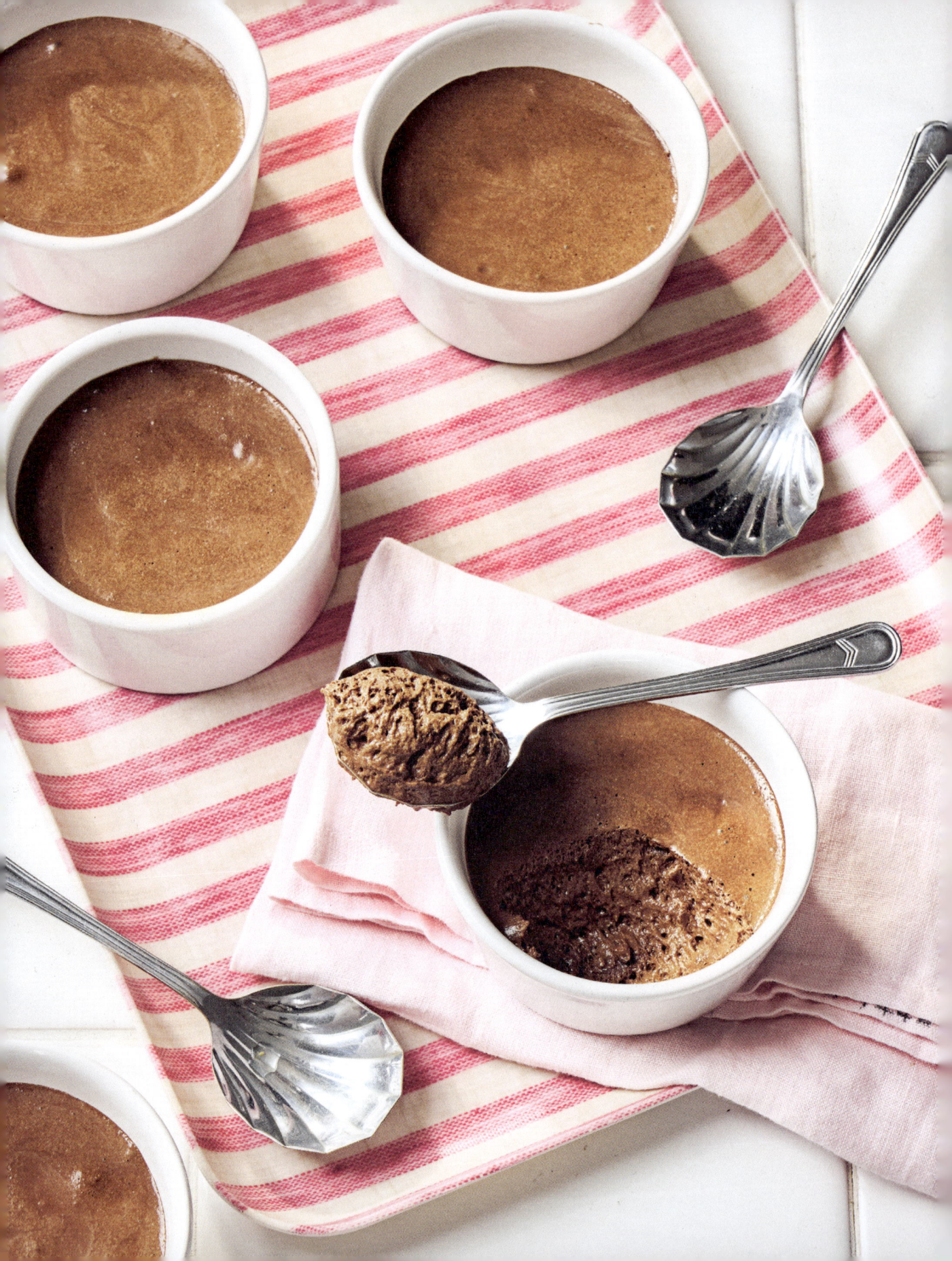

RICH CHOCOLATE MOUSSE

SERVES 6
PREP TIME 10 minutes
COOK TIME none

125g (4½oz) good-quality dark
   chocolate (70 per cent cocoa)
4 eggs, separated
pinch of salt

One of the most simple but most delicious desserts. Simply by using a good-quality dark chocolate and eggs, you can achieve a delectable mousse without the need for sugar or cream. This recipe isn't overly sweet, but it's very rich and delicious, so a little goes a long way.

1. Break up the chocolate, keeping a couple of squares back (about 15g/½oz). Melt the chocolate in the microwave (see note).

2. Whisk the egg whites in a mixing bowl with the pinch of salt until they are stiff and hold their shape. I just use a hand whisk for this and it takes me 2–3 minutes, but you can use an electric whisk if you prefer.

3. Stir the melted chocolate, then add 1 egg yolk and quickly stir it into the chocolate until you can't see any yellow remaining. Add the rest of the egg yolks and briskly stir them through until fully combined. The mixture will be quite stiff, almost like a ganache.

4. Add 2 tablespoons of the stiff egg whites to the chocolate mix and use a spatula to fold it through.

5. Fold in the remaining egg whites with a spatula: the aim now is to be gentle to try and keep some of the air in the whites, but you also want to make sure that the chocolate and eggs are fully combined.

6. Grate in half the reserved chocolate, using the finest side of a grater.

7. Divide the mousse between 6 ramekins or small bowls, then grate the rest of the chocolate over the tops. Pop into the refrigerator and leave to chill for at least 2 hours before serving.

NOTE

The 2 best ways to melt chocolate are:

Microwave method When melting chocolate in the microwave, it's best to do it in short intervals to prevent overheating and burning. Put it in a microwave-safe bowl and start with 20–30 second intervals on medium power, stirring between each. Continue microwaving and stirring until the chocolate is almost completely melted, then remove it from the microwave and stir until smooth. Be careful not to overheat the chocolate, as it can easily burn. Adjust the timing based on the amount of chocolate you're melting and the power of your microwave.

Bain marie method Also known as a double boiler, this method involves melting chocolate in a heatproof bowl set over a pot of simmering water. (Make sure the bowl does not touch the water.) The gentle heat prevents the chocolate from burning or seizing, resulting in smooth, melted chocolate.

PER SERVING

CALORIES	FAT	SAT FAT	CARBS	SUGARS	FIBRE	PROTEIN	SALT
167	12G	6.3G	6.7G	5.6G	2.3G	6.6G	0.23G

CHOCOLATE MUD PIES

MAKES 16
PREP TIME 10 minutes
COOK TIME 10 minutes

160g (5¾oz) light (reduced-fat) cream cheese
140g (5oz) light muscovado sugar
1 egg, plus 1 egg yolk
2 teaspoons vanilla extract
180g (6oz) plain flour
40g (1½oz) cocoa powder
½ teaspoon baking powder
½ teaspoon coarse salt
50g (1¾oz) milk chocolate chips

A cross between a muffin and a cookie, these tasty little chocolatey treats go down well with the whole family.

1 Preheat the oven to 210°C/190°C fan (410°F), Gas Mark 6½.

2 Put the cream cheese in a mixing bowl, add the sugar, egg, egg yolk and vanilla and mix together. Add the flour, cocoa powder, baking powder, salt and chocolate chips, then mix into a soft dough.

3 Line a large baking tray with nonstick baking paper.

4 Use your hands to shape the mixture into 16 patties (wet your hands first to prevent the mixture from sticking too much, then place on the prepared tray, allowing space between each.

5 Use a fork to gently press down on the top of each patty to create an indent. Bake for 10 minutes.

6 Allow to cool on the tray, then transfer to a wire rack with a palette knife and leave until completely cold.

NOTE

Add some finely grated orange zest to make these into chocolate-orange mud pies. You could also use dark or white chocolate chips, or a mix of the two.

PER SERVING

CALORIES	FAT	SAT FAT	CARBS	SUGARS	FIBRE	PROTEIN	SALT
120	31G	1.8G	19G	10G	1.2G	3.3G	0.31G

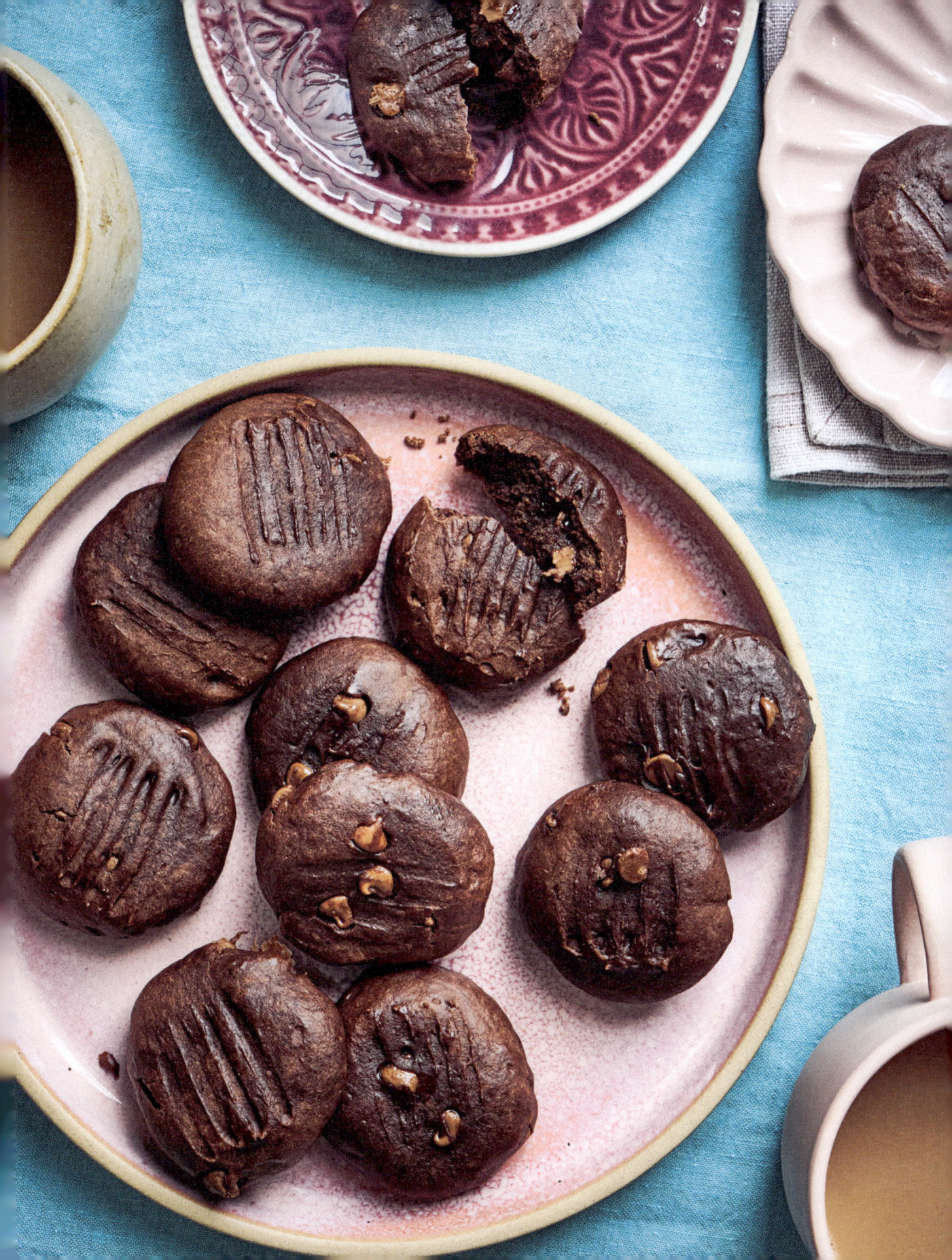

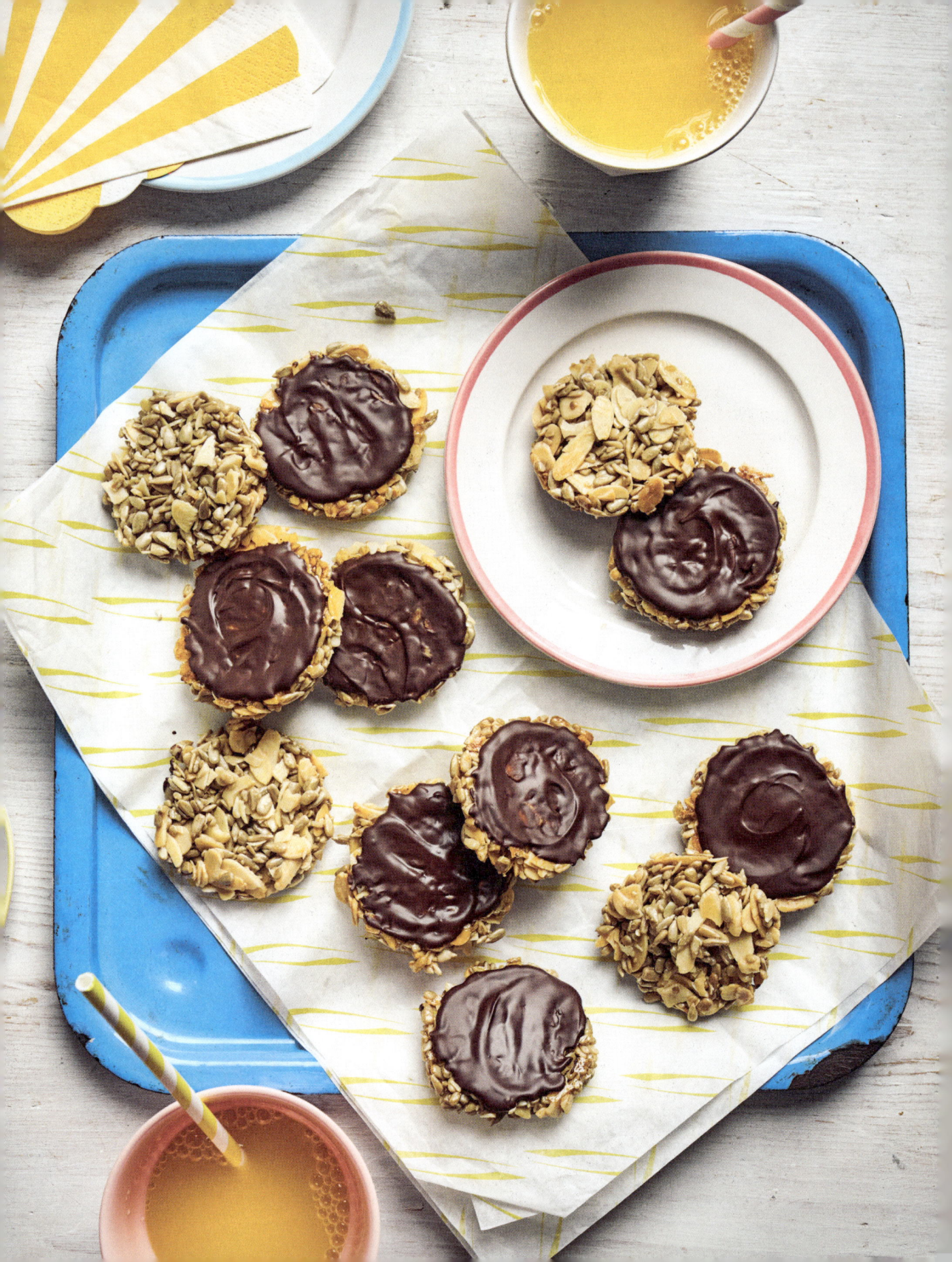

CRUNCHY CHOCOLATE CLUSTERS

MAKES 12
PREP TIME 5 minutes plus cooling
COOK TIME 20 minutes

125g (4½oz) sunflower seeds
75g (2¾oz) flaked almonds
2 tablespoons maple syrup
pinch of salt
70g (2½oz) dark chocolate

These are similar to florentines, but without the high sugar content – I find these make a lovely little treat alongside a cuppa. You can of course use milk or white chocolate instead of dark, if you prefer.

1   Preheat the oven to 180°C/160°C fan (350°F), Gas Mark 4.

2   In a small bowl, combine the sunflower seeds, almonds, maple syrup and salt. Line a large baking sheet or roasting dish with nonstick baking paper.

3   Use a small (6cm/2½ inch) plain round pastry cutter to make the clusters: place the pastry cutter on the baking paper, add a dessert spoonful of the mixture and gently push it down into the round shape. Lift the cutter slowly away to leave behind a flat disc. Repeat with all the mixture to make 12.

4   Bake on the middle shelf of the oven for 20 minutes, keeping an eye on them for the last 5 minutes, to prevent burning.

5   You now need to leave them to cool completely before the chocolate stage, because, if they are still warm when you pick them up, they are likely to crumble apart.

6   Once they have cooled, melt the chocolate using your preferred method (I melt mine in the microwave, see page 221). Use a teaspoon to swirl the melted chocolate evenly over the top of all the clusters, then leave on the baking paper to allow the chocolate to set.

7   Once the chocolate has set, you can pop them in the refrigerator to speed up the process, if you wish.

NOTE

You can customize these with different nuts and seeds, as well as different chocolate types. Try them with pumpkin seeds, chia seeds or sesame seeds, chopped cashews, pecans, hazelnuts, pistachios or walnuts.

PER CLUSTER

CALORIES	FAT	SAT FAT	CARBS	SUGARS	FIBRE	PROTEIN	SALT
142	11G	2.5G	6G	3.9G	2.2G	3.9	TRACE

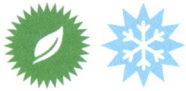

VERY BERRY COTTAGE CHEESE ICE CREAM

SERVES 4
PREP TIME 5 minutes, plus freezing
COOK TIME none

300g (10½oz) cottage cheese
170g (6oz) frozen berries (a mix of blueberries and raspberries)
25g (1oz) honey

This is a super-simple, high-protein ice cream that tastes creamy and indulgent without the need for cream. Cottage cheese may sound like an unusual base, but trust me, it blends into a smooth, delicious treat.

1　Put the cottage cheese, frozen berries and honey into a food processor or mini chopper and blend until smooth and creamy.

2　Transfer the mixture into an airtight container (I use a freezer-safe container with clip-on lid, which is 20 x 15cm/8 x 6 inches).

3　Freeze for 1½ hours, then serve and enjoy!

NOTE

For the creamiest texture, I recommend using regular cottage cheese for this recipe. Light (reduced-fat), or even fat-free versions can work, but tend to freeze harder and feel icier in the mouth.

If you plan to freeze the ice cream for longer than 1½ hours, stir it every hour while it is freezing to keep it scoopable. Otherwise, it may freeze too solid, as traditional ice cream is churned as it freezes to maintain a soft texture. If the ice cream is too firm after freezing, let it sit at room temperature for 5–10 minutes before scooping.

You can experiment with different berries or sweeteners, such as maple syrup or agave syrup, to suit your taste.

PER SERVING

CALORIES	FAT	SAT FAT	CARBS	SUGARS	FIBRE	PROTEIN	SALT
111	4.6G	2.4G	9.6G	9.6G	1.1G	7.3G	0.32G

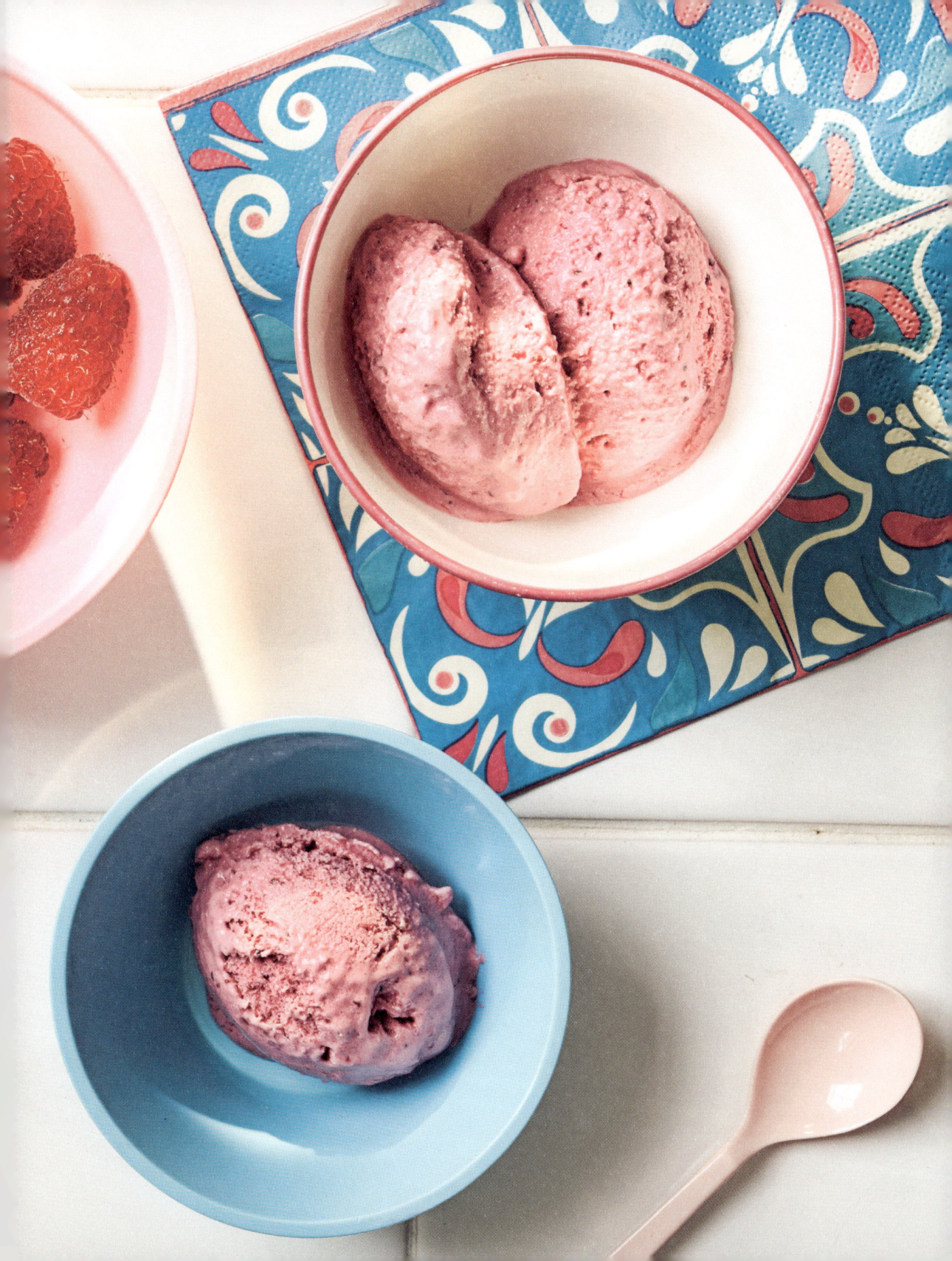

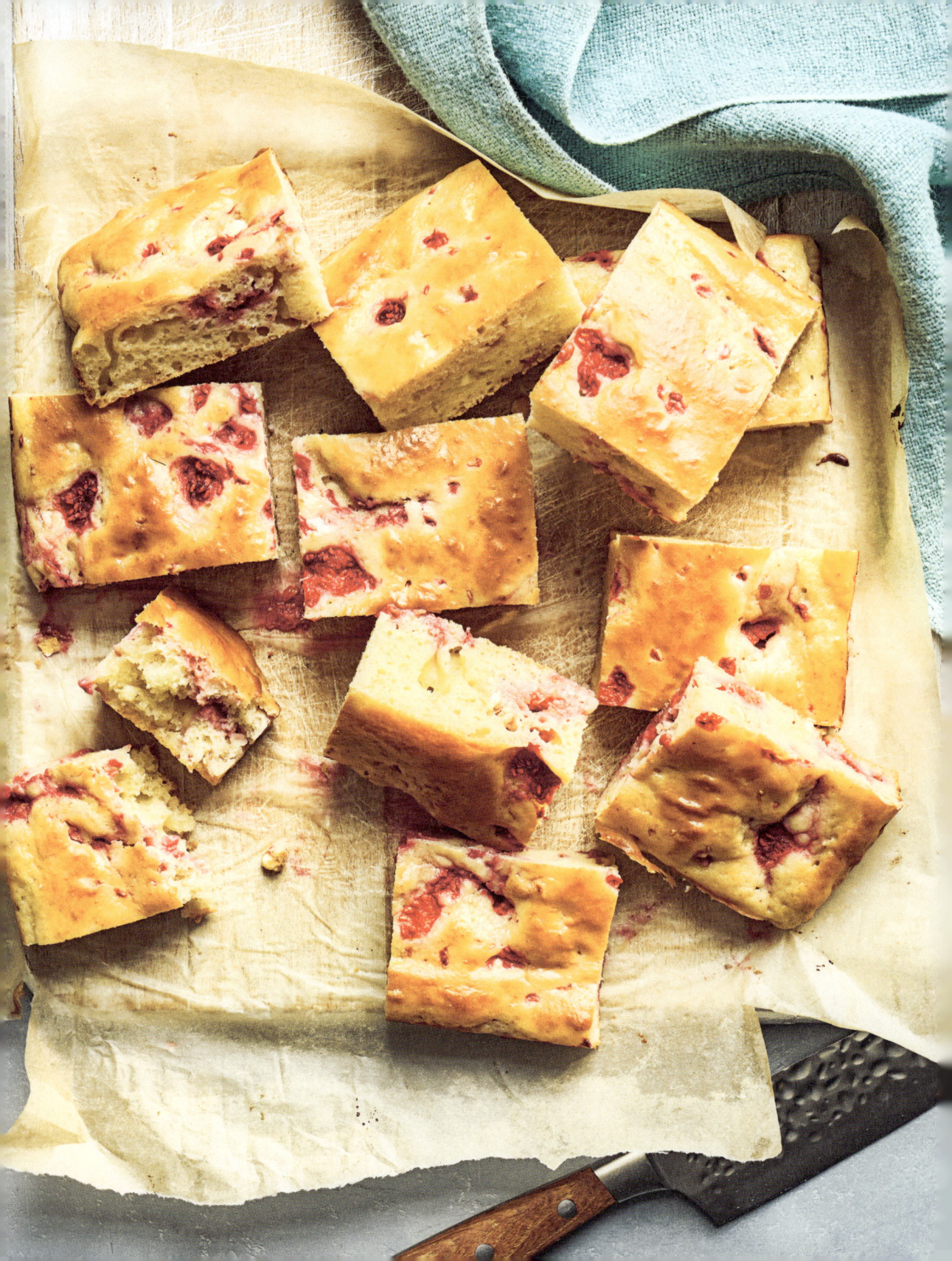

RASPBERRY & WHITE CHOCOLATE YOGURT CAKE

MAKES 12 slices
PREP TIME 10 minutes
COOK TIME 30 minutes

225g (8oz) fat-free Greek yogurt
3 eggs
100g (3½oz) caster sugar
1 teaspoon vanilla extract
200g (7oz) self-raising flour
1 teaspoon baking powder
150g (5½oz) frozen raspberries, crushed
75g (2¾oz) white chocolate chips, or white chocolate chopped into small chunks

Raspberry and white chocolate are an irresistible combination and this cake hits the spot with the whole family. Using fat-free Greek yogurt instead of butter, margarine or oil saves on calories and gives a lovely moist consistency.

1   Preheat the oven to 200°C/180°C fan (400°F), Gas Mark 6.

2   In a mixing bowl, whisk together the yogurt, eggs, sugar and vanilla extract. Fold in the flour and baking powder to form a batter, then stir through the raspberry pieces and white chocolate chips or chunks.

3   Line a 24cm (9½ inch) square cake tin with nonstick baking paper and scoop in the batter, spreading it around evenly.

4   Bake on the middle shelf of the oven for 30 minutes, until the cake is springy on top and a knife inserted into the thickest part comes out clean, without batter clinging to it. Allow to cool before serving.

NOTE

Fancy trying some different flavour combinations using this basic recipe? Why not try:

Apple & cinnamon Replace the raspberries with chopped apple and add ½ teaspoon ground cinnamon to the batter (it's up to you whether you leave in the white chocolate).

Cherry & almond Chop frozen or fresh cherries as a substitute for the raspberries, and replace the vanilla extract with almond extract.

PER SERVING

CALORIES	FAT	SAT FAT	CARBS	SUGARS	FIBRE	PROTEIN	SALT
161	3.5G	1.6G	25G	13G	1.6G	6G	0.35G

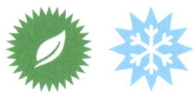

LEMON POLENTA CAKE

MAKES 16 squares
PREP TIME 5 minutes
COOK TIME 30 minutes

300g (10½oz) fat-free
    Greek yogurt
3 eggs
150g (5½oz) caster sugar
75g (2¾oz) ground almonds
75g (2¾oz) polenta
finely grated zest and juice
    of 2 lemons
1½ teaspoons baking powder
1 tablespoon demerara sugar

There's something so satisfying about the texture of a polenta cake: moist and tender, but slightly granular. Tangy lemon and ground almonds give a beautiful flavour to this recipe.

1   Preheat the oven to 170°C/150°C fan (340°F), Gas Mark 3½.

2   In a mixing bowl, whisk together the yogurt and eggs. Stir in the sugar, ground almonds, polenta, lemon zest (reserve the juice for now) and baking powder.

3   Line a 20cm (8 inch) square cake tin with nonstick baking paper and scrape in the batter. Give the tin a tap on the work surface to even out the batter, then bake on the middle shelf of the oven for 30 minutes.

4   In a small bowl, mix the lemon juice with the demerara sugar.

5   Once the cake is baked (the top should feel springy to the touch and a knife inserted into the centre should come out clean), puncture it all over with a cocktail stick or fork to create small holes. Pour the lemon mixture evenly over, using the back of a teaspoon to spread any grains of sugar around the top of the cake. Allow it to cool for 10 minutes before serving.

NOTE

You can easily substitute the lemons for oranges in this recipe.

PER SLICE

CALORIES	FAT	SAT FAT	CARBS	SUGARS	FIBRE	PROTEIN	SALT
114	3.7G	0.5G	15G	11G	0.9G	4.7G	0.2G

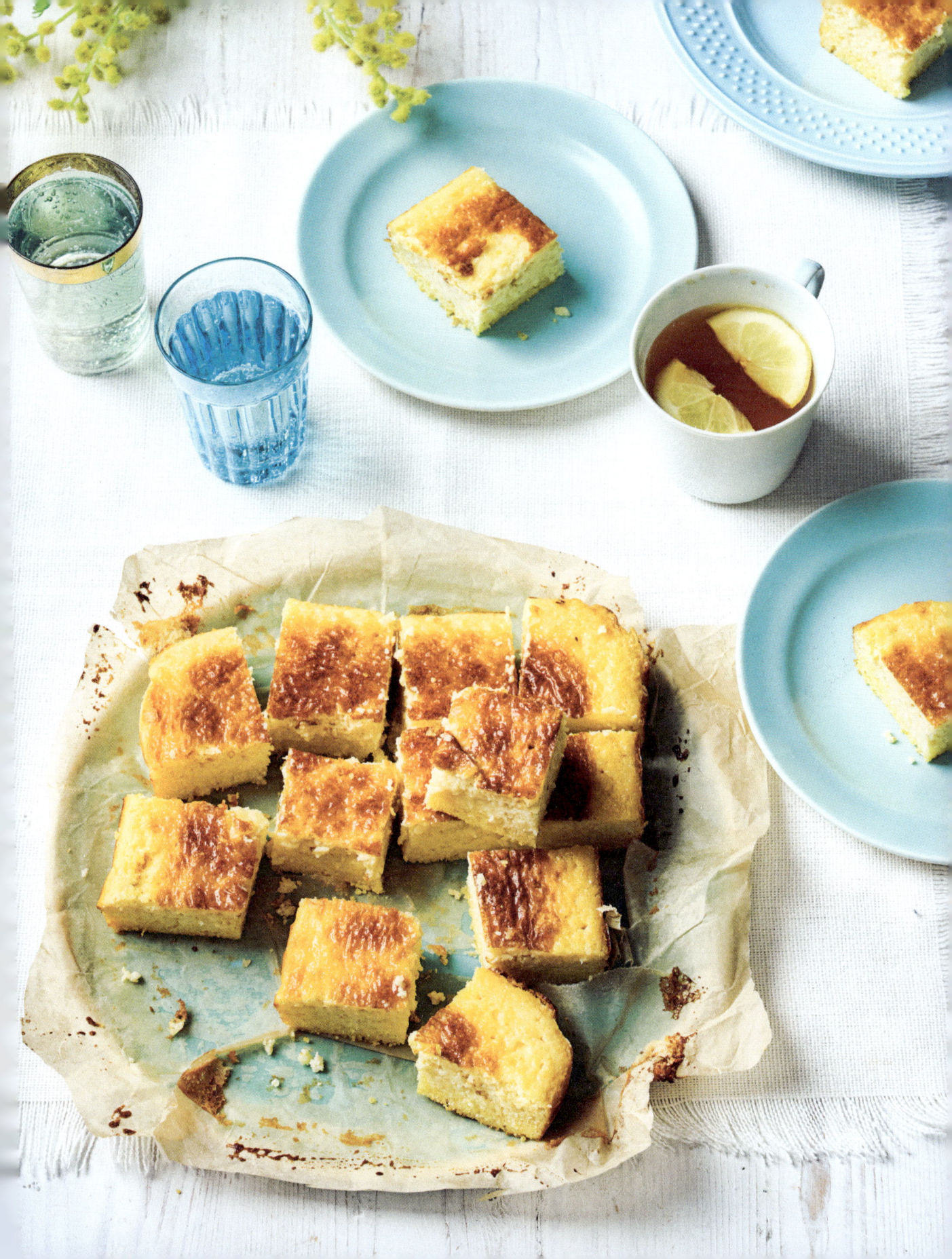

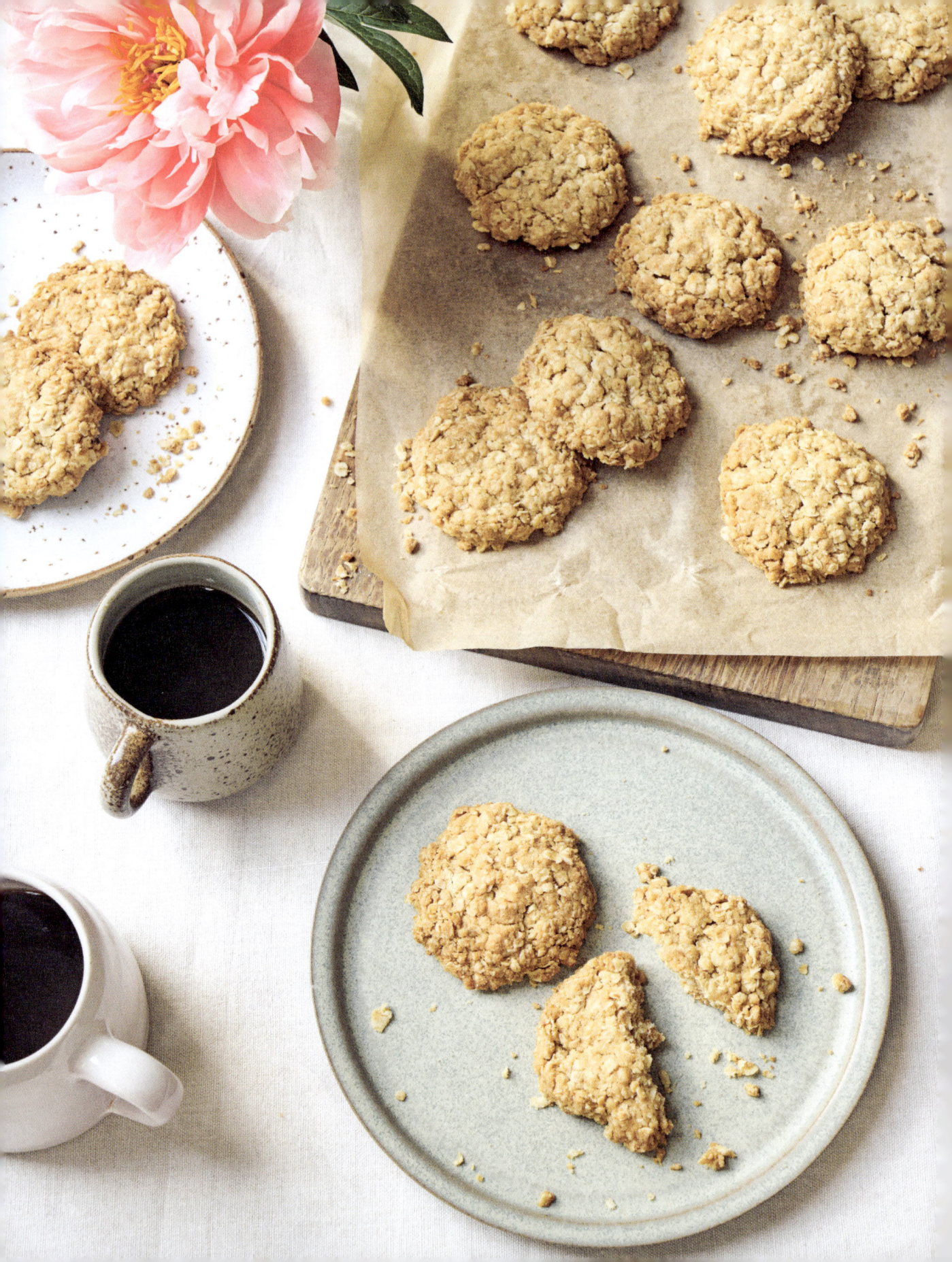

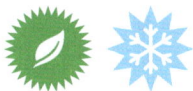

CHUNKY BUTTERY OAT BISCUITS

MAKES 16
PREP TIME 15 minutes
COOK TIME 15 minutes

50g (1¾oz) wholemeal flour
75g (2¾oz) white self-raising flour
100g (3½oz) light brown soft sugar
125g (4½oz) porridge oats
pinch of salt
100g (3½oz) butter
1 tablespoon golden syrup
1 teaspoon vanilla extract

Everyone loves these, they have a great crunch and buttery flavour. I mix brown and white flour to give them a little fibre boost. These are easy enough that children can help make them, too.

1   Preheat the oven to 180°C/160°C fan (350°F), Gas Mark 4. Line 1 large or 2 medium baking trays with nonstick baking paper.

2   In a mixing bowl, combine both flours, the sugar, oats and salt.

3   In a small saucepan, melt together the butter and golden syrup, then stir in the vanilla. Pour the butter mixture into the dry ingredients. Mix well: I use a wooden spoon for this, pressing down as I mix to help to bind the ingredients.

4   Divide into 16 balls. I try to get roughly even biscuits by dividing the mixture in half, in half again and so on. Roll into balls between your palms and place on the prepared tray or trays, flattening slightly with your palm as you place each biscuit down. Leave some space between each to allow for a little spreading as the biscuits bake.

5   Pop in the oven for 12–15 minutes (check them after 12 and leave them in for a few more minutes if they are not yet golden brown.)

NOTE

If you fancy, you can drizzle these with melted chocolate once they are baked.

PER SERVING

CALORIES	FAT	SAT FAT	CARBS	SUGARS	FIBRE	PROTEIN	SALT
134	5.9G	3.4G	17G	7.2G	1.1G	2G	0.2G

GINGERNUT THINS

MAKES 20
PREP TIME 15 minutes
COOK TIME 7 minutes

100g (3½oz) self-raising flour,
   plus more to dust
1 teaspoon ground ginger
1 teaspoon bicarbonate of soda
50g (1¾oz) dark muscovado sugar
50g (1¾oz) cold butter, chopped
   into small pieces
2 tablespoons (30g/1oz) golden
   syrup

Gingernuts have always been one of my favourite biscuits and these thin, buttery-crisp versions make a great little treat that the whole family can enjoy.

1   Preheat the oven to 210°C/190°C fan (410°F), Gas Mark 6½.

2   Put the flour, ginger and bicarbonate of soda into a mixing bowl. Add the sugar and butter, then use your fingertips to rub the butter into the other ingredients until the mixture resembles fine crumbs, making sure you aren't left with any large chunks of butter.

3   Incorporate the golden syrup with a wooden spoon, applying pressure and 'stroking' the mixture with the spoon, allowing the dry ingredients to gradually bind with the syrup, forming a cohesive dough. It might seem at first like it's not going to come together, but a little bit of patience will give you a nice smooth dough. Once it starts to come together, use your hands to bind it, then to form it into a ball.

4   Lightly flour a work surface, then roll the dough out to about 3mm (⅛ inch) thick. Use a 6cm (2½ inch) round pastry cutter to cut out the biscuits; you should get about 20 from this dough. As you cut them, place them on a large baking tray covered with nonstick baking paper. Allow some space between each biscuit as they will spread a little when baking.

5   Bake the biscuits on the middle shelf of the oven for 6–7 minutes until they are lightly golden and smelling delicious. Keep an eye on them, as they can burn very suddenly!

6   Remove the tray from the oven and allow to cool for at least 10 minutes before handling, as before they cool and set, they will be too soft to handle and will fall apart. Transfer to a wire rack with a palette knife to cool completely.

NOTE

To find these circle cutters online, search for 'plain pastry cutters'.

PER BISCUIT

CALORIES	FAT	SAT FAT	CARBS	SUGARS	FIBRE	PROTEIN	SALT
52	2.1G	1.3G	7.6G	4G	TRACE	0.5G	0.25G

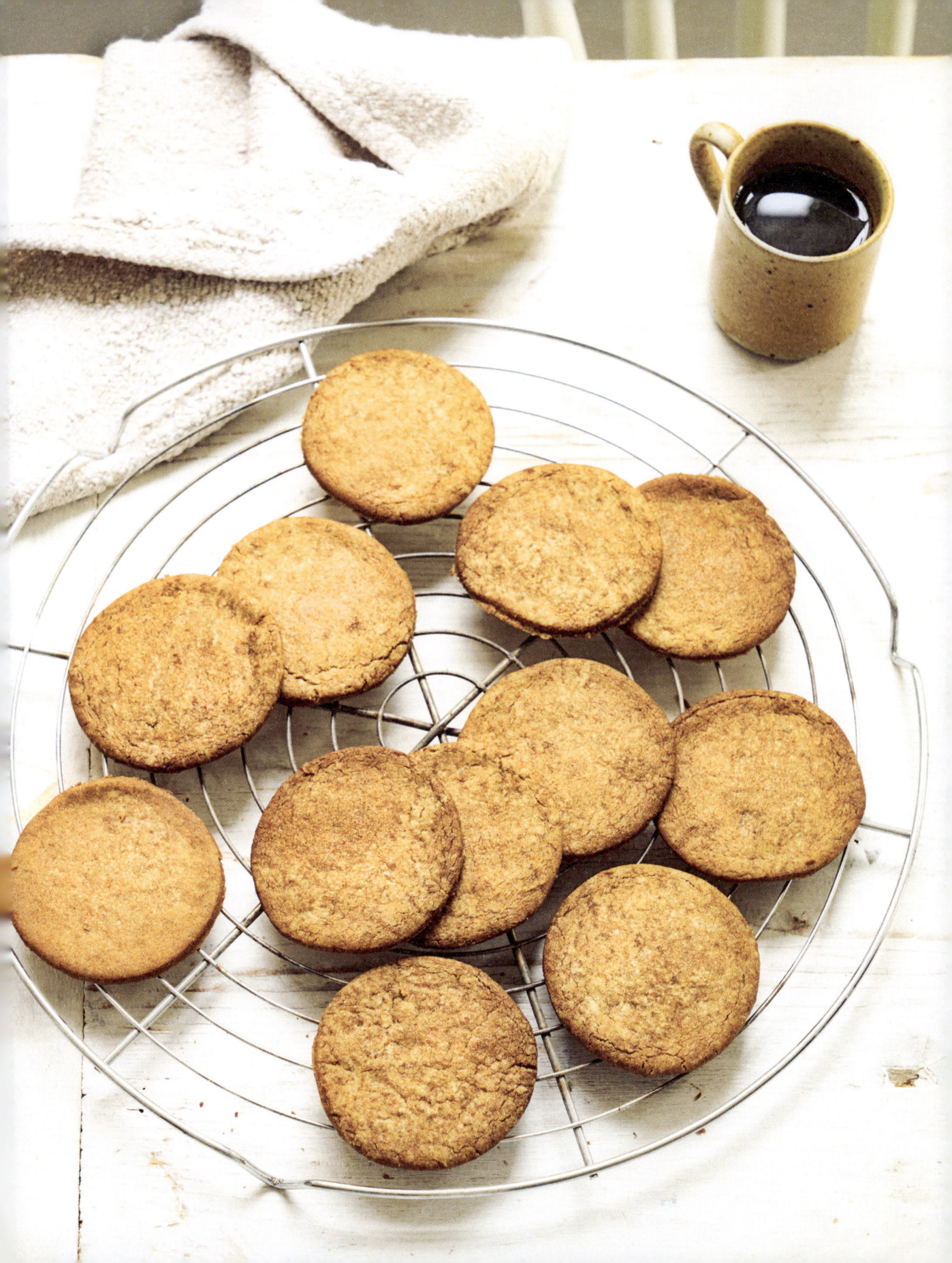

INDEX

tomatoes
- basil & chicken penne 100
- in butter chicken 166
- cheesy marinara bake 80–1
- chicken, chickpea & couscous bake 52
- in chilli con carne 21, 183
- chorizo & prawn pesto linguine 55
- curried 'shepherd's' pie 82
- in guacamole 210
- in keema curry 134
- lentil, chorizo & chilli soup 17
- marry me macaroni 119
- in meatballs 115, 175, 191
- penne Siciliana 44
- peri-peri pulled chicken 165
- in pork goulash 158
- in Provençal chicken 180
- with ras el hanout lamb 48
- in ratatouille 137
- sausage & butter bean ragu 111
- in spaghetti bolognese 142
- spicy tuna pasta bake 77
- spinach & ricotta cannelloni 85
- sun-dried, stuffed chicken breasts 63
- sweet potato & chicken curry 172
- Thai-style grain salad 51
- in three-bean chilli 179
- tomato orzo 72–3
- in two-minute salsa 209
- in veggie lasagne 169
- wedges with halloumi 129

tortillas 28, 31, 40
tuna 26–7, 76–7

W

walnuts 122, 169, 185, 225

Y

yogurt
- burger sauce 116
- in butter chicken 166
- in chicken pasanda 112
- in cinnamon buns 218
- dip for falafels 35
- in garlic bread 213
- garlic sauce 43
- in hummus 206
- in polenta cake 230
- raspberry & white chocolate cake 229
- tandoori marinade 40

GLOSSARY

UK	US
AUBERGINE	EGGPLANT
BAKING PAPER	PARCHMENT PAPER
BICARBONATE OF SODA	BAKING SODA
BUTTER BEANS	LIMA BEANS
CASTER SUGAR	SUPERFINE SUGAR
CHILLI FLAKES	CRUSHED RED PEPPER
CHIPS	FRIES
CLINGFILM	PLASTIC WRAP
CORIANDER	CILANTRO
CORNFLOUR	CORN STARCH
COURGETTE	ZUCCHINI
DEMERARA SUGAR	TURBINADO SUGAR
GAMMON	FRESH HAM
GOLDEN SYRUP	LIGHT TREACLE
GROUND ALMONDS	ALMOND FLOUR
KITCHEN PAPER	PAPER TOWELS
MARS BAR	MILKY WAY BAR
MINCED MEAT	GROUND MEAT
PLAIN FLOUR	ALL-PURPOSE FLOUR
PORRIDGE OATS	OATMEAL
PRAWNS (KING)	SHRIMP (JUMBO)
PUMPKIN SEEDS	PEPITAS
RED/GREEN PEPPERS	BELL PEPPERS
SEMI-SKIMMED MILK	2 PER CENT MILK
SPRING ONIONS	SCALLIONS
SULTANAS	GOLDEN RAISINS
TEA TOWEL	DISH CLOTH
WHOLEMEAL	WHOLEWHEAT

ACKNOWLEDGEMENTS

I can't really believe this is my sixth cookbook! I'm incredibly grateful to everyone who has supported The Slimming Foodie – whether by cooking the recipes, sharing photos, picking up a book, or engaging on social media. Your enthusiasm and interaction online are what keep me motivated and inspired every day, and I truly appreciate every bit of support.

A big thank you to Elly James and Rob Dinsdale at HHB, and a huge shout-out to Heather Holden-Brown, who retired last year after an incredible career. I was so lucky to have had the chance to work alongside you – wishing you a wonderful and fun-filled retirement! And to Lucy Bannell – thank you for your eagle eye and attention to detail in reviewing the manuscript and ensuring everything is in its best form.

I'm so thankful for the team at Octopus, whose hard work behind the scenes makes everything come together. Special thanks to Kate Fox, Natalie Bradley, Sybella Stephens, Yasia Williams, Lucy Carter and Nic Jones, Erin Brown and Karen Baker as well as everyone else at Octopus who plays a part in the process. Your dedication is greatly appreciated.

The shoot is always a highlight, and I was lucky to work again with Chris Terry and Tamsin Weston – such a talented team to collaborate with. It was also great to welcome Lizzie Harris to the team as food stylist for this book. And a special mention to Henrietta Clancy, who styled my previous books and has just welcomed a new baby – we've missed you and wish you all the very best.

To Darren, Miette and Marlie – thank you for being the heart of everything. Your love, patience, kindness, cuddles and cups of tea make this possible, and I couldn't do it without you. And to my parents – thank you for always being there when I need a hand, and for your ongoing encouragement.

Finally, thank you to Libby for helping me with the proofreading at my end, and to Sarah and Maria for all your help in managing the Facebook group. I truly appreciate everything you do to keep the community welcoming and positive.

ABOUT THE AUTHOR

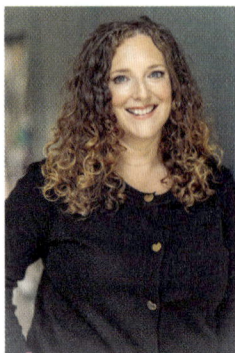

Pip Payne is behind the award-winning blog The Slimming Foodie. Her first three cookbooks were all *Sunday Times* bestsellers.

Pip's passion is creating healthy, varied recipes for the home cook, which are accessible for a kitchen novice, but tasty enough for everyone to enjoy, whether or not they are new to cooking from scratch.

Pip lives on the edge of Dartmoor, in Devon, with her husband, two daughters and their dog.

www.theslimmingfoodie.com

Instagram.com/the_slimming_foodie

Facebook.com/slimmingfoodie

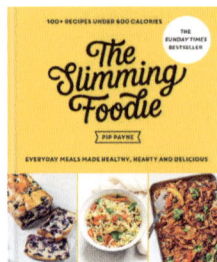

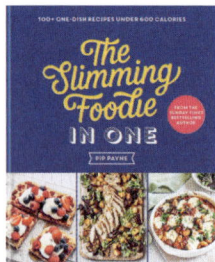

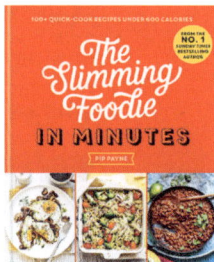

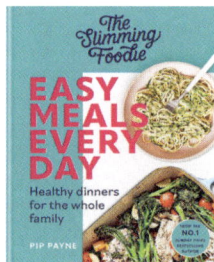

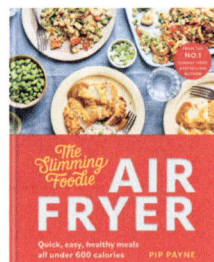